COMPUTER SCIENCE, TECHNOLOGY AND APPLICATIONS

3D IMAGING: THEORY, TECHNOLOGY AND APPLICATIONS

COMPUTER SCIENCE, TECHNOLOGY AND APPLICATIONS

Problem Solving with Delphi - CD included
Stephen John Sugden
2009. ISBN 978-1-60741-249-6

Mobile Computing Research and Applications
Kevin Y. Chen and H.K. Lee (Editors)
2009. ISBN 978-1-60741-101-7

Large Scale Computations, Embedded Systems and Computer Security
Fedor Komarov and Maksim Bestuzhev (Editors)
2010. ISBN: 978-1-60741-307-3

Performance Modelling Techniques for Parallel Supercomputing Applications
A. Grove and P.D. Coddington
2010. ISBN: 9781-60692-269-9

Data Mining and Management
Lawrence I. Spendler (Editor)
2010. ISBN: 978-1-60741-289-2

Biometrics: Methods, Applications and Analyses
Harvey Schuster and Wilfred Metzger (Editors)
2010. ISBN: 978-1-60876-412-9

Relational Databases and Open Source Software Developments
Jennifer R. Taylor (Editor)
2010. ISBN: 978-1-61668-436-5
2010. ISBN: 978-1-61668-468-6 (E-book)

Computer Animation
Jaron S. Wright and Lloyd M. Hughes (Editors)
2010. ISBN: 978-1-60741-559-6

Java Software and Embedded Systems
Mattis Hayes and Isaiah Johansen (Editors)
2010. ISBN: 978-1-60741-661-6

Computer Games: Learning Objectives, Cognitive Performance and Effects on Development
Agustin Soria and Julián Maldonado (Editors)
2010. ISBN: 978-1-60876-658-1

Computational Mechanics Research Trends
Hans P. Berger (Editor)
2010. ISBN: 978-1-60876-057-2

Design and Performance of Biometric System
John T. Elsworth (Editor)
2010. ISBN: 978-1-60692-978-0
2010. ISBN: 978-1-61668-524-9 (E-book)

Peer-to-Peer Networks and Internet Policies
Diego Vegros and Jaime Sáenz (Editors)
2010. ISBN: 978-1-60876-287-3

Agent-Based Computing
Duarte Bouça and Amaro Gafagnão (Editors)
2010. ISBN: 978-1-60876-684-0

Biometrics, Privacy, Progress and Government
Rachel B. Jefferson (Editor)
2010. ISBN: 978-1-60741-098-0

3D Imaging: Theory, Technology and Applications
Emerson H. Duke and Stephen R. Aguirre (Editors)
2010. ISBN: 978-1-60876-885-1

Computer Communication for Metropolitan and Wide Area Networks
Matthew N. O. Sadiku and Sarhan M. Musa
2010. ISBN: 978-1-61668-024-4

Peer-to-Peer Storage: Security and Protocols
Nouha Oualha and Yves Roudier
2010. ISBN: 978-1-61668-199-9
2010. ISBN: 978-1-61668-462-4 (E-book)

Persuasion On-Line and Communicability: The Destruction of Credibility in the Virtual Community and Cognitive Models
Francisco V. Cipolla-Ficarra
2010. ISBN: 978-1-61668-268-2
2010. ISBN: 978-1-61668-701-4 (Ebook)

Intuition and Computer Programming (WT)
Michael Weigend
2010. ISBN: 978-1-61668-330-6
2010. ISBN: 978-1-61668-813-4 (E-book)

Semantic Web: Standards, Tools and Ontologies
Kimberly A. Haffner (Editor)
2010. ISBN: 978-1-61668-471-6
2010. ISBN: 978-1-61668-540-9 (E-book)

Logic of Analog and Digital Machines
Paolo Rocchi
2010. ISBN: 978-1-61668-481-5
2010. ISBN: 978-1-61668-815-8 (E-book)

Wireless Sensor Networks
Liam I. Farrugia (Editor)
2010. ISBN: 978-1-61728-125-9
2010. ISBN: 978-1-61728-328-4 (E-book)

Practice and Research Notes in Relational Database Applications
Haitao Yang
2010. ISBN: 978-1-61668-850-9
2010. ISBN: 978-1-61728-460-1 (E-book)

COMPUTER SCIENCE, TECHNOLOGY AND APPLICATIONS

3D IMAGING: THEORY, TECHNOLOGY AND APPLICATIONS

EMERSON H. DUKE
AND
STEPHEN R. AGUIRRE
EDITORS

Nova Science Publishers, Inc.
New York

For permission to use material from this book please contact us:
Telephone 631-231-7269; Fax 631-231-8175
Web Site: http://www.novapublishers.com

LIBRARY OF CONGRESS CATALOGING-IN-PUBLICATION DATA

3D imaging : theory, technology, and applications / editors, Emerson H. Duke and Stephen R. Aguirre.
p. cm.
Includes bibliographical references and index.
ISBN 978-1-60876-885-1 (hardcover)
1. Three-dimensional imaging--Industrial applications. 2. Three-dimensional imaging in medicine. 3. Three-dimensional imaging in biology. I. Duke, Emerson H. II. Aguirre, Stephen R.
TA1637.A133 2009
621.36'7--dc22

2009048897

Published by Nova Science Publishers, Inc. ✢ New York

CONTENTS

PREFACE

Electron microscope tomography (EMT) has emerged as the leading technique for three-dimensional (3D) structural analysis of unique complex biological specimens. This book reviews the different computational stages involved in EMT, from image acquisition to interpretation of the 3D reconstruction. The high performance computing (HPC) techniques normally used to cope with the computational demands are also described. Moreover, combining the holographic methods with the methods for digital image processing has made it possible to develop the digital holographic interference microscope (DHIM) for real-time 3D imaging of phase microscopic objects and measurement of their morphological parameters. In this book, the classical and holographic methods of phase microobject visualization are considered. In addition, 3D imaging has become commonplace in the medical field, with its routine use in the better established institutions for pre-natal observations, diagnosis of ailments, work-up prior to surgery, recovery monitoring and many other medical procedures. This book discusses the research methodology required in the reconstruction of 3D volume and employing computer-aided diagnosis to identify various diseases. Details of the different stages of processing, along with the promising results achieved are presented. Also discussed are some considerations for future trends of 3D imaging in the medical field. Other chapters cover detailed derivations of reconstruction algorithms in 2D and modern 3D cone-beam CT (CBCT), evaluate geometric parameters of bone in 3D using CT scans or a new low-radiating device (EOS), and CT based 3D- display providing accurate preoperative visualization and computerized risk analyses for safety margins of pancreatic- and biliary- tract tumors, as well as for the assessment of abdominal aortic aneurysms (AAA).

Chapter 1 - *Background:* The advancements in medical imaging technology over the last number of years has revolutionised the management and treatment of all aspects of healthcare. Computed tomography and magnetic resonance imaging have led to the development of reconstruction software that allows internal bodily structures to be easily visualised in 3D. These developments have led to improved surgical planning and treatment. The assessment of abdominal aortic aneurysms (AAA) has benefited greatly from these advancements. There is currently much debate as when to surgically repair these life-threatening dilations of the aorta and 3D reconstructions of AAAs have led to many new diagnostic tools and rupture-prediction indices. This chapter explores some of the more recent developments in this area.

Methods: Imaging of patient-specific AAAs opens many possibilities for the surgical-planning and biomechanical examination of the diseased vessel. 3D reconstructions allow for exact measurements and dimensions of stent-grafts to be obtained. These 3D reconstructions also form the basis for all numerical modelling techniques, be it finite element analysis, computational fluid dynamics or fluid-structure interaction. Computational and experimental examination of the wall stress within a particular AAA can reveal important information regarding possible rupture sites, and relationships between wall stress and geometrical factors. 3D imaging has allowed the development of new parameters that may better assess the likelihood of AAA rupture on a patient-specific basis. Post-operative monitoring of the stent-graft also benefits from 3D imaging. The *in-vivo* pulsatile forces acting on the stent-graft, which contribute to stent-graft migration and may result in sac re-pressurisation, can be numerically determined on a patient-specific basis. The use of 3D reconstructions also allows for improved experimental testing through exact AAA replication and numerical validation models.

Results: New diagnostic tools and rupture-prediction methods have revealed that similarly sized AAAs may have significantly different rupture potentials. Experimental approaches to AAA assessment have shown that AAAs will rupture at regions of elevated wall stress and not necessarily at areas of maximum diameter. Fluid-structure interaction is a useful tool for assessing post-operative stent-graft performance, as both the haemodynamic forces acting on the stent-graft and wall stress of the aneurysm are of interest. Numerical modelling has also allowed for the design and evaluation of novel stent-graft designs such as the tapered device presented in this chapter.

Conclusion: 3D imaging has allowed engineers to aid clinicians in the management and treatment of AAAs. 3D reconstructions form the basis for many engineering techniques, both numerical and experimental, and help contribute to the decision to either surgically intervene and repair an AAA, or monitor the expansion of the AAA with regular imaging. There is a need to implement alternative factors in the clinical decision-making process and the methodologies reported in this chapter may be beneficial in future AAA rupture assessment and management.

Chapter 2 - Electron microscope tomography (EMT) has emerged as the leading technique for three-dimensional (3D) structural analysis of unique complex biological specimens. EMT makes it possible to directly visualize the molecular architectures of organelles, cells and complex viruses at close-to-molecular resolution. EMT has been crucial to reveal some of the major breakthroughs in life sciences in the last few years. EMT combines electron microscopy with the power of 3D imaging to derive the 3D structure of complex specimens. A number of computational stages are involved in a typical structural study by EMT, which range from the image acquisition with the microscope to the 3D reconstruction by means of tomographic reconstruction algorithms. Afterwards, a number of computational steps are necessary to facilitate the interpretation of the 3D data: noise reduction, segmentation and analysis of subvolumes. As the computational demands are huge in some of the stages, high performance computing (HPC) techniques are also used to make the problem affordable in reasonable time. This chapter reviews the different computational stages involved in EMT, from image acquisition to interpretation of the 3D reconstruction.

The HPC techniques normally used to cope with the computational demands are also briefly described.

Chapter 3 - Electron microscope tomography (EMT) has emerged as the leading technique for three-dimensional (3D) structural analysis of unique complex biological specimens. EMT makes it possible to directly visualize the molecular architectures of organelles, cells and complex viruses at close-to-molecular resolution. EMT has been crucial to reveal some of the major breakthroughs in life sciences in the last few years. EMT combines electron microscopy with the power of 3D imaging to derive the 3D structure of complex specimens. A number of computational stages are involved in a typical structural study by EMT, which range from the image acquisition with the microscope to the 3D reconstruction by means of tomographic reconstruction algorithms. Afterwards, a number of computational steps are necessary to facilitate the interpretation of the 3D data: noise reduction, segmentation and analysis of subvolumes. As the computational demands are huge in some of the stages, high performance computing (HPC) techniques are also used to make the problem affordable in reasonable time. This chapter reviews the different computational stages involved in EMT, from image acquisition to interpretation of the 3D reconstruction. The HPC techniques normally used to cope with the computational demands are also briefly described.

Chapter 4 - The purpose of this chapter is to provide a tutorial overview on the subject of three-dimensional (3D) imaging and processing. The authors expect the chapter to the useful for practicing engineers, medical scientists for gaining an understanding of what can and cannot be done with theory, technology, and reconstruction algorithm. Toward this end, the authors have tried to strike a balance among purely algorithmic issues, topics (tomosynthesis imaging etc.) dealing with how to generate data for reconstruction in different domains, and artifacts inherent to different data collection strategies.

This chapter is structured to cover the basics of computed tomography (CT) from x-ray modern cone-beam CT. However, the main focus of the chapter is concerned with detailed derivations of reconstruction algorithms in 2D and modern 3D CBCT systems. Since the impact of CBCT will undeniably increase in the future, 3D reconstruction algorithms are illustrated and derived in detail. A thorough analysis of CT artifacts and a discussion of practical issues, such as dose considerations, provide further insight into modern CT systems. The chapter is addressed to a wide interdisciplinary readership in an effort to explain both the fundamentals and applications of tomography. Consequently, the focus is on physics and technology, whereas radiological aspects are addressed only marginally. There is no requirement for special prior knowledge. With respect to detail problems or questions, relevant literature is referenced.

Chapter 5 - Since the 1970s, human tumor cell lines, subcutaneously implanted into immunodeficient mice, rapidly advanced to become the most important pre-clinical efficacy models. However, in recent years, doubts concerning their predictive value increased. A part of the problem may reside within the combination of tumor cell lines selected for fast growth through many rounds of passaging in 2D-petri dish cultures, with the artificial subcutaneous implantation site. Recent evidence pointed towards an important role of the stromal compartment for many aspects of tumorigenesis. Along with other groups, the authors therefore set out to implant tumor cell lines orthotopically, i.e. into the organ of their origin. This technique requires surgery, and, since the tumors don't grow visibly, a sensitive imaging system for the detection of the implanted cells. A variety of tools have been developed that provide the sensitivity required, some only applicable for experimental models, e.g. fluorescence (GFP, RFP...), and bioluminescence, others, e.g. PET/CT or MRI translatable to the clinic. Bioluminescence imaging (BLI) was our choice due to its cost-effectiveness compared to the latter, and the excellent signal to noise ratio. Tumor cells thus need to be transduced with luciferase before surgical implantation into the given organ. BLI may then be used to check implantation to the correct site, growth of the tumors, and randomization of the mice into treatment groups. Upon treatment start, the effect of the drug on primary tumor and metastases may be monitored via weekly BLI measurements. Upon termination of the experiment, organs may be investigated for metastatic tumor cells via BLI, or by homogenization followed by quantitative *in vitro* luciferase assays.

This set-up has been successfully applied to test novel treatments, or novel formulations of classical chemotherapy. It allows to distinguish between drug action against the primary tumor or metastases, yielding quantitative results.

Chapter 6 - 3D imaging has become commonplace in the medical field, with its routine use in the better established institutions for pre-natal observations, diagnosis of ailments, work-up prior to surgery, recovery monitoring and many other medical procedures. In an example such as ultrasound, the difference between 2D and 3D is dramatic as the 3D visualisation of the foetus is apparent even to the uninitiated, whereas the 2D visualisation is only discernable by experts. This chapter starts by introducing some of the common 3D equipment and the type of diagnosis for which they cater. The following section takes a retro look into examples of research work that have been undertaken in the past to produce 3D reconstructions from 2D. This is an important issue as most imaging devices still reproduce images of 3D volume as a series of 2D slice images. Description of a 3D setup for 2D ultrasound probe is provided as an example of a cost-effective means of using existing 2D equipment. The next level is to then undertake 3D processing for automatic diagnosis. This chapter discusses the research methodology required in the reconstruction of 3D volume and employing computer-aided diagnosis to identify various diseases. Details of the different stages of processing, along with the promising results achieved are presented. The chapter concludes with some considerations for future trends of 3D imaging in the medical field.

Chapter 7 - Exploration of bone using two-dimensional (2D) techniques is widely used by plain x-rays, dual x-ray absorptiometry (DXA), CT scan and magnetic resonance imaging (MRI). Evaluation of fracture risk does not depend only on the bone mineral density (BMD, g/cm^2) but also on its structure as its micro and macroarchitecture. Bone is a three-dimensional (3D) structure. Using 2D imaging systems will cause loss of information. For example BMD measured by DXA depends on bone size. Patients' height reflects bone size and therefore affects BMD results and this information should be available for a proper interpretation of the BMD results. Bone geometry (macroarchitecture) is a very important parameter in the evaluation of bone strength. It has been evaluated from DXA scans or plain X-rays. Much progress has been made in 3D imaging and 3D reconstruction from several 2D images. The authors can nowadays evaluate geometric parameters of bone in 3D using CT scans or a new low-radiating device (EOS®). The authors have also recently described a method of 3D reconstruction using 2 perpendicular DXA scans: the 3D-XA (3 Dimensional X-ray Absorptiometry). Cross-sectional area, cortical thickness, cross-sectional moment of inertia, section modulus, buckling ratio, bone size and bone diameter can be measured in vivo using 3D imaging techniques. Finite element models have also been calculated from 3D images and allows the prediction of a personalized fracture risk. The recent progress in 3D imaging has greatly improved the evaluation of bone structure. BMD, microarchitecture parameters as well as geometric parameters predict failure load and improve the calculation of an individualized risk of fracture. In vivo 3D imaging will allow longitudinal studies in animals and in humans. The effect of antiosteoporotic drugs on BMD is very heterogeneous and can't explain their antifracture effect. This can be better understood by the effect of therapeutic agents on bone micro and macroarchitecture. Three dimensional imaging of bone may contribute in the field of osteoporosis to a better prediction of a personalized risk of fracture as well as a better understanding of the mechanism of action of antiosteoporotic agents.

Chapter 8 - Multiple imaging approaches are currently used for diagnosis and surgery planning of hepatobiliary tumors and living donor liver transplantations. Conventional imaging studies remain insufficient to demonstrate the individual anatomy. Refinements in CT technology with the introduction of «multidetector-row» CT scanners and implementation of mathematical methods on computerized digital data enabled CT based 3D- visualizations. This renders preoperative surgery planning more reliable and reproducible. Since the application in oncological liver surgery has been studied previously, our interest focussed on pancreatic- and biliary tract tumors including preoperative work-up in living donor liver transplantation. CT based 3D- display provided accurate preoperative visualization and computerized risk analyses for safety margins of pancreatic- and biliary- tract tumors. In living related liver transplantation the 3D- procedure may help to recognize vascular variants and to define the splitting line. The results may have major impact on patient selection and in our opinion allow better planning of the appropriate surgical approach.

Chapter 9 - Electrical resistivity imaging (ERI) is a geophysical technique used to obtain images of geological structures from electrical measurements made at the surface or in boreholes. This technique has been widely used for environmental and engineering studies.

A 3-D electrical subsurface image can be obtained with 2-D or 3-D surveys. Since all geological structures are 3-D in nature, a fully 3-D resistivity survey using a 3-D interpretation model gives most accurate results. Here the authors describe the basic resistivity theory, compare the 3-D interpretation made from 2-D versus 3-D data sets, discuss the possible arrangements of the electrodes for a 3-D surveys, present equipment used for signal injection and automatic data acquisition and review signal processing algorithms used to process the acquired data.

The authors present the results of applying ERI in stone Cultural Heritage conservation. Two Portuguese renascence panels made of porous limestone showing severe decay phenomenon, located in the cloister of Santa Cruz Church in Coimbra, were studied in order to locate the origin of one of the most dangerous causes of stone decay – moisture.

The authors show the data acquisition system developed, which uses multichannel data acquisition boards, relays for electrode switching, DC and AC sources for current injection and LabVIEW software for data processing. The survey was carried out using a pole-pole array with electrodes arranged in a 5-by-7 rectangular grid, with the same electrode spacing in both directions (0.36 m). The electrodes were numbered consecutively from left to right and top to bottom; odd-numbered electrodes were used for potential measurement and even-numbered electrodes were used for current injection. This system, with 35 electrodes (18 potential and 17 current) provided 306 measurements in each panel and in a side masonry wall (for comparison). The data was processed using a 3-D inversion program (RES3DINV) and the resulting resistivity distributions were then displayed as volumetric 3-D tomograms.

As a non-destructive and inexpensive tool, the 3-D resistivity imaging technique allowed 1) creation of a resistivity model of the two panels and the wall, where the high levels of the moisture are clearly visible and 2) the estimation of the thickness of the panels. The resistivity is lower in the bottom half of the panels and of the wall (higher levels of moisture) showing that in this case the moisture comes from the ground, rises along the wall and reaches the stone panels.

Chapter 10 - Three-dimensional (3D) imaging is a new technology that can be applied to a broad scope of disciplines, including medicine. The application of 3D imaging research in medicine is a new and interesting topic. This type of research began in developed countries in the West and spread around the world. The status of medical 3D research in developing countries is worthy of investigation. In this brief report, the author summarizes research in medical 3D imaging in Thailand.

Chapter 11 - At the present time, the three-dimensional image has become the focus in medical imaging. It is accepted that three-dimensional images provide more information than two-dimensional images. In this brief chapter, the author reviews the concept of three-dimensional image reconstruction in medical imaging.

Chapter 12 - Three-dimensionally distributed electrical functioning is the trigger of mechanical contraction of the heart. Disturbance of this electrical flow predisposes the heart to mechanical catastrophe that hinders sufficient blood supply to the body. Because this electrical dysfunction is amenable to proper intervention, a detailed understanding of subject-specific cardiac electrophysiological conditions is of great medical interest. In current clinical practice, body surface potential recording is the standard tool for observing cardiac electrical dysfunctions. However, successful treatments require a more detailed imaging of these dysfunctions, which is normally done by laborious and invasive catheter mapping. The prospect to obtain this imaging in a less destructive and safer manner is the main motivation of our work.

The authors have developed a system approach to pursue personalized noninvasive imaging of cardiac electrical activity and tissue property of the 3D muscle of the heart wall for individual subjects. Under the guidance of existing scientific knowledge of the cardiac electrophysiological system, the authors extract the subject-specific cardiac electrical information from noninvasive body surface potential mapping and tomographic imaging data. In this way *a priori* knowledge of cardiac system leads the physiologically meaningful interpretation of personal data; at the same time, subject-specific information contained in the data identifies parameters in individual systems that differ from prior knowledge. In this framework, the authors first developed a coupled meshfree-BE (boundary element) modeling approach to represent existing physiological knowledge of the cardiac electrophysiological system on personalized heart-torso structures. Through a state space system approach and sequential data assimilation techniques, the authors then developed statistical model-data coupling algorithms for quantitative reconstruction of volumetric transmembrane potential dynamics and tissue property of 3D myocardium from body surface potential recoding of individual subjects.

Phantom experiments and real-data human studies demonstrate the potential of our framework in providing intuitive 3D visualization and quantitative understanding of volumetric cardiac electrophysiology and latent threats in the heart for individual subjects. This technique could aid in personalized diagnose, treatment planning, and fundamentally, prevention of fatal cardiac arrhythmia and cardiac arrest.

Chapter 13 - In this chapter, the authors will focus on the problem of 3D Euclidean reconstruction of structured scenes from uncalibrated images based on the property of vanishing points. Firstly, under the assumption of three-parameter-camera model with varying parameters, the authors prove that the camera projection matrix can be uniquely determined from three mutually orthogonal vanishing points under an arbitrary preassigned world coordinate system. Secondly, when multiple images of an object are present, the authors prove that a set of global consistent projection matrices can be recovered if an arbitrary reference point in space is observed across the views. In addition, the authors present some techniques to take geometric measurement from a single image, by which the authors can recover the 3D structure of the entire scene with several architectures. Compared with previous stereovision technique which is fully rely on the feature matches, the proposed method computes projection matrices from the vanishing points of parallel lines. Thus the bottleneck problem of feature matching is avoided, and more accurate, robust and realistic results are expected. Extensive experiments on synthetic and real world images validate the effectiveness of the proposed method. The proposed method is applicable to reconstruct photo-realistic and accurate model of structured scenes, especially those containing three dominate directions and some planar surfaces.

Chapter 14 - The chapter addresses the problem of estimating 3D structure and motion of non rigid object from a monocular image sequence. Many previous methods on this problem adopt the extension technique of SVD factorization based on rank constraint to the tracking matrix, where the 3D shape of nonrigid object is expressed as weighted combination of a set of shape bases. Most solutions are based on the assumption of affine camera model which may be invalid when the object is close to the camera. The chapter makes two contributions to the problem. Firstly, the authors propose a constrained power factorization (CPF) algorithm that combines the orthonormal constraint and the replicated block structure of the motion matrix directly into the iteration steps of power factorization. This algorithm overcomes the limitations of previous SVD based methods. It is easy to implement and can even deal with missing data in the tracking matrix. Secondly, the authors propose two techniques to upgrade the solutions from affine assumption to full perspective camera model. The first algorithm updates the solutions from affine to perspective projection by linear recursive estimation. The second one is based on nonlinear optimization technique by minimizing the perspective reprojection residuals. Extensive tests on synthetic and real images validate the proposed method and noticeable improvements over previous solutions are observed.

In: 3D Imaging: Theory, Technology ...
Editors: E. H. Duke and S. R. Aguirre, pp.1- 50

ISBN: 978-1-60876-885-1

Chapter 1

3D Imaging of Abdominal Aortic Aneurysms: Techniques and Applications

Barry J. Doyle, David S. Molony, Michael T. Walsh and Timothy M. McGloughlin

Centre for Applied Biomedical Engineering Research (CABER), Department of Mechanical and Aeronautical Engineering and Materials and Surface Science Institute, University of Limerick, Ireland

Abstract

Background

The advancements in medical imaging technology over the last number of years has revolutionised the management and treatment of all aspects of healthcare. Computed tomography and magnetic resonance imaging have led to the development of reconstruction software that allows internal bodily structures to be easily visualised in 3D. These developments have led to improved surgical planning and treatment. The assessment of abdominal aortic aneurysms (AAA) has benefited greatly from these advancements. There is currently much debate as when to surgically repair these life-threatening dilations of the aorta and 3D reconstructions of AAAs have led to many new diagnostic tools and rupture-prediction indices. This chapter explores some of the more recent developments in this area.

Methods

Imaging of patient-specific AAAs opens many possibilities for the surgical-planning and biomechanical examination of the diseased vessel. 3D reconstructions allow for exact measurements and dimensions of stent-grafts to be obtained. These 3D reconstructions also form the basis for all numerical modelling techniques, be it finite element analysis, computational fluid dynamics or fluid-structure interaction. Computational and experimental examination of the wall stress within a particular AAA can reveal important information regarding possible rupture sites, and relationships between wall stress and geometrical factors. 3D imaging has allowed the development of new parameters that may better assess the likelihood of AAA rupture on a patient-specific basis. Post-operative monitoring of the stent-graft also benefits from 3D imaging. The *in-vivo* pulsatile forces acting on the stent-graft, which contribute to stent-graft migration and may result in sac re-pressurisation, can be numerically determined on a patient-specific basis. The use of 3D reconstructions also allows for improved experimental testing through exact AAA replication and numerical validation models.

Results

New diagnostic tools and rupture-prediction methods have revealed that similarly sized AAAs may have significantly different rupture potentials. Experimental approaches to AAA assessment have shown that AAAs will rupture at regions of elevated wall stress and not necessarily at areas of maximum diameter. Fluid-structure interaction is a useful tool for assessing post-operative stent-graft performance, as both the haemodynamic forces acting on the stent-graft and wall stress of the aneurysm are of interest. Numerical modelling has also allowed for the design and evaluation of novel stent-graft designs such as the tapered device presented in this chapter.

Conclusion

3D imaging has allowed engineers to aid clinicians in the management and treatment of AAAs. 3D reconstructions form the basis for many engineering techniques, both numerical and experimental, and help contribute to the decision to either surgically intervene and repair an AAA, or monitor the expansion of the AAA with regular imaging. There is a need to implement alternative factors in the clinical decision-making process and the methodologies reported in this chapter may be beneficial in future AAA rupture assessment and management.

1. Introduction

1.1 Incidence and Current Opinions

Cardiovascular disease is the leading cause of morbidity and premature death of modern era medicine. It is estimated that approximately 81 million people in the United States (US) currently have one or more of the many forms of cardiovascular disease, resulting in 1 in every 2.8 deaths, or 900,000 deaths per year. 40% of all deaths in Europe are a result of cardiovascular disease in people under the age of 75, with mortality rates in Ireland reported to be as high as 43% in 1997 [Creagh et al., 2002]. Aneurysms form a significant portion of these cardiovascular related deaths and are defined as a permanent and irreversible localised dilation of a blood vessel greater than 50% of its normal diameter [Sakalihasan et al., 2005]. Although aneurysms can form in any blood vessel, the more lethal aneurysms develop in the cranial arteries, thoracic aorta and abdominal aorta, which if left untreated, will eventually expand until rupture. The vast majority of these aneurysms form in the abdominal aorta and are termed abdominal aortic aneurysm (AAA). Figure 1 shows a comparison between a healthy young male and the diseased aorta of an elderly male patient. The actual mechanisms resulting in AAA formation are still not fully understood. It is believed that these aneurysms form due to alterations of the connective tissue in the aortic wall. The degradation of the aortic wall can be attributed to risk factors such as tobacco smoking, gender, age, hypertension, chronic obstructive pulmonary disease, hyperlipidaemia and family history of the disorder [Sakalihasan et al., 2005].

With recent advancements in medical imaging technology, the recorded incidence of AAA is on the increase. It has been reported that over the last 30 years, AAA diagnosis has tripled in the Western world and this is likely to increase over the coming years as the average population age is on the rise [Bosch et al., 2001]. There are approximately 150,000 - 200,000 new cases in the US and 500,000 patients worldwide diagnosed each year. It is estimated that 1 million people worldwide are currently living with an undiagnosed AAA and that 95% of these cases could be successfully treated if detected prior to rupture. Mortality figures are also high, with a 95% mortality rate. These statistics contribute to rank AAAs as the 13th leading cause of death in the US and the 10th leading cause of death in men over the age of 55. Annually there are approximately 15,000 - 20,000 deaths in the US from AAA, and 8,000 deaths in the United Kingdom. The numbers of cases and subsequent deaths for Ireland is similar to international figures [Brosnan et al., 2009]. 30 - 50% of patients with a ruptured AAA die before they ever reach a hospital and even with surgical repair a 50 - 70% mortality rate remains. The condition is also more common in men than women, however, the disease is more lethal in women.

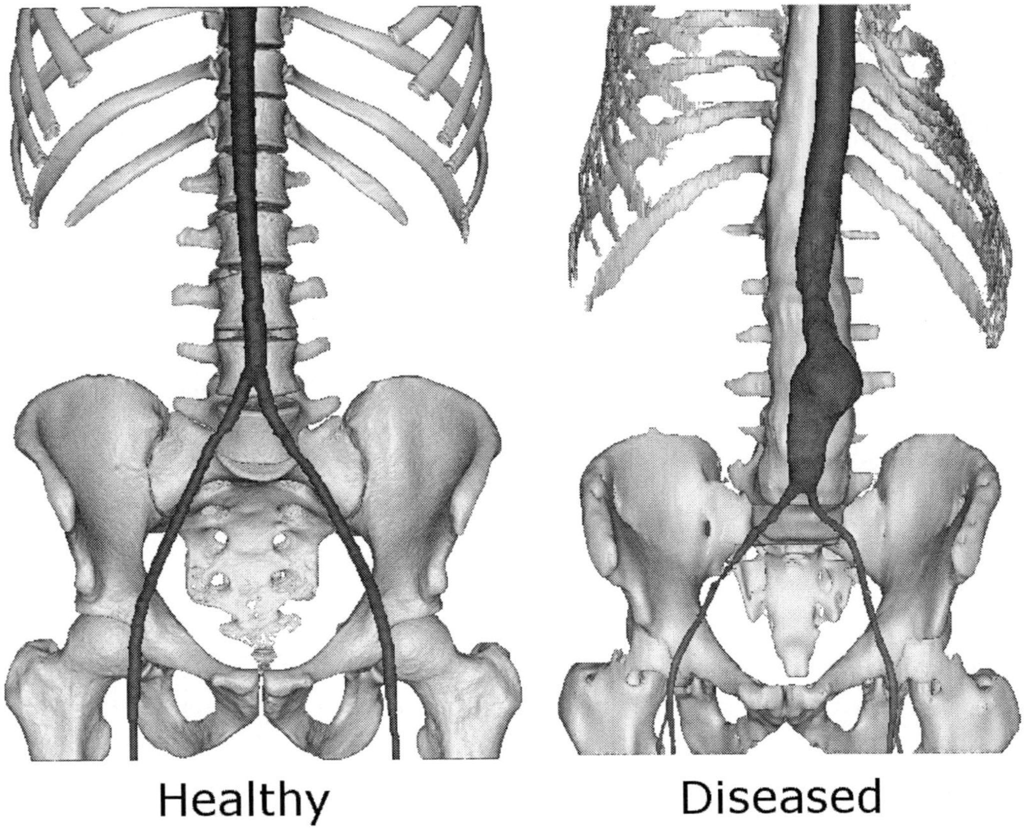

Figure 1. 3D reconstruction of a healthy (left) 28 year old male compared to a 76 year old male with an abdominal aortic aneurysm (right). The differences between the two cases are clear to see, with the diseased case showing dilation and skewing of the aorta. Notice also the differences in skeletal structure due to age between the two cases.

AAAs are typically asymptomatic and are usually detected through medical imaging as a result of unrelated health problems or screening programs of the elderly. Screening involves the use of ultrasonography to detect the AAA and the implementation of these programs is becoming increasingly common. From a theoretical screening model of a population of 100,000 it has been estimated that 1500 lives could be saved, at a cost of $78,000 per life [Quill et al., 1989; Ernst, 1993]. Measurements of AAA size determined using ultrasonography are accurate up to 6 mm [Ernst, 1993], and therefore this approach has become the most cost-effective method of AAA detection. It has been recommended that people over the age of 60 - 65 years old, in particular men, should be screened for AAA, with the recommended age reducing to 50 - 55 when there is a history of aneurysmal disease in the family as this may increase the likelihood of AAA by up to 6 times. AAA screening programs are becoming more widespread in the UK with many private institutions providing screening. The UK National Health Service (NHS) recently announced that a full screening program will be made available throughout the UK, but is unlikely to become widely available until 2013 [National Health Service, 2009]. Recently, it was suggested that AAA screening may be beneficial in Irish males aged 65 - 75 years [Brosnan et al., 2009]. According to the US Preventative Services Task Force [USPSTF, 2005], the potential benefit of screening for AAA among women over the age of 65 is low because of the number of age-related deaths in this population. The majority of AAA related deaths occur in women over the age of 80, and as there are many competing health risks at this age, any benefit of screening would be minimal [USPSTF, 2005]. Various lifestyle considerations can also affect the prevalence of AAA, such as smoking, diet and obesity; with people who fall into these categories more likely to either have or develop an AAA.

Upon detection of an AAA, there is currently much debate as how to best assess the severity and rupture risk of the patient. Currently, the trend in determining the severity of an AAA is to use the maximum diameter criteria [Cronenwett et al., 1985; Glimaker et al., 1991]. Patients with an AAA that has a maximum diameter greater than 5 - 5.5 cm are deemed a high rupture risk and are usually recommended for surgical repair [Lederle et al., 2002]. In the case of smaller AAAs where the diameter is <5 cm, the preferred approach is often careful and frequent observation using either ultrasonography or computed tomography (CT) scanning. Recent research however, has cast doubt over the suitability of surgical repair based on maximum diameter alone [Raghavan et al., 2000; Sayers et al., 2002; Fillinger et al., 2002, 2003; Vande Geest et al., 2006a; Kleinstreuer and Li, 2006; Leung et al., 2006; Doyle et al., 2009a, 2009b]. Although the diameter-criterion can be justified, as the rupture risk for an AAA is clearly related to its maximum diameter [Conway et al., 2001; Fillinger et al., 2002], surgical decision-making using the diameter-criterion alone may in fact lead to both unnecessary AAA repairs and also exclude certain cases (AAA <5 cm) from surgical repair [Darling et al., 1977; Cronenwett et al., 1985; Nicholls et al., 1998; Fillinger et al., 2002]. Nicholls et al. [1998] reported that 10 - 24% of ruptured AAAs were less than 5cm in diameter. Darling et al. [1977] also reported that of 473 non-repaired AAAs examined from autopsy reports, there were 118 cases of rupture, 13% of which were less than 5 cm in diameter. They also showed that 60% of the AAAs greater than 5 cm (including 54% of those AAAs between 7.1 and 10 cm) never experienced rupture. Vorp et al. [2008] later deduced from the findings of Darling et al. [1977] that if the maximum diameter criterion were followed for the 473 subjects, only 7% (34/473) of cases would have succumbed to rupture prior to surgical intervention as the diameter was less than 5 cm, with 25% (116/473) of cases possibly undergoing unnecessary surgery since these AAAs may never have ruptured.

Alternative methods of rupture assessment have been recently reported. The majority of these approaches involve the numerical analysis of AAAs using the common engineering technique of the finite element method (FEM) to determine the wall stress distributions. Recent reports have shown that these stress distributions have been shown to correlate to the overall geometry of the AAA rather than solely to the maximum diameter [Vorp et al., 1998; Sacks et al., 1999; Doyle et al., 2009a]. It is also known that wall stress alone does not govern failure as an AAA will rupture when the local wall stress exceeds the local wall strength. Therefore, rupture assessment is most suitable when both the patient-specific wall stress is coupled with patient-specific wall strength. A non-invasive method of determining patient-dependent wall strength was recently reported by Vande Geest et al. [2006b], with more traditional approaches to strength determination via tensile testing performed by others [Raghavan et al., 1996, 2006; Thubrikar et al., 2001a]. Newly proposed AAA assessment methods include: AAA wall stress [Fillinger et al., 2002, 2003; Venkatasubramaniam et al., 2004]; AAA expansion rate [Hirose et al., 1998]; degree of asymmetry [Doyle et al., 2009a]; presence of intraluminal thrombus (ILT)[1] [Wang et al., 2002]; a rupture potential index (RPI) [Vorp et al. 2005; Vande Geest et al., 2006a]; a finite element analysis rupture index (FEARI) [Doyle et al., 2009b]; biomechanical factors coupled with computer analysis [Kleinstreuer and Li, 2006]; growth of ILT [Stenbaek et al., 2006]; geometrical parameters of the AAA [Giannoglu et al., 2006]; and also a method of determining AAA growth and rupture based on mathematical models [Watton et al., 2004; Volokh and Vorp, 2008]. Based on these hypotheses, it is believed that an improved predictor of AAA rupture is desirable and may have clinical importance [Vorp et al., 1998; Raghavan et al., 2000a, 2000b; Sayers et al., 2002; Wang et al., 2002; Fillinger et al., 2002, 2003; Vande Geest et al., 2006b; Kleinstreuer and Li, 2006; Leung et al., 2006; Doyle et al., 2009a, 2009b].

Detection of AAAs by medical imaging leads to the clinical question: should the AAA be surgically repaired or monitored? Monitoring of AAAs, particularly smaller aneurysms, has been shown in the past to be effective, with the usual recommendations being repeat ultrasound every six months for AAAs 4 – 5 cm in diameter and every three months for larger AAAs [Ernst, 1998]. During this monitoring phase, expansion rates are also observed. If the expansion rate exceeds 0.5 cm per year, surgical intervention is often recommended. Further to aneurysm size deciding the fate of the AAA, other contraindications to elective repair are also commonly considered. These include, but are not limited to: myocardial infarction within the past six months; intractable congestive heart failure; intractable angina pectoris; severe chronic renal insufficiency, incapacitating effects from stroke, and a life expectancy of less than two years.

If the clinical outcome is to surgically repair the AAA, two approaches may be considered, both utilising a graft to exclude blood flow and pressure from the aneurysmal sac and return it to a relatively normal state. These options are either the traditional approach of open surgical repair or the minimally-invasive technique of endovascular aneurysm repair (EVAR). The gold standard in AAA repair is the open surgical method. The long-term durability of the procedure is excellent, with little need for post-operative intervention

---

[1] Intraluminal thrombus (ILT) consists of a fibrin structure incorporated with blood cells, platelets, blood proteins and cellular debris, and are found in most AAAs

[Garcia-Madrid et al., 2004; Goueffic et al., 2005; Corbett et al., 2008]. However, this procedure is highly invasive and poses serious risk of complications during the operation [Sakalihasan et al., 2005; Vogel et al., 2005; Corbett et al., 2008]. EVAR, on the other hand, is the preferred treatment in older patients and patients unfit for open repair. This procedure uses minimally-invasive techniques, entering the aorta via the femoral artery, resulting in minimal scarring, reduced blood-loss and a significant reduction in operation time. Questions have, however, been raised recently about the effectiveness of EVAR compared to open repair, in particular with regards to the biomechanical performance of the stent-graft resulting in post-operative complications such as endoleak, graft migration, and fabric tears [EVAR Trial Participants, 2005a; EVAR Trial Participants, 2005b; Corbett et al., 2008].

1.2 Medical Imaging

The term "medical imaging" commonly refers to the techniques and processes used to create images of the human body for clinical purposes or medical science. These purposes are often to reveal, diagnose or examine disease, or to study the normal anatomy and physiology of the human body. Over the last number of decades, medical imaging has advanced from the earliest forms of x-rays which began at the beginning of the 1900's to the more recent developments of sophisticated ultrasound and magnetic resonance imaging. Each imaging technique has its own strengths and weaknesses, and the method of imaging is typically defined by the desired application. For example, traditional ultrasonography is employed to image the foetus in pregnant women, as this technique is powerful enough to reveal the desired information regarding the foetus and with no health risk. More complex imaging techniques are required for the detailed examination of structures such as the cerebral arteries. In this case, magnetic resonance imaging (MRI) may be used. This imaging process allows excellent soft tissue contrast enabling detailed images of the blood vessels within the Circle of Willis to be captured. For the purpose of this chapter, medical imaging will focus on computed tomography as this is the medical imaging technique commonly employed for imaging AAAs. CT, or computed axial tomography (CAT), uses helical tomography to produce two dimensional images of the structures in a thin section of the body through the use of x-rays. The technique is a non-invasive imaging procedure that utilises non-ionizing radiation to create high-resolution 2D images of the anatomy and is capable of differentiating between a wide range of tissues. CT is the gold standard for diagnosing many abdominal diseases, such as renal stones, pancreatitis, appendicitis, diverticulitis, bowel obstruction and AAA. For an in-depth description of the underlying mathematics and theories involved with CT imaging, one can refer to Webb [1990]. A typical CT image of an AAA can be seen in Figure 2. The AAA is easily distinguishable in the image, and these 2D cross-sectional images provide valuable information to the clinician regarding size and shape of the aneurysm. One drawback of traditional CT 2D images is the difficulty in obtaining accurate wall thickness information. This problem is evident in Figure 2, as the pixel intensity, measured in Hounsfield units (HU), of the diseased AAA wall is too similar to the ILT to determine wall thickness. It is possible in certain cases to determine the wall thickness based on the thickness of the calcifications embedded in the wall, but in cases where there are negligible calcifications, the problem remains.

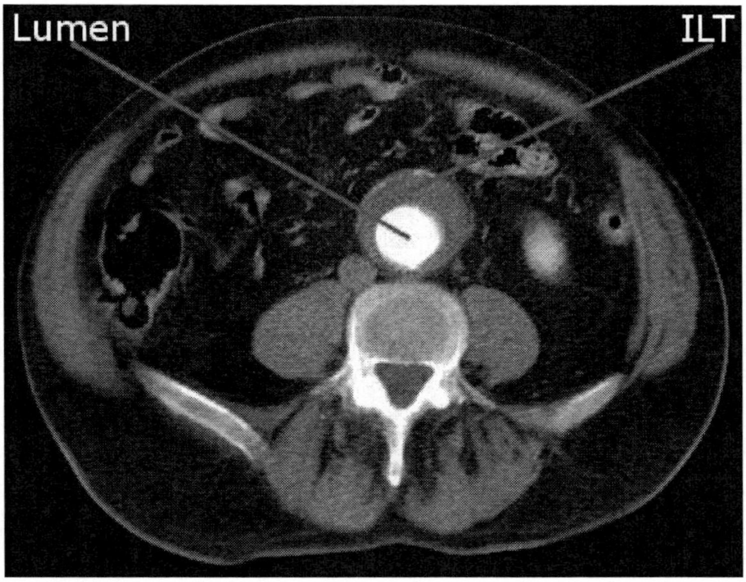

Figure 2. Typical CT scan of patient with AAA. AAAs predominantly form with ILT encapsulated between the lumen region and the diseased aortic wall.

2. 3D Reconstruction from CT Scans

Further to 2D use of CT images, recent advancements in technology have enabled the reconstruction of 3D models from the 2D images. Numerous software programs are available nowadays from freeware to commercial programs, all of which are capable of essentially generating 3D reconstructions of medical images. The reconstruction software used throughout this chapter is the commercially available software Mimics [Materialise, Belgium]. In order to actually reconstruct the 3D AAA from the 2D CT scans, many techniques are employed. Firstly, the CT scans in Digital Imaging and Communications in Medicine (DICOM) format are imported into the software. Once imported, the technique known as thresholding can be applied. The input to a thresholding operation is typically a greyscale or colour image, in this case greyscale CT scans. Thresholding is a useful method of separating out regions of an image that are of interest, from those that are background. This segmentation technique is often based on the different intensities or colours in the foreground and background regions of an image. When segmenting a CT scan, it is often useful to filter pixels whose intensity values lie within a certain range, or band of intensities. For this operation, black pixels correspond to background, and white pixels to foreground. Now, the image is segmented into regions of interest (white pixels) and background regions (black pixels). Instead of forcing foreground pixels to white, it is also possible to leave all pixels of interest as their original colour in order to preserve information.

As CT scans are complex images, they require more refinement than a simple thresholding operation. Whilst the thresholding is being performed, the software is employing an edge detection algorithm. Edge detection is a fundamental tool used in most image processing applications to obtain information from the frames as a precursor step to feature extraction and object segmentation. This process detects outlines of an object and boundaries between objects and the background in the image. The basic edge-detection operator is a matrix area gradient operation that determines the level of variance between different pixels. This edge-detection operator is calculated by forming a matrix centered on a pixel chosen as the center of the matrix area. If the value of this matrix area is above a given threshold, then the middle pixel is classified as an edge. There are many ways in which edge detection can be performed, with most being grouped into two categories; gradient and Laplacian.

The algorithm used in Mimics is the *marching squares* and *marching cubes* algorithm. Marching cubes is one of the latest algorithms of surface reconstruction used for viewing 3D data, and was first described by Lorensen and Cline in 1987. This algorithm produces a triangle mesh by computing isosurfaces from discrete data. From connecting the patches from all the cubes on the isosurface boundary, a surface representation can be obtained. This high-resolution 3D surface construction algorithm produces models with unprecedented detail. These 3D reconstructions can be generated using a variety of algorithms, but the three more commonly employed techniques are shaded surface display, maximum intensity projection, and more recently, 3D volume rendering [Calhoun et al., 1999]. Mimics utilises the 3D volume rendering approach, in particular, the OpenGL [Open Graphics Library, Silicon Graphics International] graphics language. This hardware acceleration offers high quality rendering including Gouraud shading for optimal display of the 3D objects. Gouraud shading is a method used in computer graphics to simulate the differing effects of light and colour across the surface of an object. The basic principle behind this OpenGL language is to define the volumetric data as a three-dimensional texture and render it by mapping it onto a stack of "display slices" that are orthogonal to the viewing direction [Tam et al., 1997; Cabral et al., 1994]. As a result of these algorithms within Mimics, detailed 3D reconstructions of medical images are possible. The use of additional techniques such as layering, allow reconstructions of exquisite detail to be produced. Figure 3 shows a typical reconstruction of anatomical structures from CT images, highlighting the use of layers to allow further use of the reconstructions by hiding/replacing certain regions of interest.

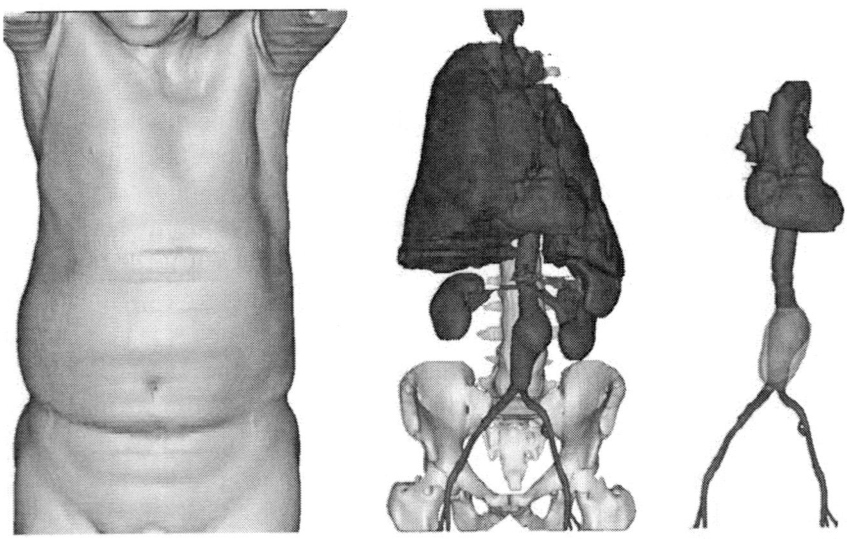

Figure 3. Full 3D reconstruction of CT scan data set. Image shows the use of layers to highlight/remove particular regions of interest such as organs and bones. Reproduced from Doyle et al. [2009c].

3. Applications of AAA 3D Reconstructions

The resulting 3D reconstructions have many applications toward the further understanding of AAA disease. Over recent years these virtual AAA models have allowed researchers to apply numerical techniques such as finite elements analysis (FEA), computational fluid dynamics (CFD) and also fluid-structure interaction (FSI) to the problem, thus highlighting regions of complex stress distributions or irregularities in the haemodynamics. 3D reconstructions also allow experimental methods to be effectively employed, as reconstructions enable the creation of *in vitro* replicas for bench-top testing. Whilst numerical techniques are the more commonly employed tools used by researchers for determining the severity of AAAs and the post-operative success of AAA stent-grafts, there remains a need for experimental methods in order to validate these numerical approaches. For the purposes of this chapter, the following work will branch into two distinct areas, that is, numerical and experimental investigations. Both avenues of research rely heavily on the 3D reconstruction method of the AAA and results can vary significantly depending on the technique used. Smoothing is essential on reconstructions to be used for further research so as to eliminate unwanted detail that will impair the quality of the results, but also ensuring that particular details are not lost due to over-smoothing. Overall, 3D reconstructions have advanced the treatment and therapy options available to patients in many areas of health and disease and now AAAs can benefit from similar advancements. The following sections of this chapter will identify and describe some of the more recent developments in the field of AAA biomechanics and 3D imaging from both a numerical and experimental viewpoint.

4. Numerical Investigations

The primary roles of numerical studies involving AAA include: 3D reconstructions of the AAA to determine the morphology and dimensions of the aneurysm for stent-graft sizing; evaluating the degree of asymmetry of the AAA and the resulting posterior wall stress; the determination of peak wall stress to assess the likelihood of rupture; examination of the fluid flow and resulting wall stress within the AAA both before and after surgical repair; the optimisation of stent-graft design in order to enhance stent-graft technology; analysis of the post-operative biomechanics of the stent-graft; and computer aided design (CAD) and computer aided manufacturing (CAM) to create experimental AAA models.

4.1 Pre-Operative Planning for EVAR

Pre-operative planning involves patient-specific 3D reconstructions of the AAA to determine the most suitable approach to EVAR. Upon reconstruction, the clinician can foresee any possible complications with the repair, in particular, problems with access sites and vessel geometry. As part of this chapter section, CT scan data was obtained from the Midwestern Regional Hospital, Limerick, and St. James's Hospital, Dublin, for 4 patients either awaiting or previously undergone surgical repair of an AAA. All patients were male with a mean age of 77.5 yrs (range 59 – 87 yrs). CT scans were obtained using a Somatom Plus 4 [Siemens AG, D-91052 Erlangen, Germany]. The mean pixel size of the CT scans was 0.675 mm with all scans taken using a 3 mm slice increment. The CT scans were imported into Mimics for

3D reconstruction. For these particular reconstructions, only the lumen regions were of clinical importance as this is the region to which the stent-graft is deployed and fixated.

Reconstruction times can range from as little as 2 minutes for a basic model where minor details are ignored, to 1 hour where all details are included such as the ILT and calcifications. The critical dimensions when concerned with EVAR stent-grafts are the neck diameter of the stent-graft, the iliac diameter, and also the length of the device. Clinician's can usually determine the neck diameter without difficulty using 2D CT scans, but problems can arise when determining length. 3D reconstruction allows the overall length to be easily measured, thus allowing the exact sizing of the medical device. The measurements are taken from below the lowest renal artery to a point in the iliac arteries where the clinician feels comfortable will maintain an adequate fixation of the device. A variety of measurements are possible from the reconstruction, as shown in Figure 4, with the clinician able to determine certain distances that can help overcome possible obstacles with the surgical repair. 3D reconstruction of one particular patient revealed an extremely tortuous proximal neck that may cause difficulties during the surgical procedure. 3D reconstruction highlighted the degree of curvature of the neck and allowed the clinician to decide on the most suitable approach before EVAR. As shown in Figure 4, the proximal neck of the AAA required special attention during the operation. As the upper portion of the stent-graft is embedded into the proximal neck, the tortuous nature of this could complicate placement and fixation of the device.

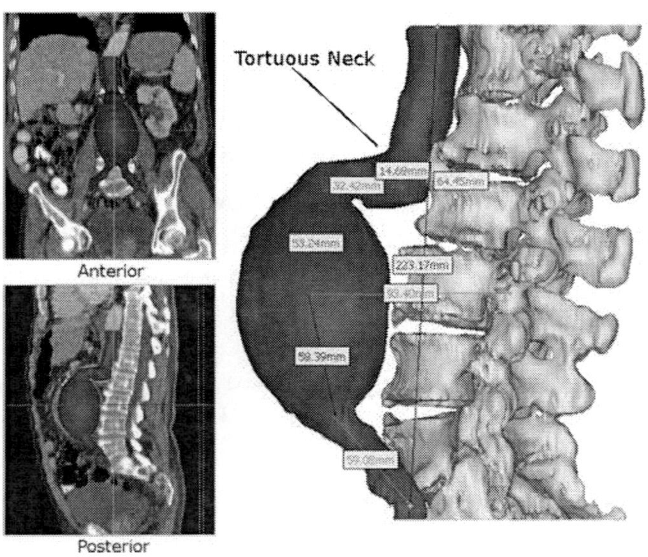

Figure 4: Example reconstruction showing measurements obtainable from reconstructions. All measurements are in millimetres (mm). The 3D reconstruction showed exactly the degree of tortuosity, allowing the clinician to decide on the most suitable means of approach during EVAR.

The patient-specific reconstruction shown in Figure 5 was a particularly extreme case. In this reconstruction, the full extent of the aneurysmal aorta was revealed. This patient had a descending thoracic abdominal aneurysm (TAA), abdominal aortic aneurysm (AAA) and also an iliac aneurysm (IA). For the case shown in Figure 5, the clinician decided to only repair the TAA with a stent-graft. This decision was solely based on surgical experience as the AAA had also exceeded the threshold for repair (diameter > 5.5cm).

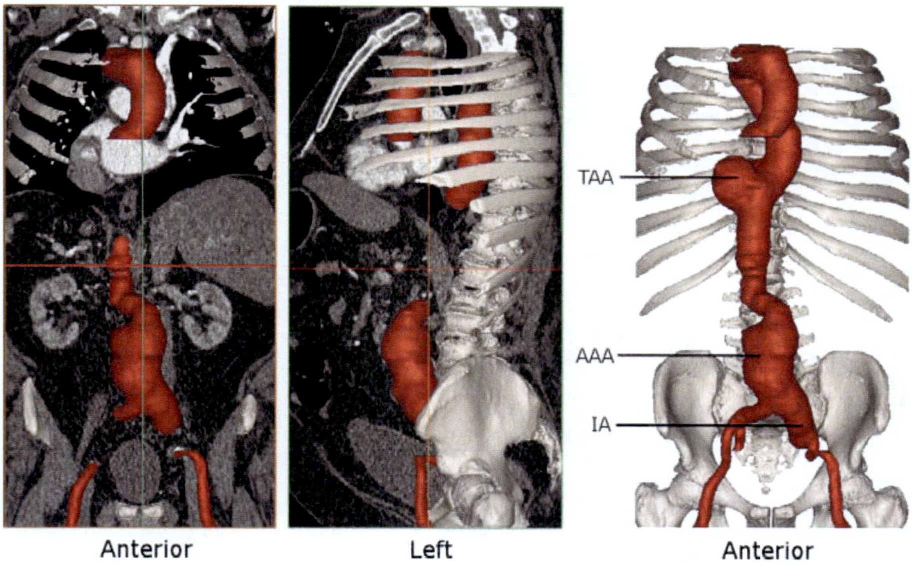

Figure 5. 3D reconstruction showing thoracic aortic aneurysm (TAA), abdominal aortic aneurysm (AAA) and iliac aneurysm (IA) from the anterior viewpoint. The patient had significant tortuosity of the aorta and aneurysms at three separate locations. The clinician decided to repair the TAA and monitor the growth of the AAA and IA.

The reconstruction of the stent-graft after placement within the TAA of Figure 5 can be seen in Figure 6. The device now excludes the region of high stress predicted using numerical tools and thus aids to return the aorta to a lower stress state that is relatively safe from rupture. This reconstruction was generated from post-operative CT scans that help to monitor the diseased aorta, and help highlight any additional aneurysm growth from endotension [EVAR Trial Participants, 2004], or further progression of the AAA. Post-operative 3D reconstructions can also aid the clinician to observe the outcome of the EVAR procedure at regular intervals. Stent-graft limbs can often become kinked, twisted or occluded by thrombosis [Corbett et al., 2008], which can complicate the flow of blood and may require further intervention by the clinician. Although these complications can be identified using 2D CT scans, 3D reconstructions allow exact visualisation of the problem and aid towards a better understanding of the overall situation of the patient. Currently, there is no institution-wide standard regarding stent-graft sizing, with many clinicians opting for their own methods of measurements, particularly lengths. There is still a degree of learning among the EVAR community when concerned with AAA morphology and stent-graft behaviour. The latest generation of the Medtronic Endurant™ graft appears to shorten more in length on deployment than its predecessor, Talent™, due to design modifications. This consequently affects the recommended measurements and sizing by the manufacturer. Ultimately, better imaging and 3D reconstructions can only add to the quality of the endovascular repair. The procedure is quick to perform and could not only help towards standardising the measurement and sizing of stent-grafts, but could also aid surgeons in improving the treatment of AAAs.

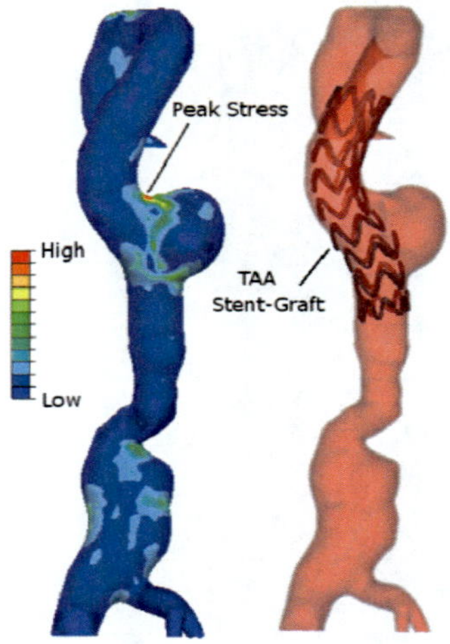

Figure 6. Illustration showing the pre-operative numerically predicted von Mises wall stress distribution *(left)*. Post-operative EVAR deployed TAA stent-graft *(right)* now excludes the TAA sac, returns blood flow in the descending aorta to a relatively normal state and reduces stress acting on the TAA wall. In this case, the clinician decided not to repair the AAA even though diameter > 5.5cm. Pre-operative wall stress somewhat validates this decision as the TAA was under significantly higher wall stress than the AAA. Transparency of the aorta in the image on the right allows easy visualisation of the medical device. Models are shown from the posterior viewpoint.

4.2 Stent-Graft Design

Further to pre-operative planning of stent-graft sizing, 3D reconstructions also greatly aid with stent-graft design. As EVAR is becoming the favoured choice for repair procedures among clinicians, much research is aimed at identifying the limitations of both EVAR and stent-grafts [Parodi et al., 1991; Egelhoff et al., 1999; Kamineni et al., 2004; Corbett et al., 2008]. The primary complications with EVAR are graft migration, endoleaks and to a lesser extent thrombotic occlusion. It has been suggested that re-designing current stent-graft devices may provide a remedy to these problems. The design of conventional grafts and stent-grafts has normally featured a constant proximal diameter with a sudden diameter reduction at the bifurcation. In the healthy aorta this is not the case as the geometry tapers smoothly into the iliac arteries [Shipkowitz et al., 1998]. The rapid cross-section area change with conventional bifurcated devices causes the flow to converge, promoting flow separation and recirculation in the iliac limbs that may be associated with graft limb thrombosis [Chong and How, 2004; Jacobowitz et al., 1999]. Occlusions are believed to be caused by thrombosis as well as kinks, even though this is not a very common problem [Corbett et al., 2008].

CFD is a numerical tool capable of modelling the haemodynamics of the arterial system. The procedure involves taking a geometrical description of the volume the fluid occupies and dividing it into a finite number of volumes. The governing equations for fluid mechanics are then solved for each volume to give a representation of the fluid flow and fluid forces acting within the volume. CFD has been used to examine stent-graft performance in the past, providing useful information on flow patterns and forces affecting the device [Li and Kleinstreuer, 2005a; Howell et al., 2007]. Drag forces, which act on stent-grafts as a result of shear and pressure forces over the pulse cycle, have been implicated in graft migration. Drag is dominated by arterial pressure and is influenced by several factors, such as iliac angle, neck angle, and neck diameter [Howell et al., 2007]. CFD can be a cost-effective method for investigating alternative stent-graft designs. Our group previously investigated the potential benefits of a newly designed tapered stent-graft that maintains an area ratio at its inlet equal to that at the bifurcation of the device [Morris et al., 2006]. This novel stent-graft design is shown compared to a conventional design in Figure 7. In an *in vitro* study, the tapered design was associated with a reduction in blood pressure compared to a conventional graft [O'Brien et al., 2008]. Further to this line of research, this novel tapered stent-graft was compared to a conventional bifurcated stent-graft using both ideal uniplanar and realistic out-of-plane model configurations.

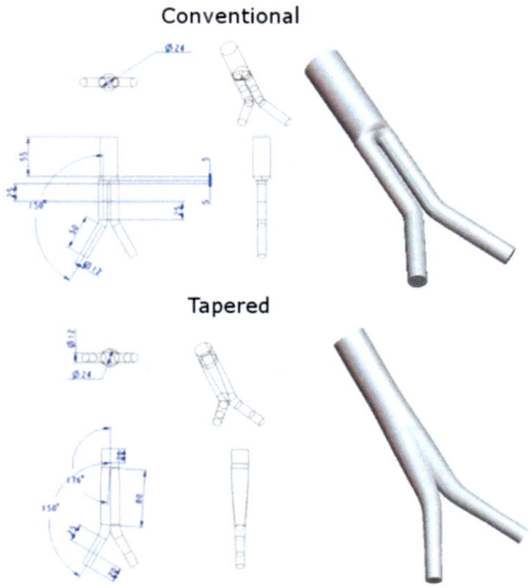

Figure 7. The conventional stent-graft design *(top)* compared to the novel tapered design *(bottom)*. The tapered stent-graft design maintains the area of the inlet throughout the bifurcation region, whereas, the conventional design has a rapid 2:1 area change at the bifurcation. This new smooth transition in area ratios has been shown to result in smoother velocity profiles and reduce secondary flows. Modified with permission from Molony et al. [2008].

The conventional stent-graft has a sudden change in area at the bifurcation point (an area ratio of 2:1 with respect to the inlet and bifurcation), while the tapered stent-graft is characterized by a tapering section from the proximal neck into the iliac limbs. The novelty of this tapered design lies in the blended transition outward as the iliac limbs separate from the trunk, which achieves a 1:1 area ratio at the bifurcation point, i.e., the same area at the entrance of the stent-graft and at the bifurcation. In order to solve the fluid equations using CFD, the fluid was assumed as laminar, incompressible, and Newtonian [Di Martino et al., 2001; Morris et al., 2004a], which is an acceptable assumption for large diameter arteries. Blood was modelled with a density of 1050 kg/m^3 and viscosity of 0.0035 Pa·s [Scotti et al., 2007]. The graft walls were considered rigid, with no slip [Morris et al., 2006]. Velocity and pressure pulses at the inlet and outlets, respectively, resembled those recorded from a typical abdominal aorta over a cardiac cycle by previous authors who had assumed laminar flow for the velocity profile [Di Martino et al., 2001; Morris et al., 2004]. By comparing the results of the conventional and tapered stent-grafts, it was apparent that the tapered design alleviated some of the problems associated with the conventional design. The new design reduced velocities by 18% and 31% above and below the iliac bifurcation, respectively. A comparison of the velocity profiles and secondary flow profiles between the two stent-graft designs are shown in Figure 8. For the full comparative study between the effectiveness of the new tapered design over the conventional stent-graft, including the application within patient-specific cases, the reader can refer to Molony et al. [2008].

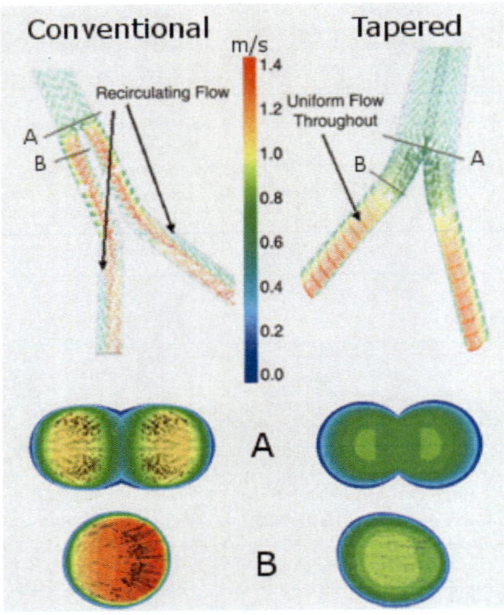

Figure 8. The axial velocity vector profiles (m/s) and cross sections showing secondary flows for the idealised models of the conventional and tapered stent-grafts. Modified with permission from Molony et al. [2008].

Based on CFD analysis, the novel tapered stent-graft improved graft haemodynamics compared to the conventional design. The tapered stent-graft reduced velocity and wall shear stress impinging on the graft wall and also resulting drag force. In the realistic scenario, the out-of-plane curvature reduces the positive impacts of the tapered design and thus, in patients with more irregular geometry, some of the benefits from the tapered design may be diminished.

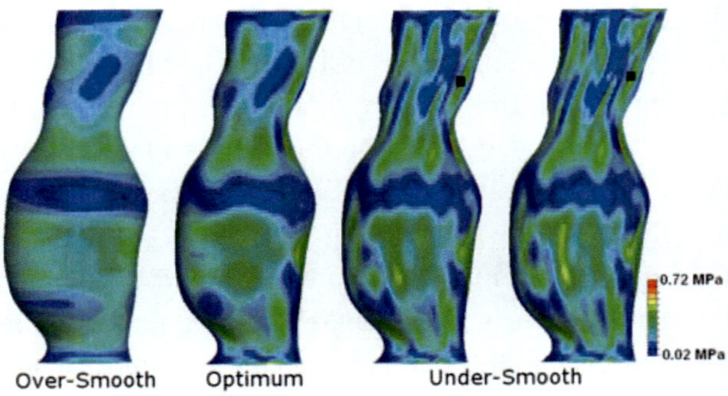

Figure 9. Axial smoothing study to determine the optimum number of control points per axial polyline. This test revealed that 20 control points per polyline is the desired level, as increasing this number over-smoothes the model, whereas, decreasing the number creates models with artificial stress distributions. The black mark in the under-smooth models indicates regions of artificially high wall stress. Reproduced from Doyle et al. [2007].

4.3 Optimum Smoothing of 3D Models

Smoothing can significantly influence the resulting stress distributions in 3D numerical models. In order to determine the optimum level of smoothing applicable for these AAA models, an axial smoothing study was performed. The CT images were thresholded and segmented within Mimics, with polylines created at the boundaries of the segmentation. These polylines were then exported in IGES file format for further processing. Four full AAA 3D reconstructions of the same case were created and exported from Mimics. Each model was created using a different smoothing level by controlling the number of control points per axial polyline. FEA was then used to determine the wall stress on each model, helping to determine the optimum smoothing level. Artificial stress contours, and unrealistically high stress regions all indicate problems with the surface of the model. As shown in Figure 9, the wall stress contours of the four models revealed that at 20 control points per polyline is the optimum level of smoothing. Smoothing levels above 20 control points may unnecessarily smooth the surface removing important local details. Whereas, under-smoothing the models with control point number in excess of 20 may result in artificially high stressed areas and incorrect stress distributions. For a full description of the effect of modelling techniques on resulting AAA wall stress the reader can refer to Doyle et al. [2007].

4.4 Determining AAA Asymmetry

Previous work [Vorp et al., 1998; Scotti et al., 2005] has identified the importance of asymmetry in idealised AAA models, and also indicated the need to investigate this aspect in realistic models. In this section, we have examined the role of asymmetry and resulting wall stress in realistic patient-specific AAA cases. Spiral CT scan data was obtained for 15 patients, comprised of 10 males and 5 females. Mean age ± standard deviation of the case subjects was 73.2 ± 6.7 years. These patient scans were obtained from the Midwestern Regional Hospital, Limerick, Ireland, and the University of Pittsburgh Medical Centre, Pittsburgh, PA, USA. All 15 patients were awaiting AAA repair, as AAA diameters had reached or exceeded the current 5 cm threshold for repair. CT scans were acquired using both the Somatom Plus 4 [Siemens AG, D-91052 Erlangen, Germany] and LightSpeed Plus [GE Medical Systems, General Electric Company] range of imaging equipment. All scans were single CT slices with a standard width x height of 512 x 512 pixels. Mean pixel size of scans was 0.742 ± 0.072 mm. The bodily structures of each subject were made visible using the non-ionic contrast dye, Optiray® [Mallinckrodt Inc., Convidien, MO, USA]. This CT data was then reconstructed using Mimics. These reconstructions allowed the computation of stress distributions within the geometries using the commercially available finite element solver ABAQUS [Dassault Systemes, SIMULIA, Rhode Island, USA]. The numerical tool of FEA involves dividing the structure into a smaller number of sub-domains, called elements. Each element is then connected via nodes. This series of elements over the surface and throughout the wall of the structure is known as a mesh. Certain constraints and boundary conditions are then applied to the model, typically to represent the conditions *in vivo*. Once adequate boundary conditions are in place, the software mathematically calculates the displacement of each node. From these displacements, stresses and strains are computed at integration points within the mesh, resulting in a full quantitative assessment of the stresses and strains within that particular AAA. Nowadays, this numerical tool is widespread among researchers in the assessment of AAA wall stress [Mower et al., 1997; Vorp et al., 1998; Raghavan et al., 2000; Di Martino et al., 2001; Thubrikar et al., 2001b; Hua et al., 2001; Wang et al., 2002; Fillinger et al., 2002, 2003; Venkatasubramaniam et al., 2004; Giannoglu et al., 2006; Leung et al., 2006; Papaharilaou et al., 2007; Speelman et al., 2007; Scotti et al., 2005, 2007; Truijers et al., 2007; Doyle et al., 2007, 2009a, 2009b, 2009c, 2009d; Rissland et al., 2009].

As CT scanning is routinely performed on AAA patients scheduled for repair, collection of this information involved no extra participation by the study subjects. All reconstructions were developed from scan positions immediately distal to the lowest renal artery to immediately proximal to the iliac bifurcation. The ILT was neglected in this study as with previous approaches [Vorp et al., 1998; Raghavan and Vorp, 2000; Thubrikar et al., 2001b; Fillinger et al., 2002, 2003; Scotti et al., 2005]. The thickness of the aorta wall is not easily identifiable from CT scans, therefore the wall was assumed to be uniform throughout the model and set to 2mm [Venkatasubramaniam et al., 2004]. This limiting assumption is one of the main concerns among researchers, as the AAA wall is known to be non-uniform in thickness, ranging from 0.23 – 4.26 mm [Raghavan et al., 2006]. All AAAs underwent the same degree of smoothing as previously reported by this author [Doyle et al., 2007]. The iliac bifurcation was omitted from this study, as in previous stress analysis work as it has been shown to not significantly affect the wall stress results of the AAA [Fillinger et al., 2002]. The AAA material was assumed to be homogenous and isotropic with non-linear realistic material properties [Raghavan and Vorp, 2000] that have been implemented in many previous publications [Sacks et al., 1999; Raghavan et al., 2000; Wang et al., 2002; Fillinger et al., 2002, 2003; Leung et al., 2005; Doyle et al., 2007; Papaharilaou et al., 2007]. The aorta is also known to be nearly incompressible with a Poisson's ratio of 0.49. The blood pressure within the AAA acts on the AAA inner wall and therefore, pressure was applied to the inner surface of the computational AAA model. A static peak systolic pressure of 120 mmHg (16 kPa) was used. In order to simulate the tethering of the AAA to the aorta at the renal junction and iliac bifurcation, the AAA model was fully constrained in the proximal and distal regions.

Most AAAs are constrained from radial expansion in the posterior direction due to the spinal column, therefore, AAAs predominantly dilate in the anterior plane. All cases studied in this analysis were naturally asymmetric in the anterior-posterior direction. In order to examine the effect asymmetry has on wall stress, the centreline of each AAA was automatically found using the reconstruction software. The centreline, which begins just below the renal arteries and ends immediately before the iliac bifurcation, passes through the centroid of each polyline slice in the series. Asymmetry is defined, in this case, as the perpendicular distance from the proximal and distal points of the centreline to a defined point on the centreline. Figure 10 shows how these asymmetry measures are obtained. Starting with the 3D AAA model in Figure 10A, a centreline is automatically created through the polyline centroids of Figure 10B, thus creating Figure 10C. Then these polylines are exported from Mimics to ProEngineer Wildfire [PTC, Lebanon, NH, USA]. Next, using the software, the end points of the centreline are connected with a straight line (Figure 10D) and a perpendicular line is extended from this connecting line, to predetermined points along the centreline (Figure 10E). The asymmetry at a specified distance along the AAA model is regarded as this perpendicular distance, and is measured in millimetres (mm). This method of determining AAA asymmetry results in a plot similar to that of Figure 10F which shows the normalised diameter plotted along the normalised length of the AAA.

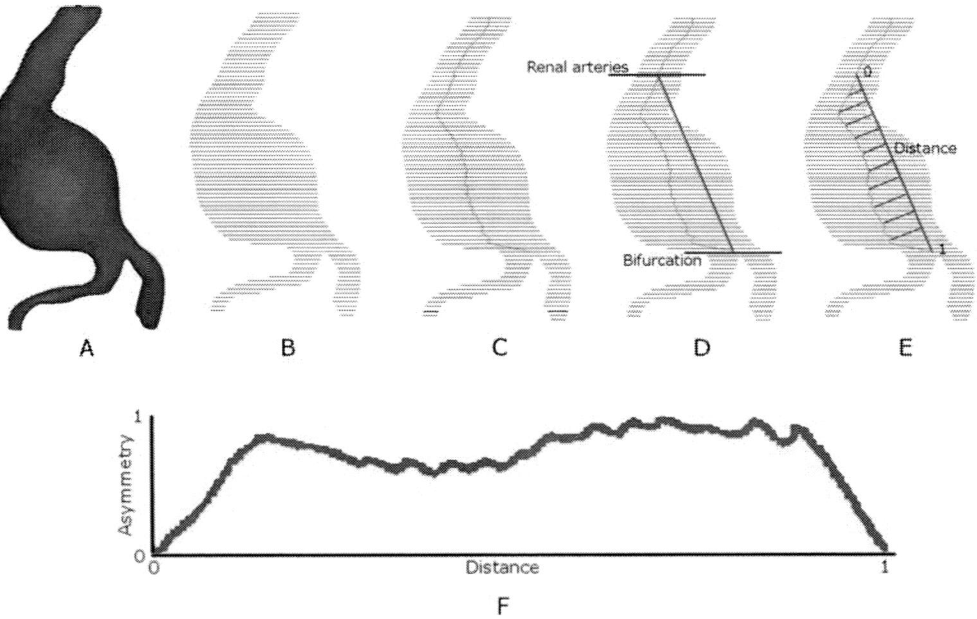

Figure 10. Illustration showing method used to obtain asymmetry measurements.

The results of this comparison revealed a strong relationship between the stress acting on the posterior wall and the degree of asymmetry in the anterior direction. In all cases studied, the relationship was evident, and as over 80% of AAAs rupture on the posterior wall [Darling et al., 1977], these findings may have clinical significance. For the full report of how posterior wall stress and asymmetry correlate, the reader may refer to Doyle et al. [2009a].

An alternative technique to measure asymmetry is also under development by the author. This tool uses the 2D CT images to directly determine asymmetry by simply comparing coordinates. The CT scan immediately below the lowest renal artery is examined, with the coordinates of the centre point of the AAA recorded. The clinician then follows through the series of CT scans until the scan revealing the most severe asymmetry is detected. This should be readily identifiable by experienced radiologists and clinicians. The coordinates of the centrepoint, or centroid, of the AAA at this region is again noted. Figure 11 shows the detection of centre points for the particular region of interest, that is, the AAA region of the CT scan. The 2D distance between these two points can then easily be determined by simply subtracting the Y-coordinates of each scan, resulting in a measurement of asymmetry in millimetres (mm). For the example shown in Figure 11, by subtracting the Y-coordinates, the resulting maximum asymmetry is approximately 25 mm. This allows the clinician to obtain a single parameter to assess the maximum degree of asymmetry of the particular AAA. The same method can be applied to each CT scan in the series if the full degree of asymmetry is desired along the length of the AAA, resulting in a plot similar to that shown in Figure 10F.

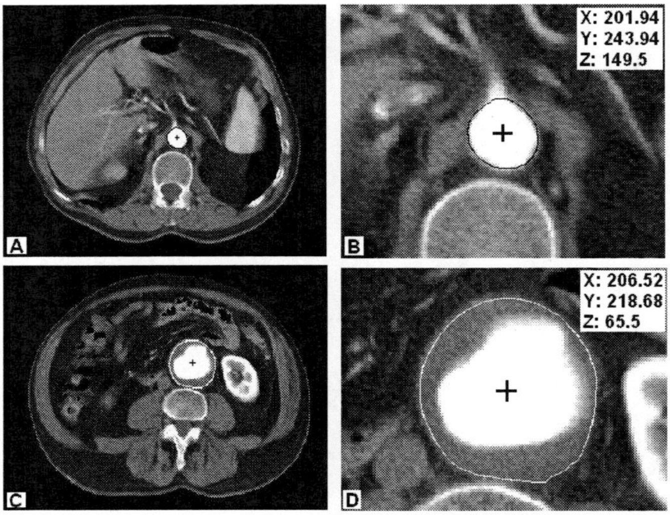

Figure 11. (A) CT scan depicting the proximal neck of the AAA with centre point identified, (B) Close-up view of region with centroid coordinates recorded, (C) Scan depicting the most severe region of asymmetry of the particular AAA, again with centroid shown, and (D) Close-up of scan with centre point coordinates recorded. Maximum asymmetry is 25 mm.

Table 1. Correlation coefficients for posterior wall stress and both asymmetry and diameter.

Patient	Asymmetry	*p*	Diameter	*p*
1	0.574	0.032	0.420	0.135
2	0.781	0.003	0.895	0.000
3	0.175	0.587	0.755	0.005
4	0.37	0.293	0.733	0.016
5	0.862	0.000	0.820	0.000
6	0.82	0.002	0.609	0.047
7	0.464	0.151	0.573	0.066
8	0.834	0.001	0.573	0.051
9	0.474	0.166	0.529	0.116
10	0.443	0.130	0.505	0.078
11	0.683	0.014	0.811	0.001
12	0.411	0.128	0.593	0.020
13	0.411	0.128	0.593	0.020
14	0.834	0.000	0.709	0.007
15	0.667	0.013	-0.132	0.668

As mentioned previously, the majority of ruptures occur in the posterior region of the AAA. Based on these findings, both the diameter and asymmetry were statistically compared to posterior wall stress along the longitudinal distance of the aneurysm for 15 cases. This analysis was performed using a Spearman's Rho correlation bivariate test with significance defined as $p<0.05$. The results of this analysis are shown in Table 1.

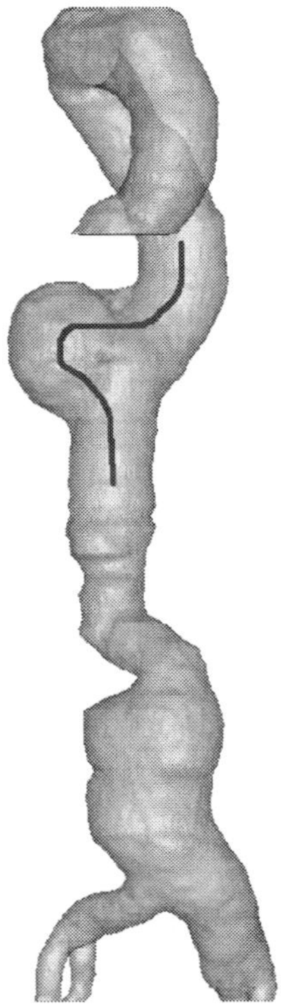

Figure 12. Image showing the centreline of a TAA which could be used to determine the level of asymmetry.

The results presented in Table 1 show how both asymmetry and diameter are comparable in their significance towards posterior wall stress. From the resulting correlations, 8/15 cases show asymmetry is significant and 9/15 cases show that diameter is significant. These results suggest that if posterior wall stress is to gain clinical acceptance as a possible high-risk rupture indicator, that both asymmetry and diameter may be as important in determining the posterior wall stress, and therefore may both equally contribute to AAA rupture. It has been previously postulated by Vorp et al. [2007] and also by Fillinger et al. [2002, 2003] that the biomechanics of the AAA may provide useful clinical guidance over the maximum diameter criteria. This present work supports this biomechanics-based approach and in particular suggests that posterior wall stress may be clinically important. The results presented also suggest that if peak wall stress is to remain the primary purpose of AAA stress analyses, then diameter remains a significant factor. It is also possible to apply this methodology to other potentially lethal aneurysms. Figure 12 illustrates how the asymmetry tool may be used to determine the asymmetrical nature of a TAA.

Although, ideally, stress analysis should be carried out on every AAA detected, the reality is that the decision to repair lies with the surgeon. The use of the maximum diameter criterion is very easy to implement for the surgeon, in that they must simply measure the maximum diameter from CT scans. The asymmetry condition described in this chapter could also be readily incorporated into the surgeon's decision making. This dilation, and ultimately asymmetry, can be identified by the clinician from basic 3D reconstruction, and could greatly aid in their decision to surgically intervene. Also, our group are developing an approach that accounts for asymmetry in all directions, and therefore the relationship between asymmetry and wall stress can be assessed in all AAAs, regardless of orientation. Once detected, the degree of bulging could be incorporated into the decision making process of the surgeon, and may refine and improve the current system of deciding on surgical intervention solely on the basis of maximum diameter.

4.5 Improving Rupture Predictions

Currently, maximum diameter is the predominant factor governing AAA rupture risk, although, it is known that rupture will occur when the wall stress exceeds the wall strength. Therefore, the AAA tissue strength must play an equal role to AAA wall stress in determining failure. A region of AAA wall that is under elevated wall stress may also have high wall strength, thus equalising its rupture potential. The purpose of this section is to examine the use of a new additional tool to assist in the assessment of AAA rupture risk. This new approach focuses on a combination of the FEM coupled with published ultimate tensile strength (UTS) data from AAA tissue reported by previous researchers [Raghavan et al., 1996, 2006; Thubrikar et al., 2001]. This new approach, which we have described as the Finite Element Analysis Rupture Index (FEARI), may be clinically useful in aiding surgeons as to the most appropriate time to surgically intervene, and may serve as a useful adjunct to both maximum diameter and asymmetry.

As part of this study, CT scan data was obtained for 10 patients (male, n = 6; female, n = 4). These patient scans were obtained from the Midwestern Regional Hospital, Limerick, Ireland, and the University of Pittsburgh Medical Centre, Pittsburgh, PA, USA. All ten patients were awaiting AAA repair at the time of CT scan, as AAA diameters had reached or exceeded the current 5 cm threshold for repair. 3D reconstructions were performed, as previously described, using the commercial software Mimics. Patient-specific wall thickness was obtained using the equation proposed by Li and Kleinstreuer [2005b]. The ILT was also included in the reconstructions as this structure has been shown to reduce wall stress [Wang et al., 2002]. The models developed by this method formed the basis for the FEM stress analysis.

In order to simulate *in vivo* wall stress in the AAA wall, realistic boundary conditions were applied to each model. The AAA wall was modelled as a homogenous isotropic hyperelastic material using the finite strain constitutive model (Eqn.1) proposed by Raghavan and Vorp [2000].

$$W = C_1(I_B - 3) + C_2(I_B - 3)^2 \quad (1)$$

Where, W is the strain energy density, I_B is the first invariant of the left Cauchy-Green deformation tensor and C_1 and C_2 are material coefficients based on population mean values (C_1 = 0.174 MPa and C_3 = 1.881 MPa). These material properties have been utilised in many previous stress analysis studies [Raghavan et al., 2000; Wang et al., 2002; Fillinger et al., 2002, 2003; Ventkatasubramaniam et al., 2004; Raghavan et al., 2005; Leung et al., 2005; Doyle et al., 2007, 2009a; Papaharilaou et al., 2007; Speelman et al., 2007]. The aorta is also known to be nearly incompressible with a Poisson's ratio of 0.49. The ILT was modelled as a hyperelastic material using the material characterisation derived from 50 ILT specimens from 14 patients performed by Wang et al. [2001] shown in Equation 2.

$$W = D_1(II_B - 3) + D_2(II_B - 3)^2 \quad (2)$$

Where II_B is the second invariant of the left Cauchy-Green deformation tensor and D_1 and D_2 are population mean material constants derived for the ILT. Each AAA was constrained in the proximal and distal regions to simulate tethering to the aorta at the renal and iliac bifurcations. The blood pressure within the AAA acts on the luminal contour of the ILT and therefore, pressure was applied to the inner surface of the computational AAA model. A static peak systolic pressure of 120 mmHg (16 kPa) was used, as employed in most AAA stress analyses [Inzoli et al., 1993; Vorp et al., 1998; Giannoglu et al., 2006; Speelman et al., 2007; Truijers et al., 2007]. It is known that patient-specific blood pressures may be higher than 120 mmHg, but for the purpose of this study a standard value was more appropriate so as to eliminate some of the unknown variables in the analysis. Mesh independence was performed by increasing the number of elements in the mesh until the difference in peak stress was less than 2% of the previous mesh [Wang et al., 2002; Truijers et al., 2007; Doyle et al., 2007, 2009a]. This method of determining wall stress distributions has been previously shown to be the most effective in computing accurate results compared with other approaches [Doyle et al., 2007].

The FEARI is defined by Equation 3. In this equation, the peak wall stress is computed using the FEM, whereas, the wall strength values are obtained from previous research on experimental testing of AAA wall specimens [Raghavan et al., 1996, 2006; Thubrikar et al., 2001].

$$\text{FEARI} = \frac{\text{FEA Wall Stress}}{\text{Experimental Wall Strength}} \quad (3)$$

This equation is based on the simple engineering definition of material failure and returns a value ranging from 0 to 1, where 0 indicates a very low rupture potential, and a value close to 1 indicates a very high rupture potential. In order to determine strength values for the AAA wall, the previous research of both Raghavan et al. [1996, 2006] and Thubrikar et al. [2001] were analysed. These publications are the most detailed reports of experimental uniaxial testing of AAA tissue. Raghavan et al. [1996] tensile tested 52 specimens of AAA tissue and found that the average UTS of this aneurysmal tissue was 0.942 MPa. Thubrikar et al. [2001] later segmented AAAs into posterior, anterior and lateral regions and tensile tested 49 tissue specimens. Average regional UTS values were shown to be 0.46 MPa, 0.45 MPa and 0.62 MPa, respectively. Raghavan et al. [2006] subsequently furthered their work, and also divided each AAA into regional sections and tested 48 samples. They showed that the UTS of AAA tissue can range from 0.336 – 2.35 MPa. They also reported that the regional variations in UTS for the anterior, posterior, left and right regions were 1.099 MPa, 1.272 MPa, 1.217 MPa and 1.224 MPa, respectively. By combining all the previously published experimental data, average regional UTS values for the four main regions of the AAA could be obtained. By subdividing the AAA into a further four sections, eight in total, more regionally accurate strength estimates were obtained, thus allowing FEARI values to be calculated. The method of dividing each AAA into regions is shown in Figure 13, with the resulting UTS values for the varying regions shown in Table 2.

Once the combined UTS values of AAA tissue were calculated, these values could be coupled with the computed wall stress results from the FEM. By recording the location of peak stress in each AAA model, the region can also be assigned a regional UTS value. FEARI was then computed for each of the ten cases. Statistical analysis was performed on all results using a Pearson's correlation test, with $p<0.05$ accepted as significant.

By observing the stress distributions computed using FEA, it was noted that the regions of elevated and peak wall stresses occurred at inflection points on the AAA surface, and not at regions of maximum diameter. This observation was also observed by previous researchers in idealised models, both experimentally [Morris et al., 2004b; Doyle et al., 2009d] and numerically [Vorp et al., 1998; Callanan et al., 2004], and also in realistic models [Doyle et al., 2007, 2009a]. Inflection points are defined as points on the AAA surface at which the local AAA wall shape changes from concave outward to concave inward. The peak wall stresses found in this study ranged from 0.3167 – 1.282 MPa, with a mean ± standard deviation of 0.6201 ± 0.2836 MPa. The results of the computational stress analysis, along with the maximum diameter and UTS for each case can be seen in Table 3. There was no statistical significance between peak wall stress and any geometrical parameters analysed here. There was however a significant relationship between both FEARI and maximum diameter ($p=0.043$), and FEARI and AAA volume ($p=0.036$). The FEARI values observed using this new predictive tool for the ten cases examined are shown in Figure 14. This figure highlights the fact that AAAs with similar diameters may have markedly different rupture potentials, implying that maximum diameter is not a "one-size-fits-all" approach to AAA management.

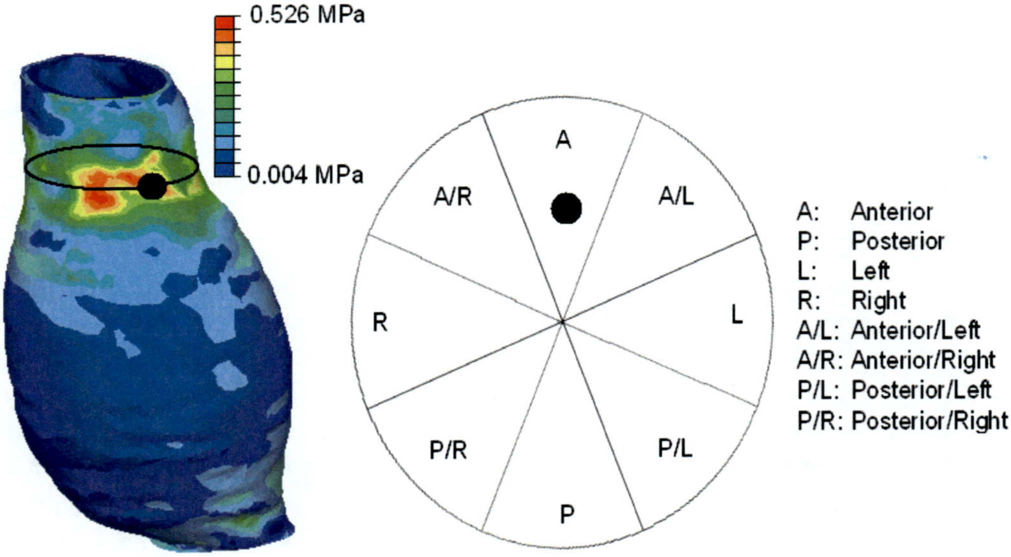

Figure 13. Illustration showing a representative AAA stress distribution for Patient 9 (ellipse passes through region of peak stress, indicated by black circle) and how each AAA model was segmented in order to determine the corresponding UTS value for the particular region of peak stress. In this case, peak stress occurs on the anterior wall of the AAA. AAA model shown in the anterior view. Reproduced from Doyle et al. [2009b].

Table 2. Regional UTS values obtained by combining and averaging previous experimental data.

AAA Region	UTS (MPa)
Anterior	0.7744
Posterior	0.8658
Left	0.9221
Right	0.9187
Anterior/Left	0.8482
Anterior/Right	0.8465
Posterior/Left	0.8939
Posterior/Right	0.8922

It is proposed that FEARI could serve as a useful adjunct to diameter-based surgical decision making. Diameter, and ultimately size of the AAA, is an obvious concern for the clinician and must remain a consideration. However, the overall geometry of the aneurysm should also play a role. Asymmetry has been shown to affect wall stress in idealised AAA models [Vorp et al., 1998; Scotti et al., 2005] and may also affect realistic cases [Doyle et al., 2009a]. Other researchers have proposed the Rupture Potential Index (RPI) [Vande Geest et al., 2006a] which uses a statistical modelling technique with the inclusion of factors such as age, gender, family history, smoking status, among others, to

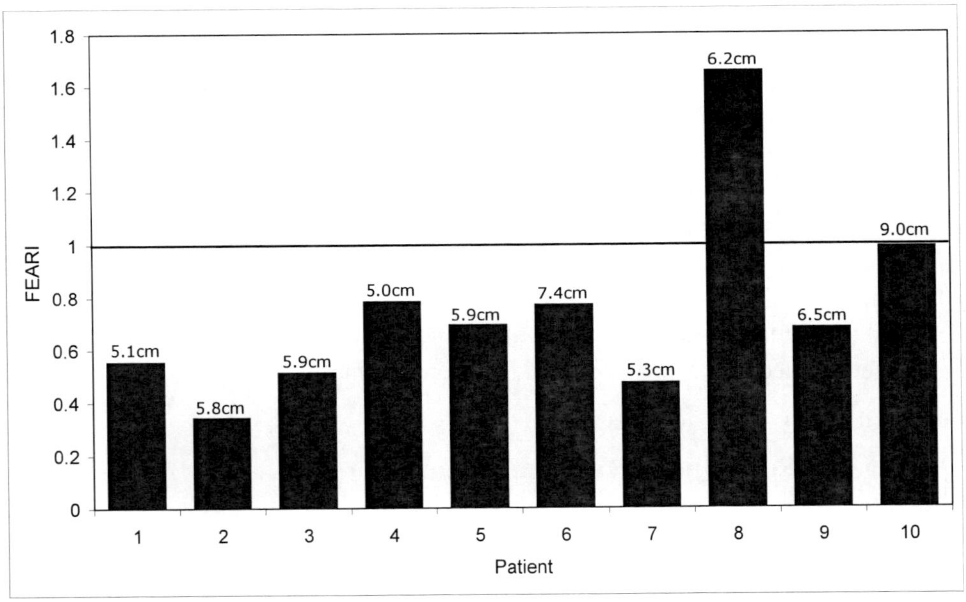

Figure 14. Graph displaying FEARI results for all ten cases. Horizontal line indicates possible AAA rupture based on the FEARI model. Diameters of each case are presented also indicating how diameter is not related to FEARI. Reproduced from Doyle et al. [2009b].

Table 3. Maximum diameter, FEA computed peak wall stress, location of peak wall stress, and UTS of peak stress region in all ten cases examined. Wall thickness was incorporated in peak wall stress calculations.

Patient	Max Diameter (cm)	Peak Wall Stress (MPa)	Location	UTS (MPa)
1	5.1	0.4291	Anterior	0.7744
2	5.8	0.3167	Left	0.9221
3	5.9	0.4346	Anterior/Right	0.8465
4	5.0	0.6641	Anterior/Right	0.8465
5	5.9	0.5866	Anterior/Right	0.8465
6	7.4	0.707	Right	0.9187
7	5.3	0.4	Anterior/Right	0.8465
8	6.2	1.282	Anterior	0.7744
9	6.5	0.5263	Anterior	0.7744
10	9.0	0.855	Posterior	0.8658

deduce patient-specific wall strength [Vande Geest et al., 2006b]. This RPI approach uses a more theoretical method of calculating wall strength, compared to the experimental approach of FEARI, and combining the two approaches may lead to improved predictions. Ultimately, the decision to surgically intervene may include a combination of factors including diameter, asymmetry, RPI and FEARI, along with clinical experience, and may determine the most suitable approach to a particular AAA. FEARI may be clinically useful due to the simplicity of the approach. Rupture occurs when the AAA tissue cannot withstand the locally acting wall stress exerted, and therefore, tissue strength must be considered when assessing AAA rupture potential. Peak wall stresses were computed, along with the location, and therefore UTS, of peak wall stress region. FEARI results indicate that surgery may not be necessary for all cases, but rather continued monitoring may suit particular patients, although, at the time of this study all cases had received either traditional open repair or EVAR. It is proposed to couple FEARI together with diameter and other important factors in AAA assessment to allow the clinician a greater understanding of the severity of an individual AAA before deciding on surgical intervention. This preliminary study of a FEARI suggests that further work into this approach may yield more interesting results, and may provide a useful adjunct to the diameter-based approach in surgical decision-making.

4.6 Pre and Post-Operative Biomechanics

Within this section, the biomechanics in a pre- and post-operative patient-specific AAA are examined. The relatively new approach of FSI was employed to determine not only the wall stresses that contribute to rupture, but also the haemodynamics involved in both the diseased vessel and post-operative stent-graft. For this particular study, CT scan data for one AAA case was obtained from the HSE Midwestern Regional Hospital, Limerick, Ireland. The pre-operative scan is used to identify the aneurysm and ILT, whereas, the stent-graft can be identified in the post-operative scan. The space between ILT and the stent-graft is assumed to consist of stagnant blood. Cross sections were segmented from just below the infrarenal aorta to the beginning of the internal iliac arteries, similar to the previously described methodology.

3D reconstructions of these geometries were then exported to Gambit [ANSYS, Canonsburg, PA, USA] for mesh generation. Here both the fluid (lumen) and structure (aneurysm wall, thrombus and graft wall) domains are meshed, with the meshes then imported to Fluent [ANSYS, Canonsburg, PA] where the solid region can then be exported to ABAQUS.

FSI is normally achieved either through a monolithic (full coupling) or partitioned approach (loose coupling) [Vierendeels et al., 2007]. The commercial software Mesh-based Parallel Code Coupling Interface (MpCCI) [Fraunhofer SCAI, Germany] was used in this work. The software is based on the loose coupling of two chosen software's, namely, Fluent (fluid) and ABAQUS (structure). This approach allows the use of familiar and mature solvers for each domain. The benefits of using mature solvers are advanced capabilities that may not be available in monolithic solvers such as the use of non-linear material models, contact and interaction of surfaces and non-Newtonian fluid models.

For this application, data was exchanged every 0.005 seconds, with Fluent sending the pressure to ABAQUS, and ABAQUS sending the deformed nodal coordinates to Fluent. Fluent uses the Arbitrary Lagrangian Eulerian (ALE) method to deal with the deforming mesh. Specifically, a remeshing technique is used where cells are remeshed based on whether they violate a user specified size and skewness criteria. Both codes share a common boundary where the data exchange occurs. MpCCI identifies nodes or elements near each other based on an association scheme and data is then transferred from one node to the other. The software also allows for non-matching meshes, useful in complex applications such as the AAA. Further information is available to the reader in the MpCCI documentation [Fraunhofer SCAI, 2008].

The ILT and AAA wall were assumed to be hyperelastic, homogenous, incompressible and isotropic. The AAA wall and ILT were modelled using the constitutive models proposed by Raghavan and Vorp [2000] and Wang et al. [2001] and presented as Equations 1 and 2 in Section 4.5. It has been shown that the use of population mean values does not significantly affect the prediction of stresses on the aortic wall [Raghavan and Vorp, 2000]. The aneurysm and ILT were assigned values of 1120 kg/m^3 and 1121 kg/m^3 for the structural density respectively [Li and Kleinstreuer, 2005a]. The stent-graft was modelled as one whole body due to the difficulty in accurately reconstructing the nitinol stents from the CT data. Future advancements in 3D imaging may alleviate this problem. A Young's Modulus of 10 MPa and a density of 6000 kg/m^3 were assumed for the stent-graft [Li and Kleinstreuer, 2005a]. The graft and artery were assumed to be tied together, simulating attachment of the stent-graft to the artery wall, thus ignoring the possibility of endoleaks and local dislodgement.

The structural model consisted of 75,849 tetrahedral elements which were used both for the aneurysm and thrombus and 19,024 hexahedral elements used for the stent-graft. The space between the ILT and stent-graft was modelled with 21,974 hydrostatic pressure elements within ABAQUS. These simulated the stagnant blood in the aneurysm sac. The aneurysm inlet and outlets were constrained in all degrees-of-freedom. For the fluid boundary conditions, a velocity inlet was assigned while at the outlets a pressure boundary was assigned. The flow rate and blood pressure were not available for this particular patient and so previously published data was used [Mills et al., 1970]. Peak systolic flow occurred at 0.305 s and the peak systolic pressure occurred at 0.4 s. Blood was assumed to be a Newtonian fluid with a density of 1050 kg/m^3 and a viscosity of 0.0035 Pas [Scotti et al., 2007]. The PISO (Pressure Implicit with Splitting of Operators) algorithm was used for pressure-velocity coupling and the QUICK (Quadratic Upwind Differencing Scheme) scheme for discretisation of each control volume. The pre-operative lumen consisted of 231,000 tetrahedral elements, while the post-operative lumen (stent-graft) had 141,000 tetrahedral elements.

The pre-operative peak wall stress was found to be 0.38 MPa, which was reduced by 92% to 0.03 MPa in the post-operative case. Figure 15 illustrates the results of the FSI simulation. Peak wall stress occurred on the posterior wall both pre- and post-operatively. The pressure of the stagnant blood in the aneurysm sac varied from 0.001 MPa to 0.0015 MPa over the course of the cardiac pulse. The maximum stress in the aneurysm was observed in the neck region where the stent-graft is in contact with the aneurysm wall. The stress in the stent-graft is much greater than the stress in the aneurysm and this is shown by the grey values of Figure 15.

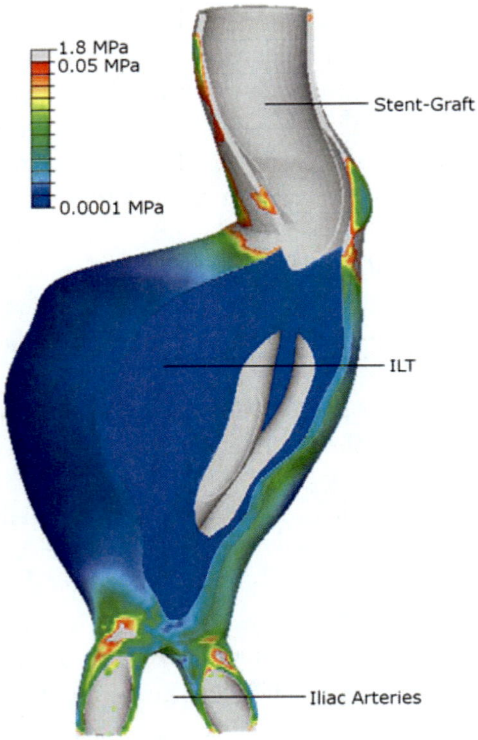

Figure 15. Cut-away view of the post-operative AAA model at t = 0.43 s of the cardiac pulse. This illustration shows how the stent-graft shields the aneurysm wall from higher stresses.

During peak systolic pressure the flow of blood has begun to decelerate, which can lead to vortex formation [Scotti et al., 2007]. The velocity pathlines and pressure contours around this time-point for the pre- and post-operative models are quite similar, as seen in Figure 16. One noticeable difference is the removal of a vortex after the graft has been implanted. This occurs just after the blood flow leaves the aneurysm neck (indicated by arrow in Figure 16). A greater pressure gradient can be seen in the post-operative model when compared to the pre-operative model. This correlates to approximately a 250 Pa greater pressure drop in the stent-graft. This large pressure gradient may be due to the curvature of the iliac limbs of the stent-graft. The drag force, which can lead to post-operative complications, is caused by pressure and viscous forces acting on the stent-graft [Morris et al., 2006a]. Peak drag force occurred prior to the peak systolic pressure with a value of 4.85 N and varied from a value of

2.85 N to 4.85 N over the cardiac cycle. Both the viscous force and pressure force followed the same trend as the velocity and pressure waveform respectively, with the majority of the force generated due to the pressure component. At peak systolic flow the viscous force was 1.1% of the total drag force, while at peak systolic pressure it was 0.35% of the total drag force.

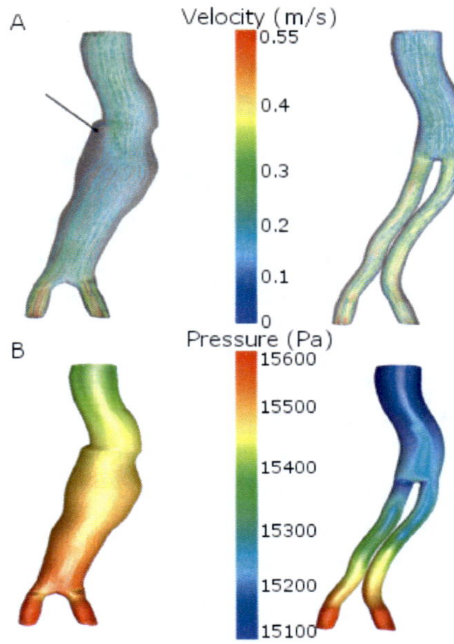

Figure 16. Velocity pathlines and pressure contours. (A) Velocity pathlines (m/s) for the pre-operative (left) and post-operative (right) cases, and (B) pressure contours (Pa) for the pre-operative (left) and post-operative (right) cases. These results are taken at the time of maximum wall stress (t = 0.4). The arrow indicates the presence of a vortex.

Fluid-structure interaction is a powerful tool available to researchers to identify both the wall stresses and haemodynamics within patient-specific AAAs. By combining both the structural and fluid elements of the AAA, the most accurate numerical predictions can be obtained. The work presented here on a pre and post-operative case study has revealed the effectiveness of EVAR as a surgical repair technique, and can also aid in highlighting any possible complications that may arise. The ability of FSI to compute the realistic drag forces acting on the stent-graft is of great benefit to clinician, as this information could help to evaluate the likelihood of graft migration which could lead to further problems such as sac re-pressurisation.

4.6 Computer-Aided Design and Computer-Aided Manufacture

In order to compliment numerical tools and ultimately validate computationally derived results, experimental models are required. Advancements over recent years in computer technology allow 3D reconstructions from medical data sets to be further developed. CAD and CAM systems now enable virtual 3D models to become a reality. Although there are a number of CAD/CAM techniques available to researchers today, this section will describe a procedure of converting 2D CT images into 3D CAD/CAM designs ready for machining.

These machined moulds can then be used with the lost-wax injection-moulding process to produce anatomically-correct experimental models. Realistic experimental models can be used, not only in stress analyses such as the photoelastic method [Morris et al., 2004b], but also for fluid dynamics studies and post-operative experimental testing, such as stent graft distraction testing. The models are created by first reconstructing a virtual AAA model, leading to mould design, and then to manufacturing via the injection-moulding technique. Previous research has examined the use of rapid-prototyping as a method of producing elastomeric replicas of arterial vessels [Seong et al., 2005]. This method, although quick and effective, does not produce the surface finish that can be achieved using the injection-moulding process. Surface finish is of paramount importance when using arterial models for experimental testing using the photoelastic method, such as that previously conducted at our laboratory [Morris et al., 2004b]. Other techniques have been employed in order to make models for use in laser-Doppler anemometry (LDA) [Loth et al., 1997] and PIV flow studies. This section describes the modelling and manufacturing processes used and to determine the effectiveness of the technique. This method of converting a standard CT scan to a patient-specific silicone model may be of value to many researchers in this field.

Polylines created in Mimics are imported into ProEngineer Wildfire. Surfaces are then recreated along these polylines. These surfaces are then split using its centreline into two exact halves, thus creating a two-piece mould set used in the manufacturing technique. Each patient-specific mould design consists of two sets of moulds. The first mould is designed to produce the casting wax model of the AAA, and the second set to produce the outer silicone model. The outer mould is approximately 2 mm larger in all regions than that of the wax mould, so as to produce a silicone model with a 2 mm thick wall. As the wall of an AAA can range in thickness from 0.23 – 4.33 mm [Raghavan et al., 2006], a wall thickness of 2 mm is a reasonable assumption and has been used in previous studies [O'Brien et al., 2005].

Each outer mould design includes supports for the inner wax cast to ensure location of the wax model inside the larger outer mould. Moulds can be designed that include or omit the iliac arteries. For experimental studies involving stress analyses, the iliac arteries are believed to be unimportant, whereas, for fluid dynamics and stent-graft testing, the iliac arteries are necessary to include. Moulds designed without the iliac arteries have cylindrical sections included both in the proximal and distal regions of the AAA, to allow attachment to experimental test rigs. Inclusion of the iliac arteries can significantly increase the complexity of the design as iliac arteries are often not on the same plane and so ensuring that the complete model is split into two exact halves with no gaps or overlaps is difficult to achieve.

Once the mould sets have been designed using CAD, the files are exported again in IGES format and imported into the software package AlphaCAM [Planit Holding Ltd., Kent, UK]. Within this software, the toolpath commands used to control the milling machine can be generated. Each mould is set-up with the same reference points so as that each mould piece fits together exactly, ensuring the resulting model has an almost negligible seamline. Machining is performed by a three-axis computer numerical control (CNC) milling machine using the machining codes generated within AlphaCAM. Moulds are machined from solid aluminium blocks (Figure 17) and are finished by hand to remove any unwanted burrs that results from the milling process. Necessary holes, guide pins, gates and vents can be added to each model during the machining procedure. For a detailed description on the CAD/CAM process see Doyle et al. [2008a].

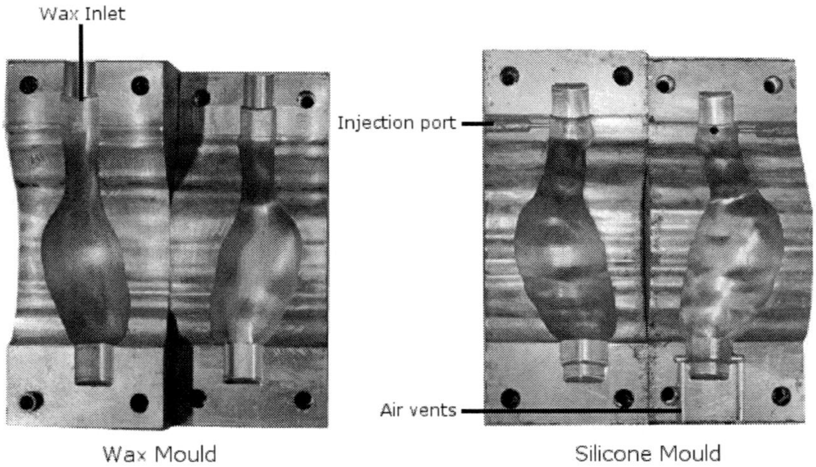

Figure 17. Example CNC-machined aluminium AAA moulds.

5. Experimental Investigations

While CAD/CAM systems are used to design anatomically-correct virtual 3D models, manufacturing techniques allows these virtual models to become a reality. This section will describe a procedure for the methodology of manufacturing bench-top models of AAAs for use in various forms of experimental testing. This chapter describes models created using silicone rubber, yet this technology is applicable to any material that can be injected in a liquid state.

5.1 *In-Vitro* Models

The procedure to actually make the experimental model is outlined as follows and detailed in full in Doyle et al. [2008a]. Over recent years the process has been refined to its current state through research into various manufacturing techniques. Initially, work began layering the silicone rubber onto an AAA phantom, a technique which has proved successful for some researchers in their efforts [Flora et al., 2002]. This method resulted in models with poor surface finish as shown in Figure 18. As surface finish is important for studies such as the photoelastic method and rupture testing, a more effective method was desired and subsequently achieved.

All mould pieces were cleaned using acetone prior to use, with the wax moulds preheated to 40°C to minimise the contraction of the wax upon pouring. A casting wax, [Castylene B581, REMET Corporation] was used to make the lumen casts. The lumen casts were then placed into the outer moulds, which were coated with mould releasing agent [Ambersil Formula 8, Chemcraft Industries Ltd, Dublin, Ireland] and then clamped tightly together. The silicone rubber was then prepared, and slowly injected into the outer mould. The mould is then placed into an oven at a temperature of 50°C and cured for 24 hours. Once cured, the model is removed and the temperature is increased to 100°C in order to melt the wax from the model. The resulting silicone model is then thoroughly cleaned, dried and inspected for defects.

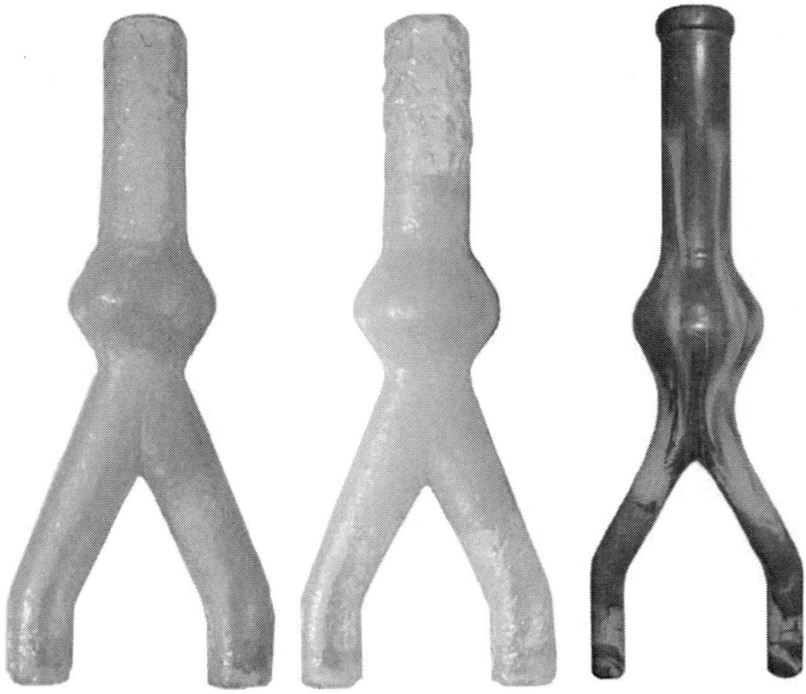

Figure 18. Evolution of the resulting silicone AAA models. Initially (*left and centre*) the material was layered onto a phantom resulting in a model with uneven and rough surface finish. Current techniques allow the creation of excellent AAA analogues (*right*), ideal for a variety of experimental studies. Notice the difference in iliac leg diameter near the bifurcation region due to the layering of the silicone.

Table 4. Averaged wall thickness measurements at four locations on the AAA wall.

		Axial Position			
		Anterior	**Posterior**	**Right**	**Left**
Patient A	Average Wall Thickness (mm)	1.87	1.97	2.09	2.55
	Standard Deviation	0.276	0.314	0.173	0.327
	Percentage Difference	6.95 %	1.78 %	4.23 %	21.47 %
Patient B	Average Wall Thickness (mm)	2.12	2.29	2.09	2.31
	Standard Deviation	0.207	0.418	0.235	0.248
	Percentage Difference	5.82 %	12.56 %	4.26 %	13.42 %
Patient C	Average Wall Thickness (mm)	2.18	2.17	2.53	2.30
	Standard Deviation	0.223	0.293	0.352	0.306
	Percentage Difference	8.08 %	7.89 %	20.99 %	13.09 %
Patient D	Average Wall Thickness (mm)	2.65	2.11	2.38	1.97
	Standard Deviation	0.653	0.282	0.414	0.281
	Percentage Difference	24.73 %	5.19 %	16.11%	1.64 %

Table 5. Averaged wall thickness measurements for each patient-specific AAA model.

	Average Wall Thickness (mm)	Average Percentage Difference
Patient A	2.12	4.24 %
Patient B	2.20	9.01 %
Patient C	2.29	12.51 %
Patient D	2.22	11.09 %

Once manufactured, models should be examined for accuracy. As part of a quality check on the resulting silicone models, four models were assessed for wall thickness, one of which included the iliac arteries (Patient D). This study was performed by cutting each model axially and measuring the wall thickness at distinct locations around the circumference of each slice. The silicone models are designed to have a uniform 2 mm wall, but due to the contraction of the wax upon solidification and the expansion of silicone upon curing, a perfectly uniform wall is difficult to achieve. Tables 4 and 5 present the wall thickness results of this study and reveal that even though deviations in wall thickness do occur, the resulting percentage differences are within acceptable limits.

These reproducible silicone models can be utilised for experimental testing of: vessel hemodynamics with LDA or PIV; wall stress analyses using either the photoelastic method or digital image correlation (DIC); and stent-graft studies by measuring dislodgement and drag forces, all of which may contribute to experimental validation of numerical work. In general, rubber models of good geometrical accuracy can be produced by sensible mould design and the use of controlled parameters in the silicone production. Models showed a maximum percentage difference of 9.21% between the designed moulds and the resulting silicone models. Overall, 3D reconstruction and CAD/CAM techniques proved to be successful in the creation of patient-specific rubber AAA models, and may help contribute to the use of patient-specific AAA models in experimental testing.

5.2 The Photoelastic Method

Following on from the previous report from our group [Morris et al., 2004b] describing the use of the photoelastic method to determine the stress and strain in the idealised AAA model, this section will briefly examine the tool when applied to realistic AAA geometries. The experimental models were manufactured as outlined Section 5.1 and Doyle et al. [2008a] using PL-3 liquid photoelastic material and PC-11 reflective coating [Vishay Measurements Group UK Ltd., Hants, UK]. For a full description of the methodology involved with the photoelastic method the reader can refer to Morris et al. [2004b]. In this study a static air pressure was applied to the internal surface of each model instead of the pulsatile cardiac loading previously used. Figure 19 compares the isochromatic fringes on the anterior wall of a patient-specific AAA under increasing loading conditions. The figure shows the fringe contours increasing as the pressure loading increases. Each fringe colour can be related to a fringe number (N) using a calibration chart, with N determining the relative stress and strain at a particular point. In Figure 19, the legend refers to the fringe number. Low fringe numbers will correspond to low stress/strain quantities. Figure 19 also reveals the complex contour distributions observed using the photoelastic method. Complex stress distributions have been witnessed in numerical stress analyses of AAAs and the use of the photoelastic method could serve as a useful technique to not only validate computational studies, but also provide researchers with an additional tool to determine the wall stress and strain of a patient-specific AAA.

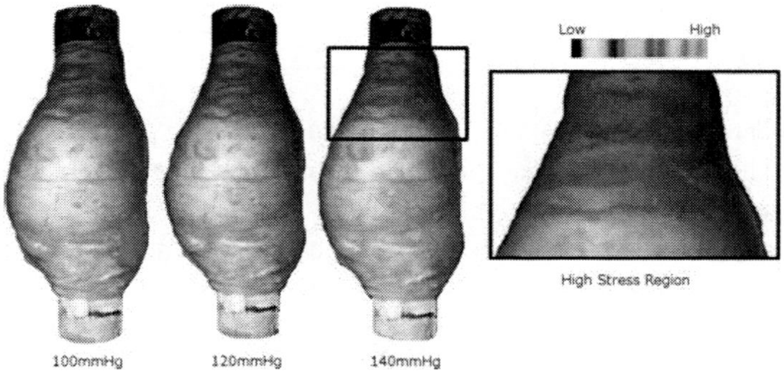

Figure 19. Isochromatic fringes on the anterior surface of a realistic AAA geometry.

5.3 Improving Experimental Materials

With the current technology in place to produce repeatable patient-specific AAA experimental models, it is desirable to improve the material analogues used to create these models. Currently, bench-top models are predominantly created using a homogenous material, often silicone, to represent the vessel wall. The diseased wall of the AAA *in vivo* is known to have a varying range of material strengths, with reports of the range in UTS to be from 0.34 – 2.35 MPa [Raghavan et al., 2006]. As AAAs are non-homogenous in UTS, AAA analogues should also be ideally non-homogenous in UTS. This section describes an effective method of creating a range of novel silicone rubbers that are linked to material strength through the colour of the material. This relationship is via calibration curves which effectively predict the strength of the silicone rubber when compared to the actual measured strength of the material.

5.3.1 Material Selection, Development and Testing

The commercially available Sylgard silicone from Dow Corning was chosen as the base material for this study, in particular, Sylgard 160 and Sylgard 170. These silicones were identified as appropriate materials as each material is easily identifiable due to its colour, and importantly, they have dissimilar material properties. Sylgard 160 is naturally grey in appearance with an UTS of 4 MPa, whereas, Sylgard 170 is naturally black in colour with an UTS value of 2 MPa. These two materials were mixed together in various ratios in order to create a range of new silicones, with gradually increasing colour intensity from grey to black and gradually decreasing failure properties from 4 – 2 MPa. The ratios of each mix were increased by 10% for each new silicone, resulting in 11 complete materials, including the original Sylgard 160 and 170.

The colour intensity of each silicone was analysed using a ColorLite sph850 Spectrophotometer [ColorLite GmbH], allowing each silicone mix to be assigned an individual colour intensity value (ΔE). Colour measurements are given in as a variation of ΔE (Eqn. 4), where pure black has a ΔE value of zero.

$$\Delta E = \left[\Delta L^2 + \Delta a^2 + \Delta b^2\right]^{\frac{1}{2}} \quad (4)$$

Uniaxial tensile testing was performed using a Tinius Olsen H25KS [Tinius Olsen, Ltd., Surrey RH1 5DZ, England] with a 1 kN load cell. Each material was formed into Type 2 dumb-bell specimens conforming to BS ISO 37. Each sample was subjected to a cross-head speed of 500 mm/min [BS ISO 37], with a preconditioning stage of 10 cycles to 20% of the gauge length. Preconditioning helps to increase repeatability of the tests by stabilising the stress-strain function of the material. The structural properties of elastomers change significantly during the first several times that the material experiences straining. This behaviour is commonly referred to as the Mullins effect [Mullins, 1969]. The primary purpose of the tensile testing in this application was to generate force-extension data, which can be converted to stress-strain data and determine the UTS of each silicone mixture.

Tear testing was performed using a modification of the trouser test pieces outlined in BS ISO 34-1. The Tinius Olsen was again used for this analysis. A cross-head speed of 100 mm/min was applied to each sample as per BS ISO 34-1. Tear testing results in tear strength (TS) values, which provide an indication of the resistance of the material to tearing, with results given in force per unit length. On failure of the specimen, the tear resistance, or tear strength, is calculated by Equation 5.

$$TS = \frac{F}{t} \quad (5)$$

Where: *TS* is the tear strength (N/mm); *F* is the maximum load (N); and *t* is the specimen thickness (mm). By relating the colour intensity of each material to its respective UTS and TS, calibration curves could be generated. These curves then allow the UTS and TS to be predicted for that particular material based on the colour intensity. These curves are shown in Figures 20 and 21 with the values tabulated in Table 6. Significant correlations between results were assessed using a non-parametric Spearman's Rho bivariate correlation test using SPSS 15.0. Correlation coefficient (CC) is shown where significant relationships were observed. Good linear relationships were shown between both ΔE and UTS (R^2=0.8082), and ΔE and TS (R^2=0.7205). It was also possible to examine how accurate these calibration curves are in predicting the material property. This was achieved by manufacturing identical batches of silicone rubber at each concentration. The colour intensity of each sample was then measured, and together with the calibration curves, could be linked to a particular strength.

In order to mechanically characterise each material so that they could be incorporated into numerical software, the experimental force-extension data from the tensile tests were converted to engineering stress and engineering strain. A 2nd order polynomial curve was applied to the data to obtain a mean experimental data curve. This mean data was then applied to the commercial FEA solver ABAQUS in order to find the most applicable strain energy function (SEF) and allow the determination of material coefficients. Material coefficients were then assessed using a Type 2 dumb-bell numerical model. The model was examined using identical boundary conditions to those applied experimentally. The stress and strain at a central node was then mapped throughout the course of the analysis and compared to the results found experimentally. The comparison between experimentally derived results and the numerical results obtained with the new material coefficients for the novel silicone rubbers is shown in Figure 22. Good linear agreement was observed between the predicted values and the measured values for both the UTS (R^2=0.8882) and the TS (R^2=0.8089). Overall, the predicted UTS and measured UTS results were significant (CC=0.945, p<0.0009), as were the predicted TS and measured TS results (CC=0.891, p<0.0009). The UTS results and tear strength results were also compared which showed a good linear trend (R^2=0.7318) and significant relationship (CC=0.9, p<0.0009) between the two material properties. This allows tear strength to be related to UTS for each varying silicone material thus giving a further insight into the relationship between the two properties. For a full description of the characterisation, SEF coefficients and development of these materials the reader can refer to Doyle et al. [2009e].

Table 6. Results of the colour analysis, tensile testing and tear testing. All results are averages of the sample size.

	Tensile Testing		Tear Testing	
Silicone Type	ΔE	UTS (MPa)	ΔE	TS (N/mm)
160	47.72	3.822	45.73	0.697
10:90	40.16	3.537	40.74	0.68
20:80	36.91	3.599	37.23	0.754
30:70	31.92	3.289	34.52	0.692
40:60	32.52	2.611	31.32	0.688
50:50	29.88	3.206	28.54	0.573
60:40	27.33	2.473	28.76	0.537
70:30	26.41	2.445	26.39	0.479
80:20	25.13	2.199	25.40	0.519
90:10	24.55	2.401	23.79	0.433
170	23.86	2.077	23.84	0.452

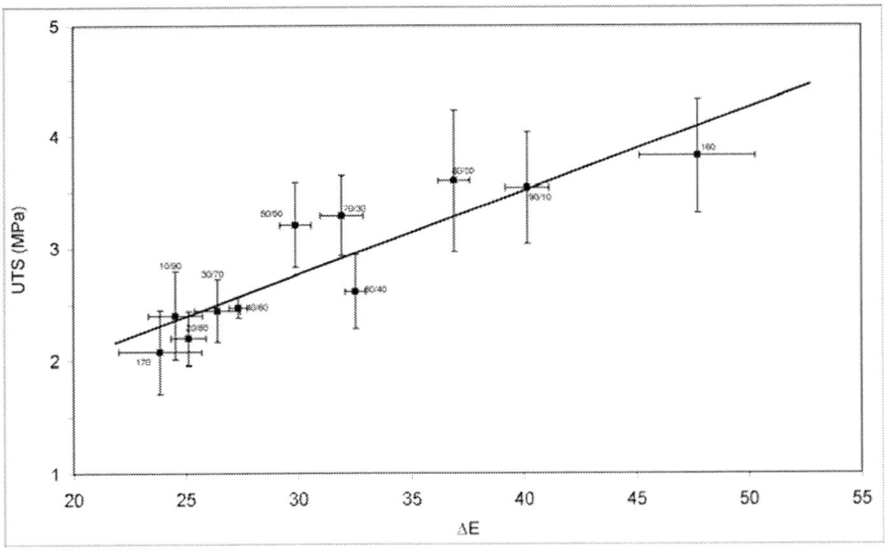

Figure 20. UTS calibration curve showing the new relationship between ultimate tensile strength and the colour of the material. Each data point is named with the corresponding material type. Reproduced from Doyle et al. [2009e].

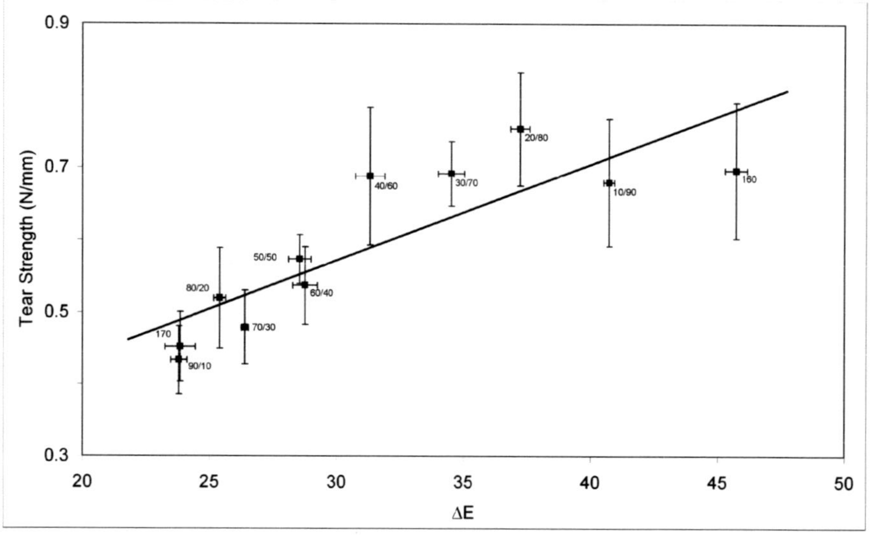

Figure 21. TS calibration curve showing the how tear strength relates to the colour of the particular material. Each data point is named with the corresponding material type. Reproduced from Doyle et al. [2009e].

5.3.2 Application to 3D Geometries

Idealised AAA silicone models were manufactured using a previously reported technique [O'Brien et al., 2005; Doyle et al., 2008a]. These analogues were designed to have realistic dimensions based on population averages obtained from the EUROSTAR data registry [Laheij et al., 2001] where the maximum outer diameter is 54 mm. This ideal AAA model has been utilised in previous research by our group [Morris et al., 2004b; Callanan et al., 2004; O'Brien et al., 2005; Doyle et al., 2008b, 2009d, 2009e]. Three models were created using Sylgard 160, three using Sylgard 170, and one model was created by randomly injecting both Sylgard 160 and Sylgard 170 through a Y-tubing connection into the wall cavity. This allowed both silicones to randomly mix via the injection process, resulting in a model of random material properties and various shades of black and grey. Examples of these models can be seen in Figure 23.

These experimental models were then used in conjunction with the non-contact strain measurement technique of videoextensometry to measure the change in diameter of each model under certain loading conditions. Each model was loaded with an internal pressure increasing from 0 mmHg to 160 mmHg in 20 mmHg increments. The models were constrained from movement at the proximal neck and iliac legs representing the attachment to the aorta *in vivo*. The diametrical change of each model was recorded with the results then averaged. These measurements were performed with the Messphysik Materials Testing Videoextensometer 1362CA [Messphysik Materials Testing, Austria] in conjunction with the Messphysik Dot Measurement for Windows software. The initial maximum diameter of each model was 54 mm and so any displacement past 54 mm at each pressure loading is recorded with the software.

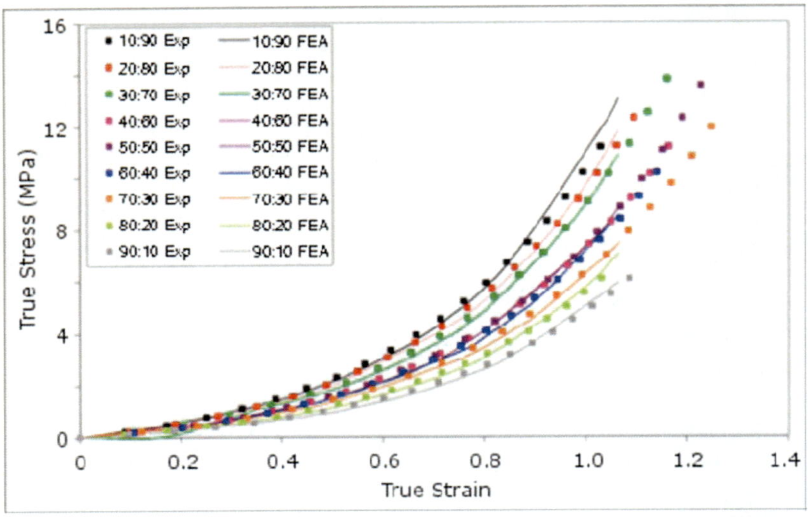

Figure 22. True stress and true strain for each of the nine novel materials developed from Sylgard 160 and Sylgard 170. Good agreement was observed between the experimental tensile result and the numerical results using the new SEF material coefficients.

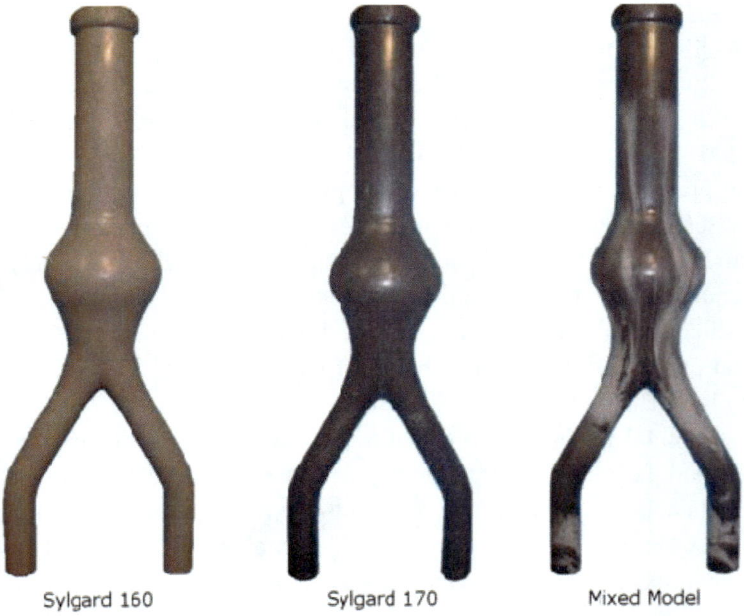

Figure 23: Example images of ideal AAAs made using Sylgard 160 (grey), Sylgard 170 (black) and a mixture of the two materials. Reproduced from Doyle et al. [2009e].

The ColorLite sph850 Spectrophotometer was used to measure the colour intensity of the mixed ideal AAA model with measurements taken at 20mm intervals along the length of the model, at the front, back, left, and right sides. These measurement locations are shown in Figure 24. The results show how the ΔE value differs depending on the concentration of either Sylgard 170 or Sylgard 160.

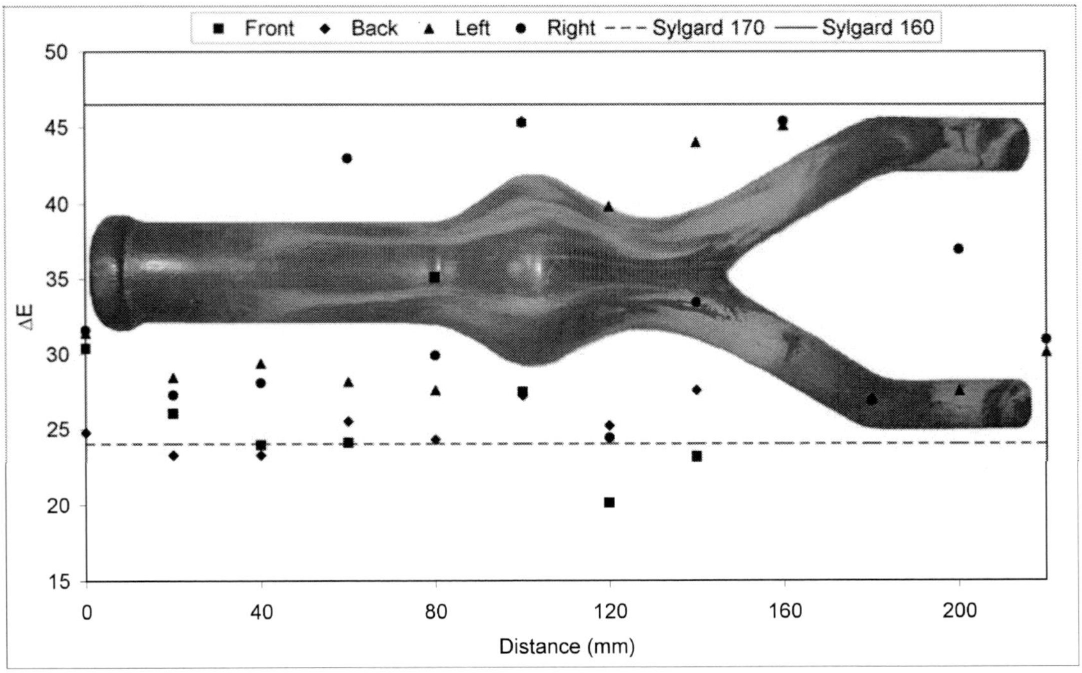

Figure 24. Colour intensity measurements along the four sides of the mixed ideal AAA model. The figure shows the random distribution of ΔE values dispersed throughout the model. Mean ΔE values for pure Sylgard 160 and Sylgard 170 are shown for comparison.

In order to assess the effectiveness of the material coefficients derived as part of this study and their applicability to 3D geometries, the videoextensometry experiment was replicated using the finite element method. The numerical model has a uniform wall of 2 mm, and was constrained from movement at the proximal neck and iliac legs, reproducing the experimental set-up. A half model was examined due to the symmetrical nature of the idealised AAA. The model was meshed using 11,443 quadratic tetrahedral 3D stress elements, with mesh independence achieved by increasing the mesh size until the difference in peak stress was <2% of the previous mesh [Wang et al., 2001; Doyle et al., 2007; Truijers et al., 2007]. The same loading conditions were applied to the inner surface of the model and the displacement of the maximum diameter region was measured at each loading. By measuring the displacement at the region of maximum diameter, the deformation of the experimental models could be compared to those observed numerically. The experimental and numerical results were statistically highly significant for the Sylgard 160 model (CC=1.0, $p<0.0009$), Sylgard 170 model (CC=1.0, $p<0.0009$) and also the mixed silicone model (CC=0.971, $p<0.0009$). Overall, there was a difference in the diameter change of 0.24% (range 0.01 - 1.78%) and 0.38% (range 0.3 - 5.27%) for the Sylgard 160 and Sylgard 170, respectively. For the mixed ideal AAA model, deformations were only measured from the front of the model, as with the experimental model, with an average percentage difference of 0.76% (range 0.25 - 5.03%). The results can be seen in Figure 25.

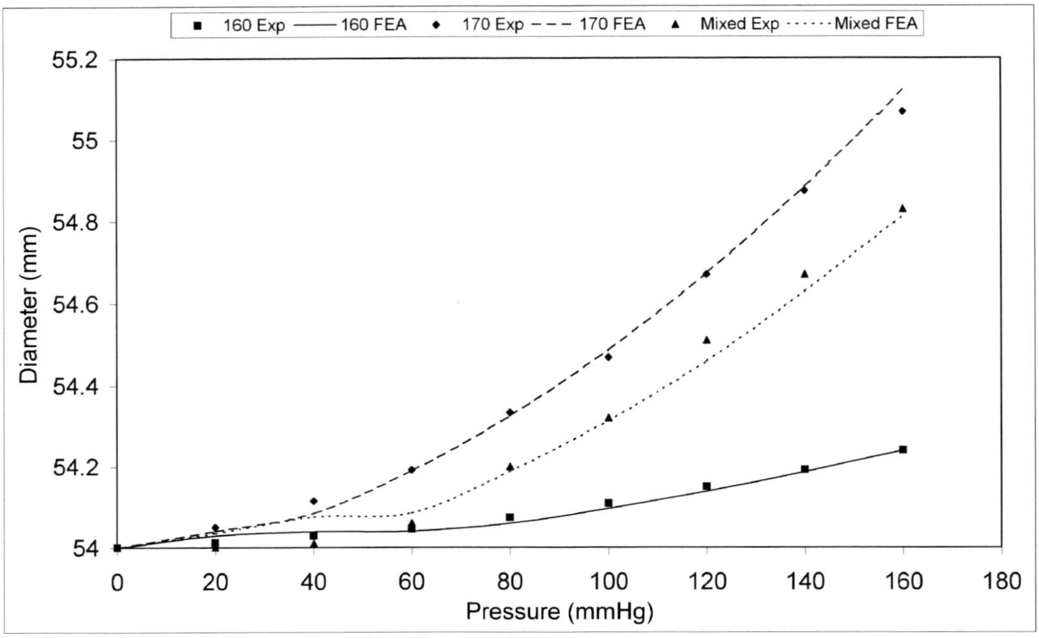

Figure 25: Experimental and numerical results for the pressure-diameter tests on the idealised AAA model. Good correlation between the two methods was observed for each model type. Reproduced from Doyle et al. [2009e].

Based on Section 5.3.1 and 5.3.2, it is now possible to create experimental AAA models with a variation of wall strengths throughout the model. Each wall strength can be effectively linked to a certain material model, which can be accurately modelled numerically.

5.4 Experimental Rupture Testing

Following on from the developments described in Section 5.3, experimental models and novel silicone rubbers can be employed in experimental rupture tests. In recent publications by Doyle et al. [2008b and 2009d], which were the first known reports on experimental AAA rupture, a methodology used to accurately capture the location of rupture was described. These articles described a technique using high-speed photography to determine exactly where an experimental model will rupture, with accurate numerical predictions computed using FEA. In these previous studies, it was shown that idealised AAA geometries rupture at inflection points on the surface of the model, with these inflection points defined as areas where there curvature changes from concave to convex. The comparison between experimental rupture and numerically predicted peak wall stress can be seen in Figure 26.

Following on from the work described thus far led to the experimental rupture technique being applied to several realistic AAA geometries using the materials developed in Section 5.3. This entailed creating 16 patient-specific AAA silicone models based on the 4 geometries shown in Figure 27. These models consisted of 8 Sylgard 160 (grey) models and 8 Sylgard 170 (black) models. A further 5 models were also created (see Figure 28) using the mixing technique described in Section 5.2.2 to produce models with randomly distributed materials with properties that can be determined using spectrophotometry.

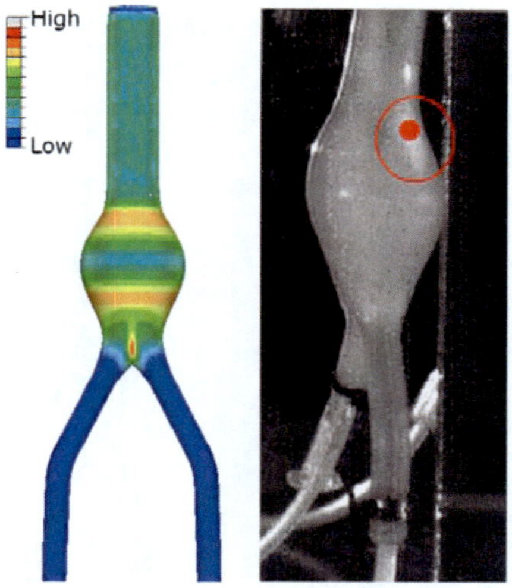

Figure 26. Numerical results compared to the experimental rupture test. Shown are the von Mises stress contours on the deformed idealised model compared to a snapshot of the moment of rupture. The numerical results show high stresses at the inflection regions with the experimental model rupturing at the proximal inflection point (marked in red). Modified from Doyle et al. [2009d].

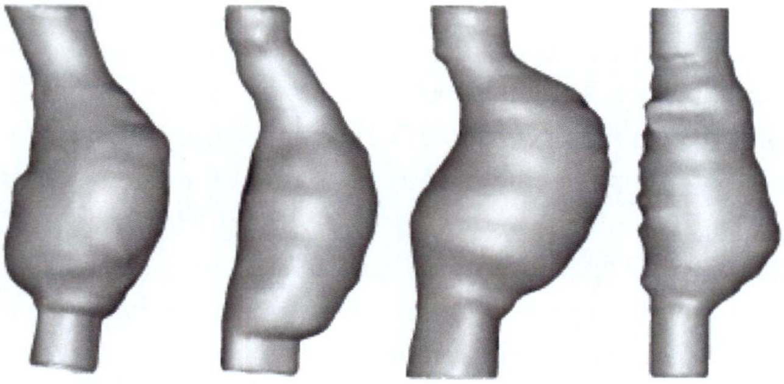

Figure 27. Realistic AAA geometries of the four patients used in the study.

An experimental test rig [Doyle et al., 2008b, 2009d] allowed each model to be connected to a pneumatic air source and inflated to the point of rupture. A high-speed camera [Photron Fastcam SA1-1, Photron USA Inc.] was used at a frame rate of 2,000 frames per second (fps) enabling the point of rupture to be accurately captured. This particular camera is capable of recording at frame rates up to 675,000 fps. The positioning of a series of mirrors surrounding the experimental model allowed a full 360° view of the model, ensuring that the position of rupture was captured by the high-speed camera. The test rig consisted of a pressure manometer, series of mirrors, pneumatic airline, pressure regulator and high-speed camera. When fully connected to the test rig, the silicone rubber model is constrained from movement at the proximal neck region, with the inside of each model dusted with calcium carbonate to ease the visualisation of the rupture. The internal pressure was increased so that the rupture of the model occurred within 240s of testing, in accordance with the standards BS ISO 1402 for burst pressure tests. Air pressure readings were also recorded in the video image for analysis post-rupture. The test set-up as viewed through the high-speed camera is shown in Figure 29. All silicone rubber models were inflated until failure with each test recorded using the high-speed camera. Significance of rupture pressures and geometrical parameters were analysed using a Spearman's Rho correlation test in SPSS 15.

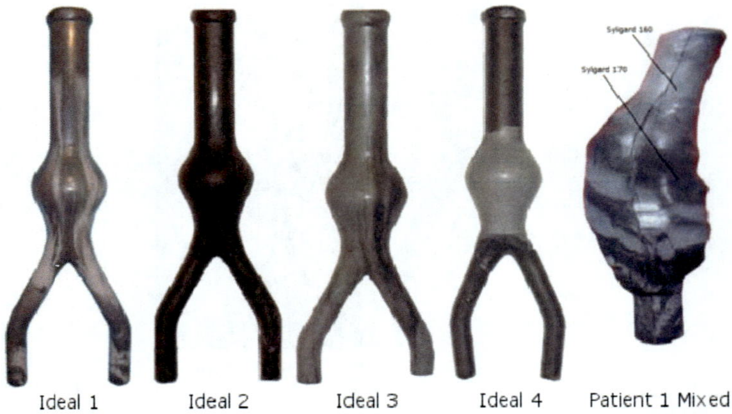

Figure 28. Illustration of the models created using the mixing technique described in Section 5.3.2. Ideal 1 is a random distribution, Ideal 2 is predominantly black, Ideal 3 is predominantly grey and Ideal 4 is a banded model with the AAA sac made using the stronger Sylgard 160 material. Patient 1 Mixed is a realistic AAA with randomly distributed materials.

The results of the experimental rupture tests revealed a large range of burst pressures for the 16 unmixed AAA models as shown in Table 7. On average, the AAA models created using the weaker silicone rubber (Sylgard 170) ruptured at lower pressures than those made using the stronger silicone type (Sylgard 160). Sylgard 160 models ruptured at a mean ± SD pressure of 650.6 ± 195.1 mmHg (range = 381.4 – 985 mmHg), whereas the weaker Sylgard 170 ruptured at a mean ± SD pressure of 410.7 ± 159.9 mmHg (range = 252.2 – 714 mmHg). All realistic AAA geometries ruptured at regions of inflection. Only the Sylgard 160 models of Patient 1 ruptured at regions near the maximum diameter, although these rupture locations experienced localised inflection as there was a sharp change in curvature over a very short length. The location of rupture in other models varied. A typical sequence of events can be seen in Figure 30, showing the frames immediately prior to rupture, through to the point of complete failure. Case shown here is Patient 4 Sylgard 160 Model 1. The model in the centre of each image in Figure 30 is the original model, with the reflected views to either side. Table 8 shows the results for the mixed material models shown in Figure 28. The colour intensities recorded at the site of rupture correlates to a specific material type in Section 5.3.1. From the results to date, mixed AAA models appear to rupture at regions of lower UTS and also at regions of inflection. Interestingly, the ideal banded model ruptured below the AAA sac and not at the inflection zones or at the material intersection. The inflection zones in this case were made of the stronger Sylgard 160, with the model rupturing at a region of Sylgard 170.

To correlate experimental and numerical results, the experiments were reproduced in the finite element solver ABAQUS. 3D reconstructions of the silicone models were used in these analyses and were reconstructed from CT images taken of each experimental model. Constraints were placed at the proximal and distal regions of each model and a uniform static air pressure was applied to the internal surface of each model. For each numerical simulation, the average rupture pressure of that material was used as the loading condition. The Gaussian surface curvature was also determined for each AAA geometry using ProEngineer Wildfire. Surface curvature revealed complex distributions of surface curvature, which has been correlated to complex stress distributions by Sacks et al. [1999]. As shown in Figure 31 using one case as an example, the experimental sites of rupture agreed well with the numerically predicted regions of elevated wall stress and the Gaussian surface curvature. A similar trend was observed for all cases examined. Figure 32 compares the numerically predicted wall stress on the anterior region of the AAA with the isochromatic fringes obtained in Section 5.2 using the photoelastic method. The qualitative agreement between the computational and experimental studies can be seen. As with the numerical model, the photoelastic method resulted in a high stress region on the proximal anterior wall, which also proved to be the rupture site for this particular geometry.

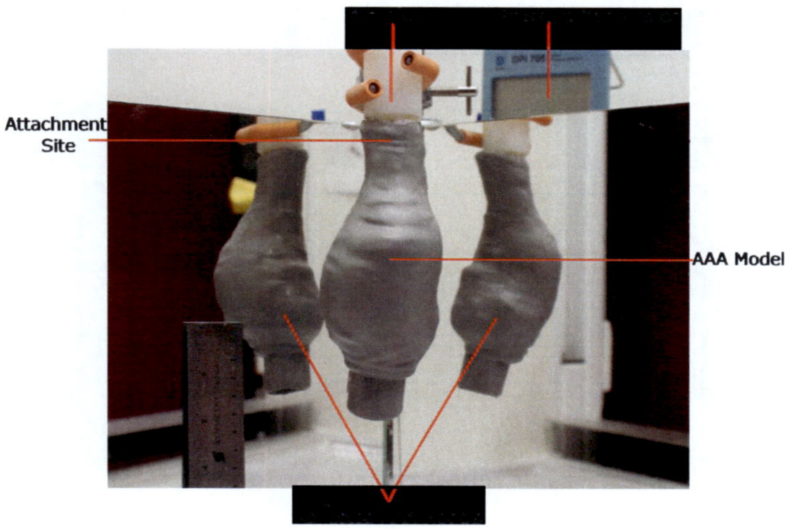

Figure 29. View through high-speed camera of test rig. Mirrors allow 360° of model to be captured. Model is constrained from movement proximally and distally. Pressure is continuously monitored with the manometer, while the model is inflated until rupture.

Table 7. Rupture pressures and wall thickness at the site of rupture for each AAA case.

	Sylgard 160			Sylgard 170		
	Model	Rupture Pressure (mmHg)	Wall Thickness (mm)	Model	Rupture Pressure (mmHg)	Wall Thickness (mm)
Patient 1	1	381.4	1.84	1	283.5	1.51
	2	985	2.03	2	309.8	1.7
Patient 2	1	909.8	1.41	1	459.3	1.41
	2	444.8	1.24	2	386.4	1.97
Patient 3	1	588.4	2.09	1	349.8	1.21
	2	629.8	1.78	2	252.2	1.57
Patient 4	1	736.9	2.34	1	320.2	2.1
	2	468	2.09	2	358.2	2.11

Table 8. Colour intensity results at the site of rupture for each model, the corresponding silicone type from previous work and the rupture pressure of each model.

Model	ΔE	Corresponding Silicone Type	Rupture Pressure (mmHg)
Ideal 1	21.76	170	440
Ideal 2	26.05	70:30	395
Ideal 3	38.37	20:80	703
Ideal 4	25.67	80:20	703
Patient 1 Mixed	23.90	170	508

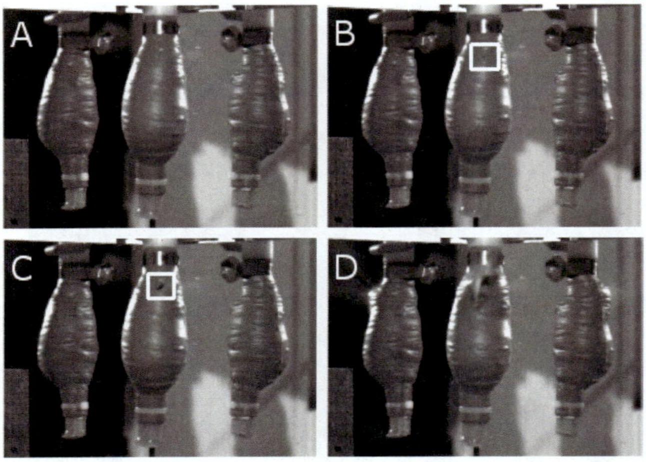

Figure 30. Typical sequence of events of rupture test. *(A)* Model is inflected with air, *(B)* silicone rubber fails (highlighted in figure), *(C)* tear develops (highlighted in figure) until *(D)* AAA model completely fails.

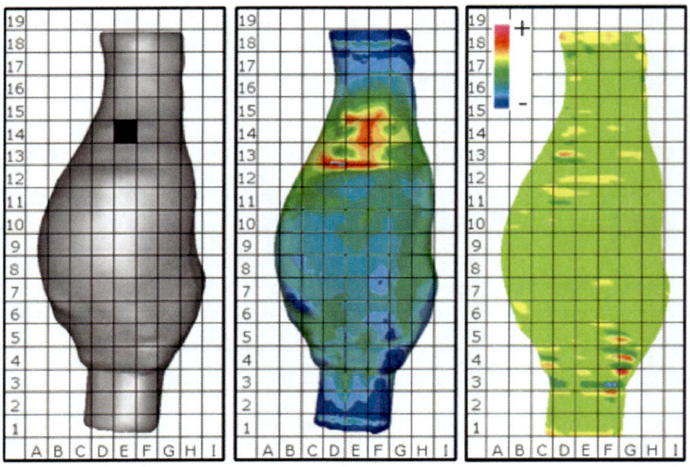

Figure 31. Comparison of experimental *(left)*, FEA *(centre)* and Gaussian surface curvature *(right)*. In the experimental results image the black mark indicates rupture site. In the FEA results image, red indicates high stress, and in the Gaussian surface curvature results, yellow/red regions indicate inflection points. Based on the three images it can be concluded that the inflection points encompass a region of high stress where the experimental model ruptured.

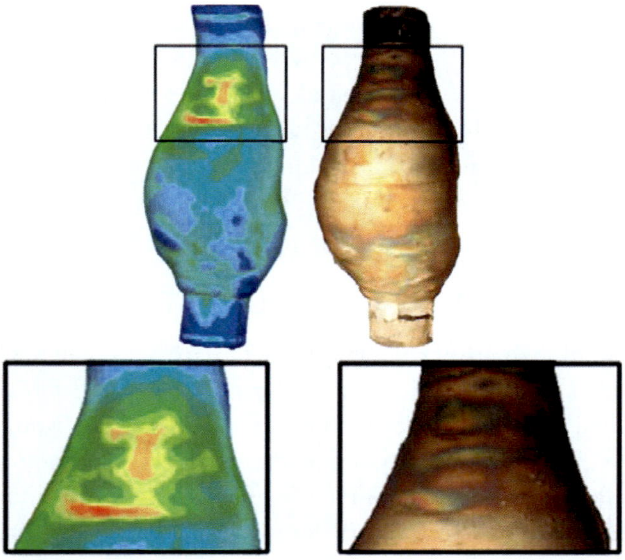

Figure 32. Comparison between FEA and the photoelastic method for a patient-specific AAA under 120 mmHg internal pressure. Model is shown from the anterior view. Good qualitative agreement was observed between the two methods.

6. Conclusion

Throughout this chapter several approaches to AAA assessment and rupture potential have been explored, with some new insights and tools also reported. In contrast to many of the published findings available in the literature indicating the ineffective nature of diameter to accurately determine an AAAs rupture potential, diameter remains the key criterion in the decision-making process of the clinician. Over the past number of years, advancements in 3D imaging have allowed new techniques to be applied to AAA assessment, with 3D reconstruction of the diseased vessels now common practice. It is widely believed that alternative methods and factors should be included in the decision to surgically repair, with several approaches described and referenced in this chapter.

In order to compliment the advancements in 3D imaging and the use of this tool to aid AAA assessment, it is believed that improvements in numerical models may yield interesting results [Watton et al., 2004; Volokh and Vorp, 2008; Humphrey and Taylor, 2008]. It has been suggested that the incorporation of growth and remodelling factors into numerical models may also provide further insights in to the possibility of AAA rupture [Humphrey and Taylor, 2008]. Alongside improvements in numerical modelling, experimental tools and techniques can also be improved. By imaging the experimental model, for example using computed tomography, prior to testing allows exact numerical reconstructions to be generated, which greatly facilitates numerical validation of experiments.

"To operate or not to operate?" still remains a the key clinical question that is predominantly answered with the maximum diameter, yet, as portrayed throughout this book chapter and in the published literature, the diameter criterion alone may not be adequate to comprehensively determine the severity of patient-specific AAAs. It is clear that 3D

reconstructions of AAAs not only compliment traditional 2D images but also provide the basis for a range of alternative assessment tools such as those described throughout this chapter. These alternative tools can be used alongside the maximum diameter criterion and will improve the current trend in AAA assessment. There is a clear need to implement alternative factors in the clinical decision-making process and the many applications of 3D reconstructions reported in this chapter may be beneficial in the future of AAA assessment.

ACKNOWLEDGMENTS

The authors would like to acknowledge (i) the Irish Research Council for Science Engineering and Technology (IRCSET) and (ii) Grant No. RO1-HL-060670 from the United States Heart Lung and Blood Institute for funding this work. We would also like to thank Prof. David A. Vorp from the University of Pittsburgh for his help and guidance over the past number of years with our AAA research. Finally, the authors would like to thank the Centre for Applied Biomedical Engineering (CABER) in the University of Limerick and the HSE Midwestern Regional Hospital for all the support.

REFERENCES

Bosch, J. L., Lester, J. S., McMahon, P. M., Beinfeld, M. T. Halpern, E. F., Kaufman, J. A., Brewster, D. C. and Gazelle, G. S. (2001). Hospital costs for elective endovascular and surgical repairs of infrarenal abdominal aortic aneurysms. *Radiology*, 220(2), 492-497.

Brosnan, M., Collins, C. G., Moneley, D. S., Kelly, C. J. and Leahy, A. L. (2009). Making the case for cardiovascular screening in Irish males: Detection of abdominal aortic aneurysms, and assessment of cardiovascular risk factors. *European Journal of Vascular and Endovascular Surgery*, 37, 300-304.

Cabral, B., Cam N. and Foran, J. (1994). Accelerated volume rendering and tomographic reconstruction using texture mapping hardware, *Proceedings 1994 ACM/IEEE Symposium on Volume Visualisation*, 91-97.

Calhoun, P. S., Kuszyk, B. S., Heath, D. G., Carley, J. C. and Fishman, E. K. (1999). Three-dimensional volume rendering of spiral CT data: Theory and method, *Radiographics,* 19, 745-764.

Callanan, A., Morris, L. G. and McGloughlin, T. M. (2004). Numerical and experimental analysis of an idealised abdominal aortic aneurysm. *European Society of Biomechanics*, S-Hertogenbosch, Netherlands.

Chong, C. K. and How, T. V. (2004). Flow patterns in an endovascular stent-graft for abdominal aortic aneurysm repair. *Journal of Biomechanics*, 37, 89-97.

Conway, K. P., Byrne, J., Townsend, M. and Lane, I. F. (2001). Prognosis of patients turned down for conventional abdominal aortic aneurysm repair in the endovascular and sonographic era: Szilagyi revisted? *Journal of Vascular Surgery*, 33, 752-757.

Corbett, T. J., Callanan, A., Morris, L. G., Doyle, B. J., Grace, P. A., Kavanagh, E. G. and McGloughlin, T. M. (2008). A review of the *in vivo* and *in vitro* biomechanical behaviour and performance of postoperative abdominal aortic aneurysms and implanted stent-grafts. *Journal of Endovascular Therapy*, 15, 468-464.

Creagh, D., Neilson, S., Collins, A., Colwell, N., Hinchion, R., Drew, C., O'Halloran, D. and Perry, I. J. (2002). Established cardiovascular disease and CVD risk factors in a primary care population of middle-aged Irish men and women. *Irish Medical Journal*, 95(10), 298-301.

Cronenwett, J. L., Murphy, T. F., Zelenock, G. B., Whitehouse Jr., W. M., Lindenauer, S. M., Graham, L. M., Quint, L. E., Silver, T. M. and Stanley, J. C. (1985). Actuarial analysis of variables associated with rupture of small abdominal aortic aneurysms. *Surgery*, 98, 472-483.

Darling, R. C., Messina, C. R., Brewster, D. C. and Ottinger, L. W. (1977). Autopsy study of unoperated abdominal aortic aneurysms. The case for early resection. *Circulation*, 56(2), 161-164.

Department of Health and Children: Dublin. (1999). *Building Healthier Hearts: The report of the cardiovascular health strategy group.*

Di Martino, E. S., Guadagni, G., Fumero, A., Ballerini, G., Spirito, R., Biglioli, P. and Redaelli, A. (2001). Fluid-structure interaction within realistic 3D models of aneurysmatic aorta as a guidance to assess the risk of rupture of the aneurysm. *Medical Engineering and Physics*, 23, 647-655.

Doyle, B. J., Callanan, A. and McGloughlin, T. M. (2007). A comparison of modelling techniques for computing wall stress in abdominal aortic aneurysms. *Biomedical Engineering Online*, 6, 38.

Doyle, B. J., Morris, L. G., Callanan, A., Kelly, P., Vorp, D. A. and McGloughlin, T. M. (2008a). 3D reconstruction and manufacture of real abdominal aortic aneurysms: From CT scan to silicone model. *Journal of Biomechanical Engineering*, 130, 034501.

Doyle, B. J., Callanan, A., Corbett, T. J., Cloonan, A. J., O'Donnell, M. R., Vorp, D. A. and McGloughlin, T. M. (2008b). The use of silicone to model abdominal aortic aneurysm behaviour. *Society of Plastics Engineers, SPE European Conference on Medical Polymers*, 115-120.

Doyle, B. J., Callanan, A., Burke, P. E., Grace, P. A., Walsh, M. T., Vorp, D. A. and McGloughlin, T. M. (2009a). Vessel asymmetry as an additional tool in the assessment of abdominal aortic aneurysms. *Journal of Vascular Surgery*, 49, 443-454.

Doyle, B. J., Callanan, A., Walsh, M. T., Grace, P. A. and McGloughlin, T. M. (2009b). A finite element analysis rupture index (FEARI) as an additional tool for abdominal aortic aneurysm rupture prediction. *Vascular Disease Prevention*, 6, 114-121.

Doyle, B. J., Grace, P. A. Kavanagh, E. G., Burke, P. E. Wallis, F., Walsh, M. T. and McGloughlin, T. M. (2009c). Improved assessment and treatment of abdominal aortic aneurysms: The use of 3D reconstructions as a surgical guidance tool in endovascular repair. *Irish Journal of Medical Science*, 178, 321-328.

Doyle, B. J., Corbett, T. J., Callanan, A., Walsh, M. T., Vorp, D. A. and McGloughlin, T. M. (2009d). An experimental and numerical comparison of the rupture locations of an abdominal aortic aneurysm. *Journal of Endovascular Therapy*, 16, 322-335.

Doyle, B. J., Corbett, T. J., Cloonan, A. J., O'Donnell, M. R., Walsh, M. T., Vorp, D. A. and McGloughlin, T. M. (2009e). Experimental Modelling of Abdominal Aortic Aneurysms: Novel Applications of Silicone Rubbers. *Medical Engineering and Physics*, 31(8), 1002-1012.

Egelhoff, C. J., Buduig, R. S., Elger D. F., Khraishi, T. A. and Johansen K. H. (1999). Model studies of the flow in abdominal aortic aneurysms during resting and exercise conditions. *Journal of Biomechanics*, 32, 1319-1329.

Ernst, C. B. (1993). Abdominal aortic aneurysm. *The New England Journal of Medicine*, 328(16), 1167-1172.

EVAR Trial Participants. (2004). Comparison of endovascular aneurysm repair with open repair in patients with abdominal aortic aneurysm (EVAR trial 1), 30-day operative mortality results: randomised controlled trial. *The Lancet*, 364, 843-848.

EVAR Trial Participants, (2005a). Endovascular aneurysm repair versus open repair in patients with abdominal aortic aneurysm (EVAR Trial 1): randomised controlled trial. *The Lancet*, 365, 2179-2186.

EVAR Trial Participants, (2005b*)*. Endovascular aneurysm repair and outcome in patients unfit for open repair of abdominal aortic aneurysm (EVAR Trail 2): randomised controlled trial. *The Lancet*, 365(9578), 2187-2192.

Fraunhofer SCAI: MpCCI Documentation. *Sankt Augustin, Germany,* 2008.

Fillinger, M. F., Marra, S. P., Raghavan, M. L. and Kennedy, F. E. (2003). Prediction of rupture risk in abdominal aortic aneurysm during observation: wall stress versus diameter. *Journal of Vascular Surgery*, 37, 724-732.

Fillinger, M. F., Raghavan, M. L., Marra, S. P., Cronenwett, J. L. and Kennedy, F. E. (2002). *In vivo* analysis of mechanical wall stress and abdominal aortic aneurysm rupture risk. *Journal of Vascular Surgery*, 36, 589-597.

Flora, H. S., Talei-Faz, B., Ansell, L., Chaloner, E. J., Sweeny, A., Grass, A. and Adiseshiah, M. (2002). Aneurysm wall stress and tendency to rupture are features of physical wall properties: an experimental study. *Journal of Endovascular Therapy*, 9(5), 665-675.

Garcia-Madrid, C., Josa, M., Riambau, V., Mestresa, C. A., Muntanab, J. and Muleta, J. (2004). Endovascular versus open surgical repair of abdominal aortic aneurysm: a comparison of early and intermediate results in patients suitable for both techniques. *Journal of Endovascular Therapy*, 28(4), 365-372.

Giannoglu, G., Giannakoulas, G., Soulis, J., Chatzizisis, Y., Perdikides, T., Melas, N., Parcharidis, G. and Louridas, G. (2006*)*. Predicting the risk of rupture of abdominal aortic aneurysms by utilizing various geometrical parameters: Revisiting the diameter criterion. *Angiology*, 57(4), 487-494.

Glimaker, H., Holmberg, L., Elvin, A., Nybacka, O., Almgren, B., Bjorck, C.G., Eriksson, I. (1991). Natural history of patients with abdominal aortic aneurysm. *European Journal of Vascular Surgery*, 5, 125-130.

Goueffic, Y., Becquemin, J. P., Desgranges, P. and Kobeiter, H. (2005). Midterm survival after endovascular versus open repair of infrarenal aortic aneurysms. *Journal of Endovascular Therapy*, 12(1), 47-57.

Hirose, Y. and Takamiya, M. (1998). Growth curve of ruptured aortic aneurysm. *Journal of Cardiovascular Surgery*, 39, 9-13.

Howell, B. A., Kim, T., Cheer, A. Dwyer, H., Saloner, D. and Chuter, T. A. (2007). Computational fluid dynamics within bifurcated abdominal aortic stent-grafts. *Journal of Endovascular Therapy*, 14, 138-143.

Hua, J. and Mower, W. R. (2001). Simple geometric characteristics fail to reliably predict abdominal aortic aneurysm wall stress. *Journal of Vascular Surgery*, 34, 308-315.

Humphrey, J. D. and Taylor, C. A. (2008). Intracranial and abdominal aortic aneurysms: Similarities, differences, and need for a new computational class. *Annual Review of Biomedical Engineering*, 10, 221-246.

Inzoli, F., Boschetti, F., Zappa, M., Longo, T. and Fumero, R. (1993). Biomechanical factors in abdominal aortic aneurysm rupture. *European Journal of Vascular Surgery*, 7, 667-674.

Jacobowitz, G. R., Lee, A. M. and Riles, T. S. (1999). Immediate and late explantation of endovascular aortic grafts: the EndoVascular Technologies experience. *Journal of Vascular Surgery*, 29, 309-316.

Kamineni, R. and Heuser, R. (2004). Abdominal aortic aneurysm: a review of endoluminal treatment. *Journal of Interventional Cardiology*, 17, 437-445.

Kleinstreuer, C. and Li, Z. (2006). Analysis and computer program for rupture-risk prediction of abdominal aortic aneurysms. *Biomedical Engineering Online*, 5, 19.

Laheij, R., van Marrewijk, C. and Buth, J. (2001). Progress report on the procedural and follow up results of 3413 patients who received stent graft treatment for infrarenal aortic aneurysms for a period of 6 years. *EUROSTAR Data Registry Centre.*

Lederle, F. A., Johnson, G. R., Wilson, S. E., Ballard, D. J., Jordan Jr., W. D., Blebea, J., Littooy, F. N., Freischlag, J. A., Bandyk, D., Rapp, J. H. and Salam, A. A. (2002). Rupture rate of large abdominal aortic aneurysms in patients refusing or unfit for elective repair. *Journal of the American Medical Association*, 287, 2968-2972.

Leung, J. H., Wright, A. R., Cheshire, N., Crane, J., Thom, S. A., Hughes, A. D. and Xu, Y. (2006). *F*luid structure interaction of patient specific abdominal aortic aneurysms: a comparison with solid stress models. *Biomedical Engineering Online*, 5, 33.

Li, Z. and Kleinstreuer, C. (2005a). Blood flow and structure interactions in stented abdominal aortic aneurysm model. *Medical Engineering and Physics*, 27, 369-382.

Li, Z. and Kleinstreuer, C. (2005b). A new wall stress equation for aneurysm-rupture. *Annals of Biomedical Engineering*, 33(2), 209-213.

Lorensen, W. E. and H. E. Cline, H. E. (1987). Marching Cubes: A high resolution 3D surface construction algorithm, *Computer Graphics*, 21(4), 163-169.

Loth, F., Jones, S. A., Giddens, D. P., Bassiouny, H. S., Glagov, S. and Zarins, C. K. (1997). Measurements of velocity and wall shear stress inside a ptfe vascular graft model under steady flow conditions. *Journal of Biomechanical Engineering*, 119(2), 187-194.

Mills, C., Gabe, I., Gault, J., Mason, D. and Ross, J. (1970). Pressure-flow relationships and vascular impedance in man. *Cardiovascular Research*, 4, 405-417

Molony, D. S., Callanan, A., Morris, L. G., Doyle, B. J., Walsh, M. T. and McGloughlin, T. M. (2008). Geometrical enhancements for abdominal aortic stent-grafts. *Journal of Endovascular Therapy*, 15, 518-529.

Morris, L., Delassus, P., Walsh, M. and McGloughlin, T. (2004a). A mathematical model to predict *in vivo* pulsatile drag forces acting on bifurcated stent grafts used in endovascular treatment of abdominal aortic aneurysms (AAA). *Journal of Biomechanics*, 37, 1087-1095.

Morris, L., O'Donnell, P., Delassus, P. and McGloughlin, T. (2004b). Experimental assessment of stress patterns in abdominal aortic aneurysms using the photoelastic method. *Strain*, 40, 165-172.

Morris, L., Delassus, P., Grace, P., Wallis, F., Walsh, M. and McGloughlin, T. (2006a). Effects of flat, parabolic and realistic steady flow inlet profiles on idealised and realistic stent graft fits through abdominal aortic aneurysm (AAA). *Medical Engineering and Physics*, 28, 19-26.

Morris, L., McGloughlin, T., Dellasus, P., Walsh, M., O'Brien, T. and Callanan, A. (2006b). A vascular graft. *International Patent WO* 2006/103641 A1.

Mower, W. R., Quinones, W. J. and Gambhir, S. S. (1997). Effect of intraluminal thrombus on abdominal aortic aneurysm wall stress. *Journal of Vascular Surgery*, 26, 602-608.

Mullins, L. (1969). Softening of rubber by deformation. *Rubber Chemistry and Technology*, 42, 339-62.

National Health Service, (2009). *National Screening Program for Abdominal Aortic Aneurysm* [online] available: http://aaa.screening. nhs.uk [accessed 9 Feb 2009].

Nicholls, S. C., Gardner, J. B., Meissner, M. H. and Johansen, H. K. (1998). Rupture in small abdominal aortic aneurysms. *Journal of Vascular Surgery*, 28, 884-888.

O'Brien, T., Morris, L., O'Donnell, M., Walsh, M. and McGloughlin, T. (2005). Injection-moulded models of major and minor arteries: The variability of model wall thickness owing to casting technique. *Proceedings of the International Mechanical Engineers, Part H: Journal of Engineering in Medicine*, 219.

O'Brien, T., Morris, L. and McGloughlin, T. (2008). Evidence suggests rigid aortic graft increase systolic blood pressure: results of a preliminary study. *Medical Engineering and Physics*, 30, 109-115.

Papaharilaou, Y., Ekaterinaris, J. A., Manoussaki, E. and Katsamouris, A. N. (2007). A decoupled fluid structure approach for estimating wall stress in abdominal aortic aneurysms. *Journal of Biomechanics*, 40, 367-377.

Parodi, J. C., Palmaz, J. C. and Barone, H. D. (1991). Transfemoral intraluminal graft implantation for treatment of abdominal aortic aneurysms. *Annals of Vascular Surgery*, 5, 491-499.

Quill, D. S., Colgan, M. P. and Sumner, D. S. (1989). Ultrasonic screening for the detection of abdominal aortic aneurysms. *Surgical Clinics of North America*, 69, 713-720.

Raghavan, M. L., Kratzberg, J., de Tolosa, E. M. C., Hanaoka, M. M., Walter, P. and da Silva, E. S. (2006). Regional distribution of wall thickness and failure properties of human abdominal aortic aneurysm. *Journal of Biomechanics*, 39(16), 3010-6.

Raghavan, M. L. and Vorp, D. A. (2000). Toward a biomechanical tool to evaluate rupture potential of abdominal aortic aneurysm: identification of a finite strain constitutive model and evaluation of its applicability. *Journal of Vascular Surgery*, 33, 475-482.

Raghavan, M. L., Vorp, D. A., Federle, M. P., Makaroun, M. S. and Webster, M. W. (2000). Wall stress distribution on three-dimensionally reconstructed models of human abdominal aortic aneurysm. *Journal of Vascular Surgery*, 31, 760-769.

Raghavan, M. L., Webster, M. W. and Vorp, D. A. (1996). Ex vivo biomechanical behaviour of abdominal aortic aneurysm: assessment using a new mathematical model. *Annals of Biomedical Engineering*, 24, 573-582.

Rissland, P., Alemu, Y., Einav, S., Ricotta, J. and Bluestein, D. (2009). Abdominal aortic aneurysm risk of rupture: Patient-specific FSI simulations using anisotropic model. *Journal of Biomechanical Engineering*, 131, 031001.

Sacks, M. S., Vorp, D. A., Raghavan, M. L., Federle, M. P. and Webster, M. W. (1999). *In vivo* three-dimensional surface geometry of abdominal aortic aneurysms. *Annals of Biomedical Engineering*, 27(4), 469-479.

Sakalihasan, N., Limet, R. and Defawe, O. D. (2005). Abdominal aortic aneurysm. *The Lancet*, 365(9470), 1577-89.

Sayers, R. D. (2002). Aortic aneurysms, inflammatory pathways and nitric oxide. *Annals of the Royal College of Surgeons England*, 84(4), 239-246.

Scotti, C. M. and Finol, E. A. (2007). Compliant biomechanics of abdominal aortic aneurysms: a fluid-structure interaction study. *Computers and Structures*, 85, 1097-1113.

Scotti, C. M., Shkolnik, A. D., Muluk, S. C. and Finol, E. (2005). Fluid-structure interaction in abdominal aortic aneurysms: effect of asymmetry and wall thickness. *Biomedical Engineering Online,* 4, 64.

Seong, J., Sadasivan, C., Onizuka, M., Gounis, M. J., Christian, F., Miskolczi, L., Wakhloo, A. K. and Lieber B. B. (2005). Morphology of elastase-induced cerebral aneurysm model in rabbit and rapid prototyping of elastomeric transparent replicas. *Biorheology*, 42(5), 345-361.

Shipkowitz, T., Rodgers, V., Frazin, L. and Chandran, C. B. (1998). Numerical study on the effect of steady axial flow development in the human aorta on local shear stresses in abdominal aortic branches. *Journal of Biomechanics*, 31, 995-1007.

Speelman, L., Bohra, A., Bosboom, E. M. H., Schurink, G. W. H., van de Vosse, F. N., Makaroun, M. S., Vorp, D. A. (2007). Effects of wall calcifications in patient-specific wall stress analyses of abdominal aortic aneurysms. *Journal of Biomechanical Engineering*, 129, 1-5.

Stenbaek, J., Kalin, B. and Swedenborg, J. (2000). Growth of thrombus may be a better predictor of rupture than diameter in patients with abdominal aortic aneurysms. *European Journal of Vascular and Endovascular Surgery*, 20, 466-469.

Thubrikar, M. J., Labrosse, M., Robicsek, F., Al-Soudi, J. and Fowler, B. (2001a). Mechanical properties of abdominal aortic aneurysm wall. *Journal of Medical Engineering and Technology*, 25(4), 133-142.

Thubrikar, M. J., Al-Soudi, J. and Robicsek, F. (2001b). Wall stress studies of abdominal aortic aneurysm in a clinical model. *Annals of Vascular Surgery*, 15, 355-366.

Truijers, M., Pol, J. A., SchultzeKool, L. J., van Sterkenburg, S. M., Fillinger, M. F. and Blankensteijn, J. D. (2007). Wall stress analysis in small asymptomatic, symptomatic and ruptured abdominal aortic aneurysms. *European Journal of Vascular and Endovascular Surgery*, 33, 401-407.

United States Preventative Services Task Force (USPSTF). (2005) Screening for abdominal aortic aneurysm: Recommendation statement. *Annals of Internal Medicine,* 142(3), 198-202.

Vande Geest, J. P., Wang, D. H. J., Wisniewski, S. R., Makaroun, M. S. and Vorp, D. A (2006a). Towards a non-invasive method for determination of patient-specific wall strength distribution in abdominal aortic aneurysms. *Annals of Biomedical Engineering*, 34(7), 1098-1106.

Vande Geest, J. P., Di Martino, E. S., Bohra, A., Makaroun, M. S. and Vorp, D. A. (2006b). A biomechanics-based rupture potential index for abdominal aortic aneurysm risk assessment. *Annals of the New York Academy of Science,* 1085, 11-21.

Venkatasubramaniam, A. K., Fagan, M. J., Mehta, T., Mylankal, K. J., Ray, B., Kuhan, G., Chetter, I. C. and McCollum, P. T. (2004). A comparative study of aortic wall stress using finite element analysis for ruptured and non-ruptured abdominal aortic aneurysms. *European Journal of Vascular and Endovascular Surgery*, 28, 168-176.

Vierendeels, J. D., Lanoye, L., Degroote, J. and Verdonck, P. (2007). Implicit coupling of partitioned fluid-structure interaction problems with reduce order models. *Computers and Structures*, 85, 970-976

Vogel, T. R., Nackman, G. B., Crowley, J. G., Bueno, M. M., Banavage, A., Odroniec, K., Brevetti, L. S., Ciocca, R. G. and Graham, A. M. (2005). Factors impacting functional health and resource utilisation following abdominal aortic aneurysm repair by open and endovascular techniques. *Annals of Vascular Surgery*, 19, 641-647.

Volokh, K. Y. and Vorp, D. A. (2008). A model of growth and rupture of abdominal aortic aneurysm. *Journal of Biomechanics*, 41(5), 1015-21.

Vorp, D. A. (2007). Biomechanics of abdominal aortic aneurysm. *Journal of Biomechanics*, 40(9), 1887-1902.

Vorp, D. A., Raghavan, M. L. and Webster, M. W. (1998). Mechanical wall stress in abdominal aortic aneurysm: influence of diameter and asymmetry. *Journal of Vascular Surgery*, 27(4), 632-639.

Vorp, D. A. and Vande Geest, J. (2005). Biomechanical determinants of abdominal aortic aneurysm rupture. *Arteriosclerosis, Thrombosis and Vascular Biology*, 25, 1558-1566.

Wang, D. H. J., Makaroun, M. S., Webster, M. W. and Vorp, D. A. (2002). Effect of intraluminal thrombus on wall stress in patient-specific models of abdominal aortic aneurysm. *Journal of Vascular Surgery*, 36, 598-604.

Wang, D. H. J., Makaroun, M., Webster, M. W. and Vorp, D. A. (2001). Mechanical properties and microstructure of intraluminal thrombus from abdominal aortic aneurysm. *Journal of Biomechanical Engineering*, 123, 536-539.

Watton, P., Hill, N. and Heil, M. (2004). A mathematical model for the growth of the abdominal aortic aneurysm. *Biomechanics and Modelling in Mechanobiology*, 3(2), 98-113.

Webb, S. (1988). *The Physics of medical imaging. 1st ed.* London: Institute of Physics Publishing.

In: 3D Imaging: Theory, Technology … ISBN: 978-1-60876-885-1
Editors: E. H. Duke and S. R. Aguirre, pp.51- 92

Chapter 2

3D Imaging of Phase Microscopic Objects by Digital Holographic Method

T. V. Tishko, D. N. Tishko and V. P. Titar
Laboratory of Holography, Kharkov National University, Ukraine

Abstract

Combining the holographic methods with the methods for digital image processing has made it possible to develop the digital holographic interference microscope (DHIM) for real-time 3D imaging of phase microscopic objects and measurement of their morphological parameters. The instrument integrates holographic interference microscope with digital processing of interferograms. For the first time it has become possible to obtain optically 3D images of native cells. In this chapter the classical and holographic methods of phase microobject visualization are considered. Experimental results of DHIM application for experimental study of the 3D morphology of biological and technical phase microscopic objects are presented. They are human blood erythrocytes and thin films. It is demonstrated that, in addition to hematological diseases, the diseases of various genesis and external factors serve as the reason for the morphological modification of blood erythrocytes. It is detected that morphologic modifications are nonspecific. It is proved that erythrocyte 3D morphology reflects the state of a living organism and the level of its biological response on different external factors influence. The proposed 3D model of erythrocyte makes it possible to quantitatively estimate the effect of morphological modifications of blood erythrocytes on their functionality with respect to oxygen transfer. It is demonstrated that the observed morphological modifications of erythrocytes lead to a significant decrease in the blood oxygen capacity and can serve as a reason for hypoxia. It is demonstrated that DHIM can also be successfully used for transparent thin films (with thicknesses less than the wavelength of the light being used) 3D imaging and quantitative investigation.

Introduction

A lot of objects of wildlife and nonliving matter are microscopic objects. They are invisible for human eye. A. Leeuwenhoek was the first, who created a microscope. Since that time microscopes are used for investigation of microscopic objects. Most of microscopic objects are phase objects that do not change the intensity of the radiation transmitted through them and are inaccessible to direct observation by optical microscope. They are cells and tissues of human organism, thin films, etc. To observe such phase microscopic objects it is necessary to convert phase changes inserted by them into the light wave into intensity changes. Special methods must be used for phase microscopic objects visualization. For the first time this problem was solved by F. Zernike [1]. For the phase-contrast method and the phase-contrast microscope he won Nobel Prize in physics in 1953. But classical microscopy methods allow only two-dimensional visualization of phase microscopic objects, measurement of their morphological parameters is impossible. The interference contrast method allows quantitative measurements, but this method can be used only for thin films thickness measurements. So, the problem of 3D visualization of phase microscopic objects has not been solved in classical microscopy. Till recently, electron microscopy was the only method for the 3D imaging of microscopic objects. However, this high-resolution method necessities long preliminary treatment of the sample, this renders study of native cells impossible. In addition, such a treatment affects cells and the reliability of the results of electron microscopy can be debated. Moreover, this method does not make it possible to measure morphological parameters of the microscopic objects. Improving resolution of electron microscopy, D. Gabor proposed the method of holography (Nobel Prize in Physics in 1971) [2]. Though Gabor's idea has not realized in microscopy, the advent and development of holography as the method for the record and reconstruction of the wave phase and amplitude resulted in the appearance of holographic analogs of the classical microscope methods [3-5]. The holographic analogs of classical methods exhibit several advantages. The development of computers and the methods for the digital data processing has led to a new stage in microscopy. The problem of 3D visualization of phase microscopic objects has been solved by combining the holographic methods with the methods for digital image processing [6, 7]. The first digital holographic interference microscope (DHIM), which allows the real-time 3D imaging of phase microscopic objects and the quantitative measurements of their morphological parameters, has been created at the Laboratory of Holography, Kharkov National University, Ukraine. The first 3D images of the native human blood erythrocytes were obtained using the microscope in [8]. Due to the topicality of the problem, several digital holographic microscopes were proposed for the 3D visualization of phase microscopic objects [9, 10].

1. Classical and Holographic Methods of Phase Microobjects Visualization

In this chapter a comparative theoretical and experimental analysis of classical and holographic methods for solving the problem of phase microscopic objects 3D imaging is given. The classical Zernike phase-contrast and interference contrast methods, and the holographic phase-contrast method and the method of holographic interferometry in fringes of finite width are considered; the description of the digital holographic interference microscope and experimental results of its application for phase microscopic objects 3D imaging are presented.

1.1 Classical Methods of Phase Microscopic Objects Visualization

As light travels through a microobject, interaction with this microobject causes its amplitude and phase to change in a way which depends on properties of the microobject. If the microobject absorbs light, it causes changes of intensity of light passing through it and it is accessible for observation in a usual optical microscope. But there are such microobjects which practically don't change the intensity of light transmitted through them and insert only phase shifts. They are inaccessible to observation because neither eye nor any other radiation detector senses such phase changes. To visualize phase microscopic objects, it is necessary to convert the phase shifts inserted by them into the transmitted light wave into intensity changes. Interference is the single phenomenon in which the phase difference of two interacting waves can be converted into changes of the resulting intensity. Two methods based on the interference phenomenon are used in classical microscopy for the phase microscopic objects visualization: F. Zernike phase-contrast method and interference contrast method [1].

1.1.1 Zernike phase-contrast method

The transmission function of phase object takes the form:

$$F(x,y)=\exp[i\varphi(x,y)],$$

where $\varphi(x,y)$ is the phase shift inserted by the phase microscopic object into transmitted light wave. When a phase microscopic object is observed, the intensity of the image is not modulated in the image plane of the microscope by the phase relief of the microobject, and it is invisible.

Staining of the sample is used when such microobjects are studied in biology and medicine, and this alters the properties of the microobjects being investigated. Moreover, such a method does not make it possible to obtain 3D images of microobjects or to measure their parameters.

Electron microscopy makes it possible to obtain an image of phase microobjects with high resolution. However, this method requires special sample preparation and does not make it possible to study untreated microobjects. Biological specimens break down when they are studied by electron microscopy. Therefore, a given specimen cannot be repeatedly studied, but only a similar specimen. Moreover, this method does not make it possible to determine morphological parameters of the microobjects.

The main drawback of non-optical methods of studying phase microobjects is that an effect is produced on the test microobject itself.

Another approach to the study of phase microobjects consist of producing an effect not on the test specimen but on a light wave transmitted through it. To do this, it is necessary to use special methods that can convert phase changes into intensity changes.

The well known phenomenon in which phase differences are converted into intensity changes is interference. To interfere, the waves must be coherent. The main equation of interference of two coherent waves has the form [18]:

$$I=I_1+I_2+2\sqrt{I_1I_2}\cos(\phi_2-\phi_1), \qquad (1)$$

where I_1, I_2 are the intensity of waves, ϕ_1,ϕ_2 are the phase of the waves. So, the resulting intensity is modulated by the phase difference of the waves. If the waves have equal intensity, i.e. $I_1 = I_2 = I_0$, then

$$I = 2I_0[1+\cos(\phi_2 - \phi_1)]. \tag{2}$$

E. Abbe was the first who formulated the wave theory of microscopic imaging (1872), which is based on the idea that the microscopic image is the result of interference of the wave diffracted on the microobject and the zeroth-order wave (the direct, non diffracted wave) [11]. The diffracted wave is shifted in phase by $\frac{\pi}{2}$ relative to the phase of the zeroth-order wave and has low intensity by comparison with the intensity of the zeroth-order wave.

Using E. Abbe's theory as a basis, F. Zernike proposed a method of phase microobject visualization that became known as phase-contrast method [1, 11, 18].

The essence of the method is that it is possible independently affect the diffracted and direct waves changing their phase relationship. So a special phase plate that retards or advances the phase of the zeroth-order wave by $\frac{\pi}{2}$ is placed in the microscope in zeroth order of diffraction. As a result, a phase shift equal 0 or π is created between the zeroth order wave and the diffracted wave. The waves in the former case are in phase (addition of waves), and this strengthens the intensity of the image by comparison with the background, whereas they are anti-phased in the latter case (subtraction of waves), and this weaken the intensity of the image by comparison with the background. The effect of the phase plate, situated in the back focal plane of the microscope objective, is described by the transmission function:

$$A = a \cdot e^{i\alpha}; \quad a \le 1,$$

where a is the transmission coefficient of the phase plate, α is the phase shift inserted by this plate. In this case the intensity in the image plane of microscope has the form [11]:

$$I(x',y') = |c|^2 \left\{a^2 + 2\left[1 - a\cos\alpha - \cos\varphi(x,y) + \cos(\alpha - \varphi(x,y))\right]\right\}, \tag{3}$$

where c is a constant. We suppose that $\varphi(x,y)$ is small, the phase inserted by the plate $\alpha = \pm\frac{\pi}{2}$. Then the intensity in the microobject image in the image plane of the microscope is modulated by the phase shift $\varphi(x,y)$ inserted by the microobject into the transmitted wave:

$$I(x',y') = |c|^2 \cdot \left(a^2 \pm 2a\varphi(x,y)\right), \tag{4}$$

where $|c|^2$ is the intensity of the zero order wave (direct wave).

So, the phase shifts, inserted by the microobject into the light wave transmitted through it, are converted into intensity changes in its image, which are proportional (with an accuracy up to the constant) to the phase shifts. If the phase of the zeroth-order wave lags behind the phase of the diffracted wave (the sign "+" in the formula (4)), then the image of the microobject is brighter than the background. This is so called *bright phase contrast.* It the phase of the zeroth- order wave leads phases of diffracted waves (the sign "–" in the formula (4)), then the image of the microobject is darker than the background. This is so called *dark phase contrast.*

The contrast of the image is determined by the ratio of the second term in the brackets of the formula (4) to the first and it is equal $\frac{2\varphi(x,y)}{a}$. It follows that the higher the absorption of the plate, the higher the contrast of the image. So, the satisfactory contrast is achieved by absorption of the direct light, and as a result, the decrease of total intensity takes place.

Thus, in Zernike's phase contrast method, the phase shift inserted by a microobject into a wave transmitted through it is converted by means of interference into an intensity change of its image. However, since waves of different intensity interact in the phase-contrast method, adding and subtracting the waves does not provide high image contrast, and consequently the method does not achieve high sensitivity. Absorbing phase plates are used to increase the image contrast, increasing the sensitivity of the method while reducing the overall illumination. The phase-contrast method is based on the possibility of separate acting on the direct light without changing the light diffracted at the microobject. Consequently, it can only be used for observing small objects, in the other case the direct light will be mixed with the diffracted light.

Thus, the phase-contrast method operates the more successfully, the smaller the phase microobject in optical thickness and dimensions.

1.1.2 The method of interference contrast

This method is also based on the phenomenon of interference of two waves. The interference contrast method can be realized in two main variants: interferometry in an infinitely wide fringe and interferometry in fringes of finite width.

The method of interferomertry in an infinitely wide fringe

The interferometry in an infinitely wide fringe solves the same problem as the phase-contrast microscopy. But in this case phase objects become visible due to the interference of two waves of equal intensity, one of which passes through the object under study. In two-beam interferometer [1] two compared waves are formed simultaneously, but propagate in different ways, then are combined and interfere. The resulting image intensity I_{im} in the case of interference of two coherent waves of equal intensity passed two identical channels of the interferometer and which differ only by the phase shifts inserted by the object under study is determined by the main interference equation:

$$I_{im}(x',y') = 2I_0\left\{1+\cos\left[\Phi_2-\Phi_1+\varphi(x,y)\right]\right\}. \quad (5)$$

And the background intensity I_b is equal to:

$$I_b(x',y') = 2I_0\{1+\cos(\Phi_2 - \Phi_1)\}, \tag{6}$$

where I_0 is the intensity of each of the interacting waves; Φ_1 and Φ_2 are the phase of the waves; $\varphi(x,y)$ is the phase shift inserted by the object under study into the wave transmitted through it.

From the expression (5) and (6) it follows that the image intensity differs from the background intensity and depends on the phase shift inserted by the object.

Let us estimate the effects of different phase shifts on the intensities of the image and the background. Suppose that such a phase difference of the beams can be achieved by adjusting the interferometer to make $\Phi_2 - \Phi_1 = 0$.That means that interacting waves are in phase (addition of waves). Then

$$\begin{aligned} I_{im+}(x',y') &= 2I_0[1+\cos\varphi(x,y)], \\ I_{b+}(x',y') &= 4I_0. \end{aligned} \tag{7}$$

It follows that while the phase shift $\varphi(x,y)$ is increasing, the image intensity is decreasing compared with the background intensity. In the point $\varphi(x,y) = \pi$ the image intensity becomes equal zero. So, in the case of the wave addition we obtain dark images against the bright background.

If the interferometer is adjusted so that $\Phi_2 - \Phi_1 = \pi$; it means that interfering waves are anti-phased (subtraction of waves). Then

$$\begin{aligned} I_{im-}(x',y') &= 2I_0[1-\cos\varphi(x,y)], \\ I_{b-}(x',y') &= 0. \end{aligned} \tag{8}$$

So, in the case of subtraction of the waves we obtain bright images against the dark background.

Thus, the phase object is observed as dark on a bright background in the case of addition of the waves, whereas it is observed as bright on the dark background in the case of subtraction. The intensity in the image of the object is modulated by the phase shifts introduced by the object into the transmitted wave. This method is equivalent to the phase-contrast method. However, although both methods are based on the interference of waves transmitted through a phase object and bypassing it, they have the difference that waves of equal intensity interact in the interference-contrast method. This makes it possible to maximize the image contrast and consequently the sensitivity of the method. Besides, the method is applicable for objects of every size.

However, the advantages of the interference-contrast method are reduced by the complexity of the apparatus and the difficulty of adjusting the interferometer. An especially complex problem in classical interferometry is the problem of obtaining two identical wave fronts. Moreover, interferometry in an infinitely wide fringe is impossible when strong objectives are used. And this method is not used in classical microscopy for phase microobject imaging.

The method of interferometry in fringes of finite width

The method of interferometry in fringes of finite width involves the interaction of the waves between which there is a certain angle θ. In this case instead of homogeneous field, a line field is obtained, with uniform alternation of intensity maxima and minima. In this case in accordance with the main interference equation (1), the intensity distributions in the image of the object I_{im} and in the background I_b have the form:

$$I_{im}(x',y') = 2I_0\{1+\cos[\Phi_2 - \Phi_1 + \varphi(x,y) - 2\pi x/T]\},$$
$$I_b(x',y') = 2I_0[1+\cos(\Phi_2 - \Phi_1) - 2\pi x/T]. \quad (9)$$

where $T = \lambda/\sin(\theta/2)$.

T is the period of the background interference fringes; I_0 is the intensity of each of the interacting waves, λ is the wavelength of the radiation being used; Φ_2, Φ_1 are the phase of the interacting waves, $\varphi(x,y)$ is the phase shift inserted by the object under study into the transmitted wave.

The equation of dark interference fringes has the form:

$$\Phi_2 - \Phi_1 + \varphi(x,y) - \frac{2\pi xx}{T} = (2m+1)\pi \quad (10)$$

And the equation of bright interference fringes is

$$\Phi_2 - \Phi_1 + \varphi(x,y) - \frac{2\pi x}{T} = 2m\pi, \quad (11)$$

where $|m| = 0,1,2,...$

One can see that the phase shifts inserted by the object under study into the wave transmitted through it result in change of the initial interference picture, what is manifested in deviations of the background interference fringes in the place of the location of the image of the object. Thus a phase silhouette of the object shows up in kinks of the interference fringes. As it follows from equations (10) and (11) the deviation h of the image interference fringe in some point is proportional to the phase shift $\varphi(x,y)$ inserted by the object, i.e.

$$h(x',y') = \frac{T\varphi(x,y)}{2\pi}. \quad (12)$$

So, measuring the deviations of the image interference fringes and the period of the background interference fringes, it is possible to determine the phase shifts.

Thus, the method of interferometry in fringes of finite width gives the possibility not only to visualize the phase object, but also to measure the phase shifts inserted by the object into the light wave transmitted through it.

But realization of the interferometry methods in classical microscopy meets some difficulties. In the first place, this is the mentioned above difficulty of creation of two identical wavefronts, and, as a result, high requirements to the quality of optics, complexity of the adjustment of the microinterferometer and high prices.

Though theoretically methods of interferometry have some advantages for phase microobject visualization compared to the Zernike phase-contrast method, practically the classical interference microscopes are used only for thin films thickness measurements. There are a few types of classical interference microscopes [1]. They generally differ by the methods of separation and combining the light beams.

1.2 Holography as the Method of Recoding and Reconstruction of Waves

Holography is the method of wave recording and reconstruction which is based on registration of an interference pattern, produced by two coherent waves: the object wave and reference one. The recorded interference pattern is called a hologram. The processes of hologram recording are described in many works [13-15]. Let us consider the optical arrangement for recording holograms of transparent objects. The optical layouts for recording and reconstruction of holograms are presented in Figure. 1.

The beam of coherent light (Figure 1a) from the laser 1 is broadened by the lenses 2 and 4.The semitransparent mirror 5 divides the broader beam in the two beams: the object beam and the reference beam. The reference beam B_2 is directed to the mirror 6 and is reflected in the direction of the holographic plate 8.The object beam B_1 passes through the object under study 7 and is also directed to the holographic plate 8. The beams are coherent. They interfere and their intereference pattern (hologram) is recorded on the holographic plate 8.

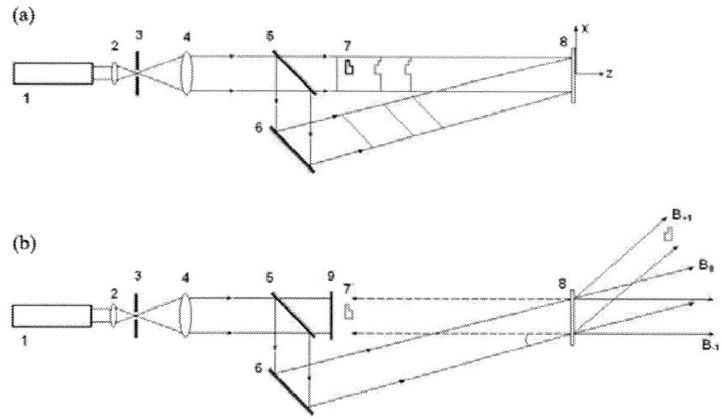

Figure 1. The optical layout for recording (a) and reconstructing (b) holograms of transparent objects. 1– laser; 2, 4 – lenses; 3 – diaphragm; 5 – semi-transparent mirror; 6 – mirror; 7 – object; 8 – hologram; 9 – opaque screen.

Let us express this mathematically. The hologram is produced by the interference of the object wave B_1 transmitted through the transparent object 7 and the reference wave B_2. Suppose that $A_1(x,y)$ is the complex amplitude of the object wave $B_1$and $A_2(x,y)$ is the complex amplitude of the reference wave B_2 in the plane of the photoplate 8:

$$A_1(x,y) = a_1(x,y)\exp[-\varphi_1(x,y)];$$
$$A_2(x,y) = a_2(x,y)\exp[-\varphi_2(x,y)], \tag{13}$$

where $a_1(x,y)$ and $\varphi_1(x,y)$ are the amplitude and the phase of the object wave; $a_2(x,y)$ and $\varphi_2(x,y)$ are the amplitude and the phase of the reference wave.

The complex amplitude of the resulting wave in the plane of the hologram 8 is equal:

$$A(x,y) = A_1(x,y) + A_2(x,y)$$

and, consequently, the intensity is equal to:

$$I(x,y) = A(x,y)A^*(x,y),$$

where $A^*(x,y)$ is the complex conjugate value.

Suppose that the wave transmitted through the object is directed on the holographic photoplate at the right angle, and the object change only the phase along the x axis:

$$a_1(x,y) = a_1,\ \varphi_1(x,y) = \varphi_1(x).$$

Suppose that the reference wave is directed on the photoplate at the angle θ_2:

$$a_2(x,y) = a_2,\ \varphi_2(x,y) = \frac{2\pi}{\lambda} x \cdot \sin\theta_2,$$

where λ is the wavelength of the used light.

Then the intensity in the interference pattern, produced by the waves, interacting in the plane of the photoplate 8, is determined by the main interference equation:

$$I(x) = a_1^2 + a_2^2 + 2a_1a_2\cos\left[\frac{2\pi}{\lambda}\cdot x\sin\theta_2 - \varphi_1(x)\right]. \tag{14}$$

where a^2_1 is the intensity of the object wave, a^2_2 is the intensity of the reference wave. From this formula one can see that the interference pattern is the alternation of dark and bright fringes. The positions of the dark and bright interference fringes depend on the phase $\varphi_1(x)$ of the object wave as follows:

$$x_{\max} = \frac{[2m\pi + \varphi_1(x)] \cdot \lambda}{2\pi \sin\theta_2}$$

$$x_{\min} = \frac{[(2m+1)\pi + \varphi_1(x)] \cdot \lambda}{2\pi \sin\theta_2}, \qquad (15)$$

where $|m| = 0, 1, 2....$

So, the information on the phase of the object wave is coded in the arrangement of the interference fringes recorded on the holographic plate.

Information on the amplitudes of the waves is coded in contrast v of the interference fringes:

$$v = \frac{I_{\max} - I_{\min}}{I_{max} + I_{\min}}, \qquad (16)$$

where $I_{\max}, I_{\min}$ are the maximal and minimal values of interference fringes intensity.

Using the expression (14) we can get:

$$v = \frac{2a_1 a_2}{a_1^2 + a_2^2}.$$

So, the amplitude of the object wave a_1 is uniquely determined if the amplitude of the reference wave a_2 is constant.

Thus, the recorded pattern of interference of the object and the reference waves (a hologram) contains information on the phase and amplitude of the object wave.

The methods of recording holograms can be different. The hologram can be recorded as variations of the absorption coefficient (amplitude holograms), or as variations of the refractive index (phase holograms). The hologram can be recorded on a surface (two-dimensional recording) or in a volume (holograms in the three-dimensional medium).

The object considered above is very simple (it changes the phase only in one direction). But the results of the consideration are suitable for very complicated objects. As the result, the recorded hologram will be also very complicated.

Let us consider the reconstruction process (Figure 1b). The hologram 8 (the developed holographic plate) is illuminated by the same reference wave which was used in the process of the hologram recording, when the object beam is screened by the opaque screen 9.Due to the process of light diffraction on the interference structure of the hologram, we obtain the three beam : the direct beam B_0 and the two diffracted beams B_{-1} и B_{+1}`.The two diffracted beam are responsible for the reconstruction of the 3D image of the object .

Let us describe mathematically the process of the reconstruction. We are going to consider the case, when the distribution of the intensity in the interference pattern is recorded as the variations of the absorption coefficient. Such situation occurs under recording holograms on the industrial holographic plates. In this case the amplitude of the wave transmitted through the hologram depends on the amplitude transmission of the hologram τ_a. In the case of the linear dependence of the amplitude transmission of the hologram from the light intensity

$$\tau_a = \kappa I(x,y),$$

where κ is constant and $I(x,y)$ is the intensity distribution in the recorded interference pattern (hologram).So, if the hologram 8 is illuminated by the wave, which is identical to the reference wave, then the complex amplitude of the transmitted wave is equal to:

$$A^{'}(x,y) = \tau_a A_2 = \kappa I(x,y) A_2. \tag{17}$$

Substituting the expressions (13) and (14) into equation (17), we obtain:

$$\begin{aligned} A'(x) = k_1 a_2 \exp\left[-i\frac{2\pi}{\lambda}x\cdot\sin\theta_2\right] + k_2 a_1 \exp\left[-i\varphi_1(x)\right] + \\ + k_2 a_1 \exp\left[i\varphi_1(x) - 2i\frac{2\pi}{\lambda}x\cdot\sin\theta_2\right], \end{aligned} \tag{18}$$

where $k_1 = \kappa\left(a_1^2 + a_2^2\right);\ k_2 = \kappa\cdot a_2^2$

This equation can be considered as the main holography equation. The first value corresponds to the direct waveB_0 in Figure 1b; the second value corresponds to the diffracted wave B_{-1}, which forms the virtual image (the reconstructed object wave); and the third value corresponds to the diffracted wave B_{+1}, which forms the real image. As it can be seen from the equation (19), the phase φ_1 of the wave B_{+1} differs by the value $-2i\frac{2\pi}{\lambda}x\sin\theta_2$ from the phase of the original object wave, and that's why the real image is deformed.

Thus the holographic method allows recording and reconstructing the amplitude and the phase of the object wave; the reconstructed virtual image is the replica of the original object wave. So, holography allows 3D imaging f objects.

According to relative position of object and reference light beams, one can obtain different types of holograms, which have some distinctive features. The inventor of holography D. Gabor suggested an optical scheme in which the interfering waves travel in one direction (axial holograms) [2]. E. Leith and J. Upatnieks (1964) contrived an optical arrangement for hologram recoding , in which two interfering waves are directed on the photoplate at some angles (off-axis holograms) [12]. Yu. Denisyuk (1967) proposed to record holograms in contra-directional waves [13]. Thick photoemulsion is needed for recording such holograms, and the holograms can reconstruct images in white light.

1.3 Holographic Methods of Phase Microscopic Objects Visualization

1.3.1 History of holographic microscopy

Holography was proposed by D. Gabor [2] as the method for electron microscope improvement. He proposed to record the hologram by an electron beam and reconstruct it in the optical range. The main magnification in the method is achieved without application of optics and determined by the ratio $\frac{\lambda_{opt}}{\lambda_{el}}$, where λ_{el} is the wavelength of the reconstructing wave in the optical range; λ_{opt} is de Broglie wavelength of the recording wave. D. Gabor based the proposed method theoretically and demonstrated holographic process of recoding and reconstruction of an image in the optical range. Because of the absence coherent source of electron beams this method has not found the application in the electron microscopy. But holography has opened up new possibilities for optical microscopy.

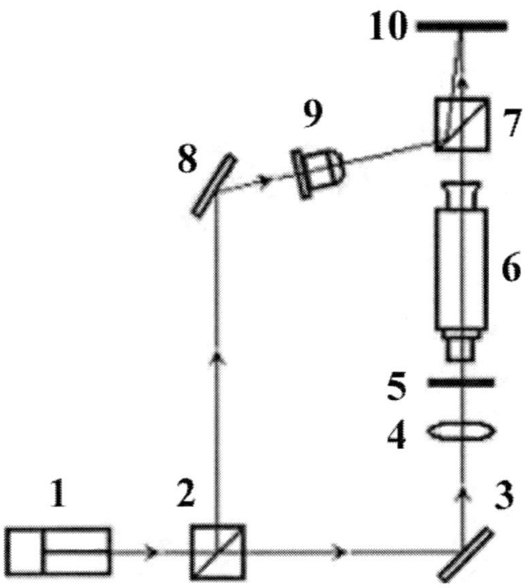

Figure 2. The optical layout of the holographic microscope. 1 – laser; 2 – beam splitter; 3, 8 – mirrors; 4, 9 – collimators; 5 – microobject under study; 6 – microscope; 7 – beam connector; 10 – hologram.

When optical lasers were developed, E.N. Leith and J Upatnieks proposed the off-axis optic scheme for hologram recording and the optical layout of the optical holographic "lensless" (without an objective) microscope [12]. Though it was impossible to reach the high magnification in the microscope, these promoted using holography in the optical microscopy.

The first holographic microscope using an optical microscope in its scheme was described by R.F. van Lighten and G. Ostenberg in 1966 (Figure 2). The image of the microobject magnified by the optical microscope was recorded on the hologram. Holograms of brain neural net with the optical resolution about 1 μm were obtained using the microscope [17].

An optical resolution is the main characteristics of a microscope. The optical resolution of classical microscope is determined by two quantities: the wavelength λ of the radiation being used and by the quantity of the numerical aperture of the objective $n \sin u$. In the case when non coherent radiation is used, the minimal resolved element of an object is determined by the formula [18]:

$$d \geq \frac{0.61 \cdot \lambda}{n \cdot \sin u},$$

where u is the aperture angle, n is the refractive index of the ambient media. Using immersion liquid, it is possible to increase the quantity of the numerical aperture to 1.35; and the minimal resolvable distance between two elements of the microobject under study can be about half of the wavelength of the radiation being used. The coherent laser radiation is used in the holographic microscope to illuminate the microobject under study. In this case the optical resolution of the microscope is determined by the formula:

$$d \geq \frac{\lambda}{n \cdot \sin u}.$$

Thus, the minimal resolvable distant between two details of the microobject under study is of the order of the wavelength. Decrease of the optical resolution of holographic microscopes is the principle shortcoming of the holographic method.

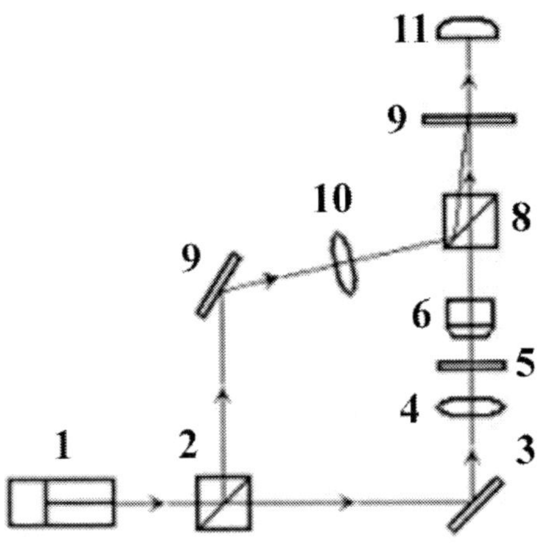

Figure 3. The optical layout of the holographic microscope, proposed by G. W. Ellis. 1 – laser; 2 – beam splitter; 3,9 – mirrors; 4,10 – collimators; 5 – microobject under study; 6 – microobjective; 8 – bean connector; 9 – hologram; 11 – eyepiece.

The next step in the development of holographic microscopy involved increasing the field of vision and the depth of the recorded scene. G. W. Ellis [19] proposed to place the hologram between the objective and eyepiece of the microscope (Figure 3). The reconstructed image is studied through the eyepiece which can be moved along the depth and all over the field of vision of the recorded scene. The general magnification of the microscope, which is determined either by the objective, or by the eyepiece, is maintained.

The main advantage of the holographic microscope lies in the possibility of a posteriori study of the reconstructed image, to which all the known methods of the optical and digital processing can be applied. That is very important in the case of short-living and moving microobjects.

The Zernike phase-contrast method began to be used with the appearance and evolution of holographic microscopy for observing the images of phase microobjects reconstructed from a hologram. The images of the phase microobject against dark and bright background were obtained by placing a plate into zeroth order of the diffraction spectrum of the microobject.

A problem associated with the use of high-coherent radiation sources arises in holographic microscopy. This is the coherent noise speckle structure of holographic images, which produce more noise, the smaller the microobject under study. Speckle structure and coherent noise produce a falloff of contrast and a reduction of image quality. So, Zernike phase-contrast method is not effective for application in holographic microscopy; and the problem of phase microobjects visualization has remained open.

Method of holographic microinterferometry was proposed practically simultaneously in a few works [14-16, 20]. Holography allows easily overcome the difficulties of classical microscopy, described above. The image, reconstructed from a hologram, is a copy of the initial object wave, and the problem of obtaining two identical waves is completely removed. By contrast to the classical interferometry, waves that are transmitted along the same path but in different instants of time interfere in holographic interferometer.

Holographic interferometry is used in two variants: real time and two exposure interferometry. In the real time interferometry only one object wave is recorded on the hologram using the reference wave. The interference pattern (an interferogram) is the result of interference of two object waves: the real wave and reconstructed from the hologram. This method allows observing the time history of the object under study. If the "empty" object wave is recorded on the hologram, then real time interferometry allows obtaining real-time interferograms of the phase objects. In the two-exposure method two object waves, characterizing object state in different moment of time, are recorded on a hologram. Such method allows recording and comparing two states of the object under study.

The holographic interferometry method allows performing measurements, and it is applied in science and technique for solving different problems, generally, for investigation of different deformations and processes. Holography has given the possibility to use the method of interferometry in fringes of infinite width for phase microobjects study [14].

1.3.2 Holographic phase-contrast method (the method of holographic addition and subtraction in an interference fringe)

As it was shown above, the interference-contrast method in an infinitely wide fringe is efficient for visualization of phase microobjects. If the advantages of the method are neutralized in the classical microscopy by the difficulties of obtaining two identical waves and adjustment of the interferometer, the use of holography removes these problems. This is because the wave which is a copy of the object wave can be recorded and reconstructed from a hologram. However, because of certain difficulties, the method of holographic interferometry in an infinitely wide fringe has not been used for obtaining images of phase microobjects. The difficulty consisted of providing the holographic addition and subtraction of the waves.This problem is easy to solve theoretically. The possibility of subtracting waves to obtain a difference image was already predicted in the early papers of D. Gabor. The phase of the wave recorded and reconstructed from an amplitude hologram (the negative of the initial interference pattern), is shifted by π relative to the phase of the initial wave. Therefore, the object wave and its anti-phased copy reconstructed from the hologram must quench each other when they are observed simultaneously (subtraction of waves). If one of the waves was transmitted through a phase microobject, then its bright image must be observed on the dark background. Such holographic subtraction can be realized in the real-time interferometry. On the other hand, when the unperturbed object wave and the object wave perturbed by a microobject are recorded on a single hologram, then the addition of waves must be observed, because the phases of both waves will be shifted by π relative to the phase of the initial wave. And a dark image of the microobject must be observed on the bright background. The holographic addition of waves can be realized by the method of two-exposure interferometry. However, because of phase shifts that arise when the holographic emulsion is processed and the very high sensitivity to of the method to vibrations, it was not possible earlier to obtain addition and subtraction of the waves in such an experiment. And the problem of obtaining in-phase and anti-phase waves remained open, like the problem of accomplishing phase contrast in holographic microscopy.

The problem of realizing phase contrast in holographic microscopy was solved for the first time in the author's works [3, 5], in which the method of adding and subtracting waves in an interference fringe was proposed. The proposed method was called the holographic phase-contrast method. In this method the two object waves interfere: the unperturbed "empty" object wave and the perturbed by the microobject object wave. The "empty" wave is the wave which is transmitted through the optical elements of the microscope in the absence of microobject under study. The real object wave is the wave transmitted through the optical elements of the microscope when the microobject is placed in front of the objective. The essence of this method is that a small angular shift is introduced between the interacting "empty" object wave and object wave, one of which is recorded and reconstructed from a hologram, so that the period of the resulting interference pattern significantly exceeds the size of the microobject image. When this is done, the conditions for waves to be anti-phase (subtraction of the waves) are automatically created within a dark interference fringe, and bright images of the phase microobjects are observed on a dark background, while the conditions for the wave to be in phase (addition of the waves) are created within a bright interference fringe, and dark images of the microobjects are observed on a bright background.

In accordance with (7, 8), the intensity in the phase microobject image $I_{im}(x', y')$ and the intensity of the background I_b in the case of addition of waves (a bright interference fringe) are determined by the expressions:

$$I_{im+}(x',y')=2I_0\left[1+\cos\varphi(x,y)\right],$$
$$I_{b+}(x',y')=4I_0; \tag{19}$$

and in the case of the subtraction of waves (a dark interference fringe) by the expression:

$$I_{im-}(x',y')=2I_0\left[1-\cos\varphi(x,y)\right];$$
$$I_{b-}(x',y')=0, \tag{20}$$

where $\varphi(x,y)$ is the phase shift inserted by the microobject into the wave transmitted through it; I_0 is the intensity of each of the two waves. As it follows from the expressions (19), (20) the dependences of the images intensities on the phase shifts inserted by the microobject are antiphased. The minimal intensity in the microobject image in the case of the wave addition corresponds to the maximal intensity in the image in the case of the wave subtraction and vice versa, so the contrast of the images is inverted.

To obtain contrast images of phase microobjects one of the two object waves (the "empty" one or the transmitted through the microobject) must be recorded on the hologram. Both these variants are used depending on the type of the problem being solved.

The variant of obtaining contrast images of phase microobjects recorded and reconstructed from a hologram can be used for study of alive moving microobjects or in the cases when the microobjects are accessible for observation during a short period of time. In this case the microobject under study is placed in front of the microscope objective, and its hologram is recorded using the reference wave for a short exposure time or even in the pulse mode of laser radiation. The processed hologram is placed into its initial position. The interferogram of the microobject is produced by the intereference of the object wave, reconstructed from the hologram, and the "empty" real wave. Changing the angle between the two waves (by shifting the hologram from its initial position) it is possible to reach the situation when the period of interference fringes on the interferogram of the microobject is considerable more than the dimensions of the microobject. In this case dark image of the microobject in the bright interference fringe, and bright image of the microobject in the dark interference fringe are observed. In this variant a separate hologram is recorded for every microobject under study.

In the variant of obtaining contrast images of phase micoobjects in real time the "empty" object wave (when the microobject under study is absent in front of the microscope objective) is recorded on the hologram using the reference beam. The microobject is placed in front of the objective. The interferogram of the microobject is produced by the interference of the reconstructed from the hologram "empty" object wave and the real object wave, transmitted through the microobject. It is obvious that in this case we can observe the dynamic of the microobject changes. In this variant of the method one hologram can be used to study different microobjects. But every objective of the microscope needs it own hologram.

The details of the practical realization of the holographic phase-contrast method will be described in the Chapter 1.4, devoted to the description of the digital holographic interference microscope and its operation.

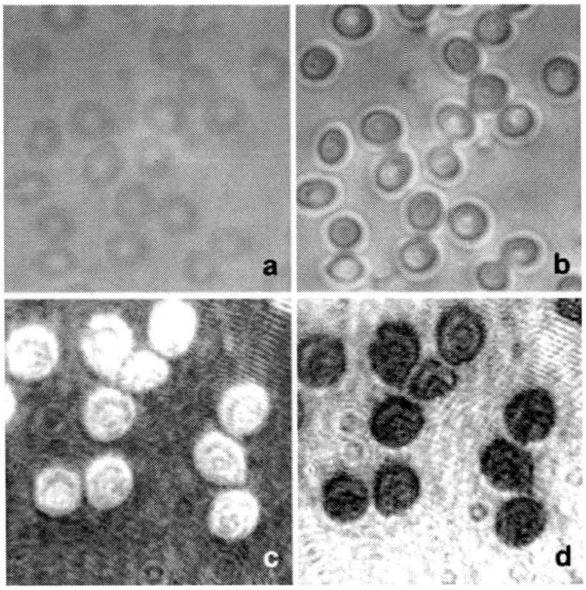

Figure 4. The images of human blood erythrocytes, obtained by the classical and holographic methods (x 400): a – using the "Lumam" microscope in the white light; b – by F. Zernike method using the phase-contrast attachment in the microscope "Lumam"; c – by the method of holographic subtraction; d – by the method of holographic addition using the digital holographic interference microscope.

Experimental studies using the digital holographic interference microscope confirmed that the proposed method is effective for obtaining contrast images of phase microobjects. Untreated blood smears on glass slides were used as test objects. The experimental results [23] allow one to compare the classical and holographic phase-contrast methods for visualization such microobjects as human blood erythrocytes (Figure 4). A He-Ne laser with radiation wavelength equal to 0.63 μm was used as a source of light in the digital holographic interference microscope to obtain the images. Different blood smears were used for obtaining the optical and holographic images, presented in Figure 4. The images illustrate the efficiency of the holographic phase-contrast method for obtaining contrast images of phase microobjects. The contrast of the images obtained when the holographic subtraction and addition were applied, are maximal. But coherent noises caused by diffraction of laser radiation on grains and in homogeneity of the substrate and optical elements of the microscope worsen the image quality.

The intensity of images on the interferograms of microobjects is modulated by the phase shifts, inserted by the microobject into the transmitted wave. According to the expression (19) and (20) the phase shift is equal:

$$\varphi(x,y) = \arccos[\pm(1 - \frac{I_{im\mp}(x',y')}{2I_0})], \tag{21}$$

where $I_{im\mp}(x',y')$ is the intensity of the microobject image; I_0 is the intensity of each of the two interfering waves; the sign "+" corresponds to the case of wave subtraction; the sign "–"

corresponds to the case of wave addition. In accordance with the formula (19), $I_0 = \frac{I_{b+}}{4}$, where I_{b+} is the background intensity in the case of wave addition. Then

$$\varphi(x,y) = \arccos[\pm(1 - \frac{2I_{im\mp}(x',y')}{I_{b+}})]. \qquad (22)$$

So, measuring the intensities in the holographic image of phase microobject and the background intensity in the case of holographic addition of waves it is possible to reconstruct the phase relief of the microobject under study.

The intensity variations on the interferogram of the phase microobject are caused by the phase increment of the transmitted wave through the entire thickness of the microobject,

$$\varphi(x,y) = \frac{2\pi}{\lambda}\int_{z_1}^{z_2}\Delta n(x,y,z)dz,$$

where $\Delta n(x,y,z)$ is the difference of the refractive indices of the microobject and the ambient medium. If the microobject has a homogeneous refractive-index distribution, i.e. $\Delta n(x,y,z) = const$, we get

$$\varphi(x,y) = \frac{2\pi}{\lambda}t(x,y)\Delta n, \qquad (23)$$

where $t(x,y) = z_2 - z_1$ is the thickness of the microobject in the point (x, y). From this,

$$t(x,y) = \varphi(x,y)\frac{\lambda}{2\pi\Delta n}.$$

Taking into consideration the expression (22) we get the expression for the thickness of the phase microobject:

$$t(x,y) = \frac{\lambda}{2\pi\Delta n}\arccos[\pm(1 - \frac{2I_{im\mp}(x',y')}{I_{b+}})], \qquad (24)$$

where λ is the wavelength of the radiation being used, Δn is the difference of the refractive indices of the microobject and ambient medium, $I_{im\mp}(x',y')$ is the intensity in the corresponding point of the microobject image on its interferogram, I_{b+} is the background intensity when the waves are added. The + sign corresponds to the case of subtraction of waves, the – sign corresponds to addition of waves.

Thus, the method of holographic addition and subtraction of wave make it possible to determine physical thickness of the phase microobjects in every point and reconstruct its 3D image. With the development of methods of computer processing of images, the possibility appeared of solving the problem of 3D imaging of phase microobjects, which was achieved earlier only by the method of electron microscopy.

The following algorithm can be used for computer reconstruction of the 3D image of a phase microobject from its interferogram, obtained when the holographic method of phase contrast is used.

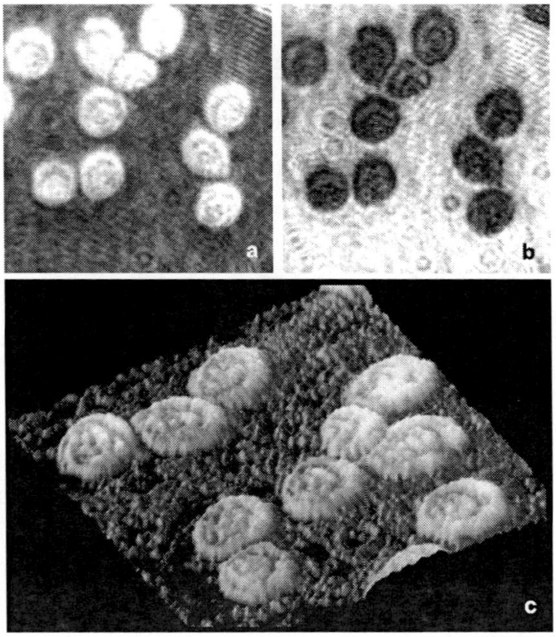

Figure 5. Computer 3D imaging human blood erythrocytes: a – the interferogram of a segment of an untreated blood smear with subtraction of waves, b – with addition of waves, c – the reconstructed 3D image of erythrocytes from these interferograms.

The image is transformed into an array of intensities I_{im} at each of its point. The mean background intensity I_{b+} (the mean intensity in a segment chosen by the operator or by the program itself) and the initial intensity $I_0 = I_{b+}/4$ are found. Next the phase shifts are calculated from the formula (22) for each point of the image, and an array is formed corresponding to the phase relief of the wave transmitted through the microobject. If the microobject has a homogeneous refractive-index distribution and the phase increment is consequently a linear function of the thickness of the microobject, the algorithm for constructing a 3D image regards the array of values of the phase increment as an array of values of the third coordinate (the height), taking into account equation (24).

Human blood erythrocytes are phase microobjects with the homogeneous refractive-index distribution. Dry blood smears on glass slides were used in our experiment, thus Δn is the refractive-index difference of the erythrocytes and air. The refractive index of blood was determined by means of an Abbe refractometer using a He-Ne laser and equal 1.352, the refractive index of air equal 1. These values were used in formula (24).

Figure 5 shows 3D image of blood erythrocytes obtained by the holographic phase-contrast method using the digital holographic interference microscope [25].

1.3.3 The method of holographic interferometry in fringes of finite width

In the holographic method of interferometry in fringes of infinite width (the method of holographic addition and subtraction of waves) the phase shifts inserted by the microobject into the wave transmitted through it modulate the intensity in the microobject image, and it becomes visible. As it is shown above, the method of interferometry in fringes of finite width involves the interaction of waves between which there is a certain angle. In this case, instead of homogeneous field, a line field is obtained, with uniform alternation of intensity maxima and minima. So, in the method of interferometry in fringes of finite width the system of background interference fringes is modulated by the phase shifts inserted by the microobject into the wave transmitted through it, and this manifests itself in curvatures of the interference fringes. As it follows from equations (10) and (11) the deviation of the interference fringe in some point of the interferogram is proportional to the phase shift $\varphi(x, y)$ in the corresponding point of the object, i.e.

$$h(x', y') = \frac{T\varphi(x, y)}{2\pi}, \qquad (25)$$

where T is the period of the system of the background interference fringes.

The main difference of the holographic method of interferoimetry in fringes of finite width from the classical one consists in the following. The system of the reference interference fringes in the classical interferometer is produced by the interference of two waves transmitted simultaneously along two paths and re-joined. The system of reference interference fringes in the holographic interferometer is produced by two waves transmitted along the same path but in different instants of time. One of these waves is recorded and reconstructed from a hologram. The holographic interferometer is a single arm interferometer as opposite to the classical interferometer which is a two-arm interferometer. Because the recorded and reconstructed from the hologram wave is a copy of the initial object wave, the problem of obtaining the two identical object waves, which is the main problem of classical interferometry, is completely removed [4-7, 21, 22].

As it was mentioned above, the phase shifts introduced by the microobject into the wave transmitted through it manifests itself in deviations of the reference interference fringes from their initial positions in the place of the microobject image. So, measuring the deviations of the interference fringes on the interferogram of the microobject it is possible to determine the phase shifts inserted the microobject into the transmitted wave and reconstruct the phase profile of the phase microobject. Then from (25)

$$\varphi(x, y) = \frac{2\pi h(x', y')}{T}, \qquad (26)$$

where $h(x',y')$ is the deviation of the interference fringe from its initial position in the corresponding point, T is the period of the system of reference interference fringes. If the microobject has a homogeneous refractive-index distribution (23), then the thickness of the microobject at a point is equal:

$$t(x,y) = \frac{\lambda h(x',y')}{T\Delta n}, \tag{27}$$

where $h(x',y')$ is the deviation of the interference fringe in the corresponding point, T is the period of the system of reference interference fringes, λ is the wavelength of the radiation being used, Δn is the difference of refractive indices of the microobject and the ambient medium.

Thus, measuring the deviations of the interference fringes from their initial positions on the interferogram of the microobject it is possible to determine the thickness of the microobject in each its point and reconstruct its 3D image.

The algorithm for the mathematical processing the interferogram obtained by the method of holographic interferometry in fringes of finite width consist of interpreting the deviations of the interference fringes as the heights of the microobject in accordance with equation (27), followed by 3D visualization of the microobject, as well as the determination of its morphological parameters.

A problem of this type has no exact mathematical solution. However, an approximation algorithm may be used, provided that the error that it introduces does not exceed the error introduced into the image by the fundamental deficiencies of the physical experiment (coherent noise, speckle structure, etc.). Moreover, the problem of reducing the influence of such noise on the image quality can also be solved by computer-processing the interferograms.

Experiments have confirmed the efficiency of the using the method of holographic interferometry in fringes of finite width for study of the phase microobjects. 3D images of phase microobjects were obtained for the first time when investigating the erythrocytes of patients suffering from hemolytic anemia [8].

Figure 6 shows interferograms in fringes of finite width of individual erythrocytes and images of the erythrocytes reconstructed from the interferograms [6, 7].

Figure 7 shows a segment of an interferogram of an untreated blood smear in fringes of finite width and a reconstructed three-dimensional image of this segment. These results were obtained using the digital holographic interference microscope. Notice that there is blood plasma apart from erythrocytes in the native blood smears. When water vaporizes from the plasma, the substances contained in it (in general, proteins) form space structures which are also phase microobjects and are observed on the reconstructed three-dimension images of blood smears. These elements of the plasma form some fibers (figure 7) that is connected with the method of the smear preparing (expansion of a blood drop along the glass substrate).

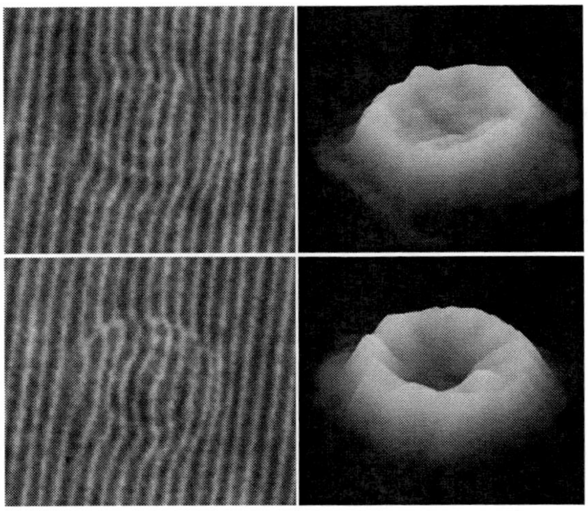

Figure 6. Interferograms of individual erythrocytes (at the left) and images reconstructed from them (at the right).

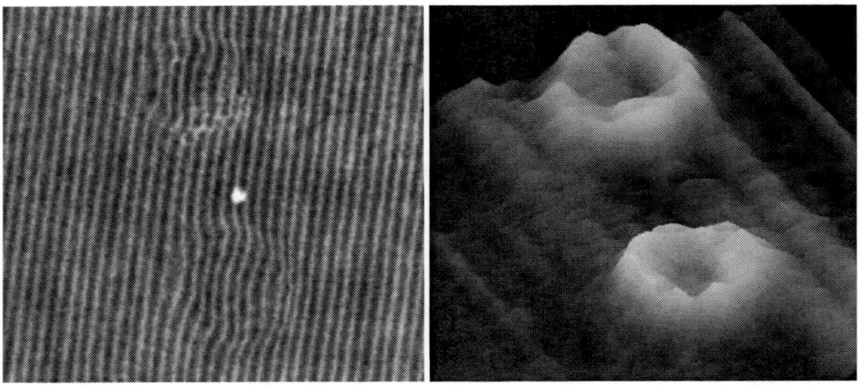

Figure 7. Segment of an interferogram of an untreated blood smear in fringes of finite width (at the left) and the reconstructed three-dimensional image (at the right).

1.3.4 Comparison of the possibilities of the holographic methods for solution the problem of obtaining 3D images of phase microobjects

The carried out theoretical and experimental investigations have shown that the method of holographic addition and subtraction of waves (Figure 5) and the method of holographic interferometry in fringes of finite width (Figures 6, 7) together with the methods of computer processing images can be used for 3D imaging phase microscopic objects. The 3D images of phase microobjects not only give clear qualitative information concerning the shape of these objects, but they also make it possible to make various quantitative measurements of such geometrical parameters of these microobjects as the linear sizes, the spericity coefficient, the surface area, and the volume.

To compare the methods, interferograms of the same microobject were obtained by the holographic phase-contrast method and by the method of holographic interferometry in fringes of finite width. The results are shown in Figure 8. The high level of correspondence of the images obtained by the methods (Figure 8d and 8e) makes it possible to conclude that the computer-processing methods that were used adequately reflect the experimental information and are quite suitable for solving such general problems.

Each method has its own advantages and disadvantages for solving problem of three-dimensional visualization of phase microscopic objects.

When the method of addition and subtraction in an interference fringe is used, fairy simple exact processing algorithms can be used for computer processing of the interferograms. However, since absolute intensities are used in this method, it is necessary for the transfer function of the image-recording unit to be linear in order to obtain adequate three-dimensional visualization.

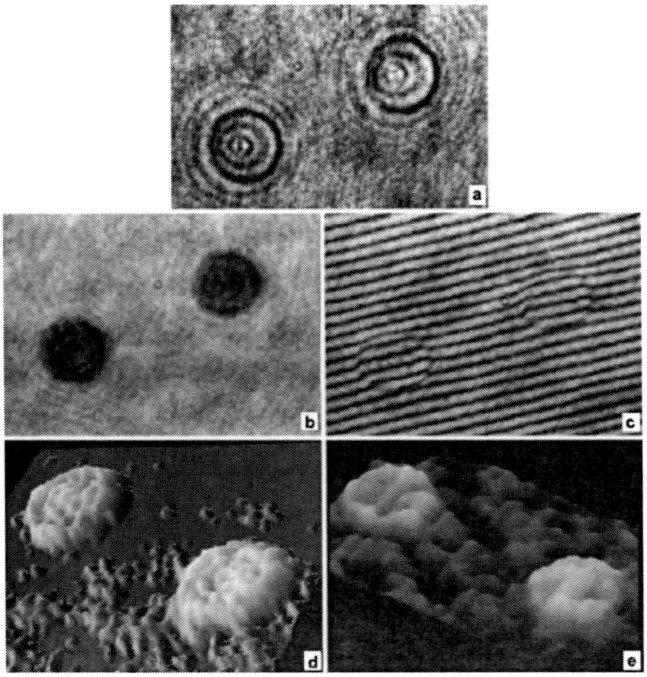

Figure 8. Comparison of the holographic methods of phase microobject 3D imaging. Photograph of erythrocytes (a), image of erythrocyte in the case of waves addition (b), interferogram of erythrocytes in fringes of finite width (c), images of erythrocytes reconstructed from the interferograms (d and e).

At the stage of recording the interferogram, this method imposes very high requirements on the vibration stability of the interferometer.

The problem of three-dimensional visualization of phase microobjects when the method of interferometry in fringes of finite width is used has no exact mathematical solution. However, it is allowable to use approximate processing algorithms, provided that the error that they introduce does not exceed the error introduced by the fundamental drawback of the physical experiment (speckle structure, coherent noise). Moreover, computer processing makes it possible to use supplementary algorithms to reduce the effect of these drawbacks (filtering of the speckle defects, averaging of the coherent noise). There are no high requirements on the vibration stability of the apparatus at the interferogram- recoding stage, and the interferometer can operate without any special vibration-proofing measures in such a regime. Thus, the method of holographic interferometry in fringes of finite width is best suited for phase microobjects investigation.

It has been shown that holographic methods have a number of advantages over classical method when solving the problem of the three-dimensional visualization of phase microscopic objects. Experimental investigations of the holographic method of addition and subtraction in an interference fringe and the method of interferometry in fringes of finite width have confirmed that they are effective for computer 3D visualization such objects.

1.4 Digital Holographic Interference Microscope

Combination of holographic microscopy and the methods of digital image processing makes it possible to realize the 3D visualization of phase microobjects. The first digital holographic interference microscope (DHIM), which allows the real time 3D imaging of phase microobject and the quantitative measurements of their parameters, has been created in the Laboratiry of Holography, Kharkov National University. The first 3D images of the native human blood erythrocytes were obtained using microscope in [8]. All experimental results presented in this article were obtained using the DHIM.

One advantage of holographic methods of studying phase microobjects is that the method of holographic subtraction and addition of waves and the method of interferometry in fringes of finite width can be implemented in the same apparatus.

The DHIM consists of three main units: holographic microinterferometer, digital video camera and computer. The interferograms of the microobjects under study obtained using the holographic microinterferometer are recorded by the digital camera. The digital interferograms are computer processed using the mathematical algorithms that makes it possible to reconstruct the 3D images of microobjects and to measure their geometrical parameters.

The optical layout of DHIM is shown in Figure 9.

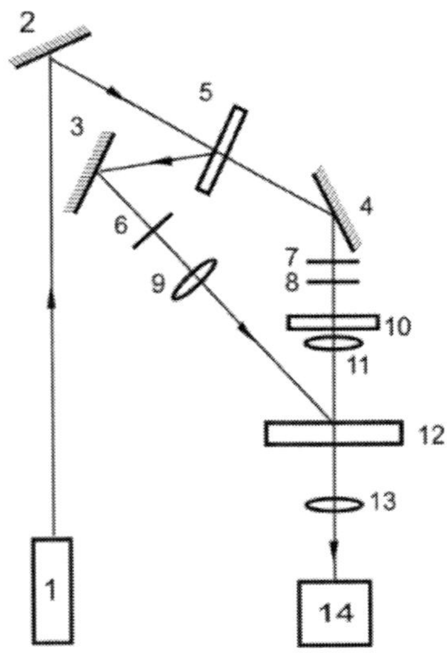

Figure 9. Optical layout of a digital holographic interference microscope. 1 – laser; 2 ,3 and 4 – mirrors; 5 – semitransparent mirror; 6, 7 and 8 – polarizers; 9 – collimator; 10 – test specimen; 11 – objective; 12 – hologram; 13 – eyepiece; 14 – image-recording unit.

A He-Ne laser that emits at 0.63 μm is used as a coherent radiation source. The radiation of laser *1* is divided into two beams by semitransparent mirror *5*: the object beam and the reference beam. The object beam passes through microscope objective *11* and is directed to holographic plate (hologram) *12*.The reference beam passes through collimator *9* and also is directed to hologram *12*. Mirrors *3* and *4* are introduced into the system to rotate the rays. The reference beam plays an auxiliary role in the system. It is needed for recording and reconstructing the object wave from the hologram.

A hologram of the "empty" object wave is recorded on holographic plate *12* in the absence of the specimen with microobjects under study in front of the microscope objective. The developed and fixed hologram is returned to its original position and serves as an optical element of the microscope. A special holder makes it possible to displace the hologram relative to its original position. Hologram *12* is placed between objective *11* and eyepiece *13*. Since an unfocused image is recorded on the hologram, such a placement of the hologram makes it possible to increase the field of view of the microscope because of the possibility of displacing the eyepiece in a plane orthogonal to the observation direction, and to carry out additional focusing over the depth of the observed scene. The test specimen *10* is placed in front of the microscope objective *11*. When the "empty" object wave reconstructed from the hologram by means of the reference beam and the perturbed real object wave transmitted through the microobject under study propagate simultaneously, their interference pattern, i.e. the interferogram, can be observed by means of eyepiece *13*. The necessary period of the background interference fringes for obtaining an interferogram in an infinitely wide fringe or in fringes of finite width is formed by transversely shifting the hologram *12* from its initial position by means of the micrometer screws of the holder.The hologram recorded for the given objective can be used permanently when working with the given objective.

As it well known, the quality and contrast of holograms and interferograms are determined by such a quantity as the modulation depth of the interference pattern, $\mu = \dfrac{2\sqrt{\alpha}\cos\beta}{(1+\alpha)}$, where α is the intensity ratio of the interfering waves, while β is the angle between the directions of linear polarization of these waves. As follows from this expression, we obtain the maximal value of $\mu = 1$ when the interfering waves have identical intensities and polarizations. Polarizes *6, 7*, and *8* are introduced into the system to equalize the intensities and polarizations of the interacting waves. Polarizes *6* and *8* give identical directions of the plane of linear polarization of the interacting waves, while the intensities of the interacting waves are equalized by rotating the plane of polarization of polarizer *7*.

Interferograms of the microobjects being investigated are recorded by means of image-recording unit *14,* containing digital camera.

A 40 x 0.65 objective and 10X eyepiece were used in the experiments. The holograms were recorded on PFG - 03 plates. Developer GP - 2 was used for processing the holograms.

Figure 10 shows 3D image of a fragment of an untreated human blood smear with a leukocyte and two erythrocytes obtained using the DHIM.

Figure 11 shows 3D image of a fragment of a rabbit blood smear with pathological erythrocytes.

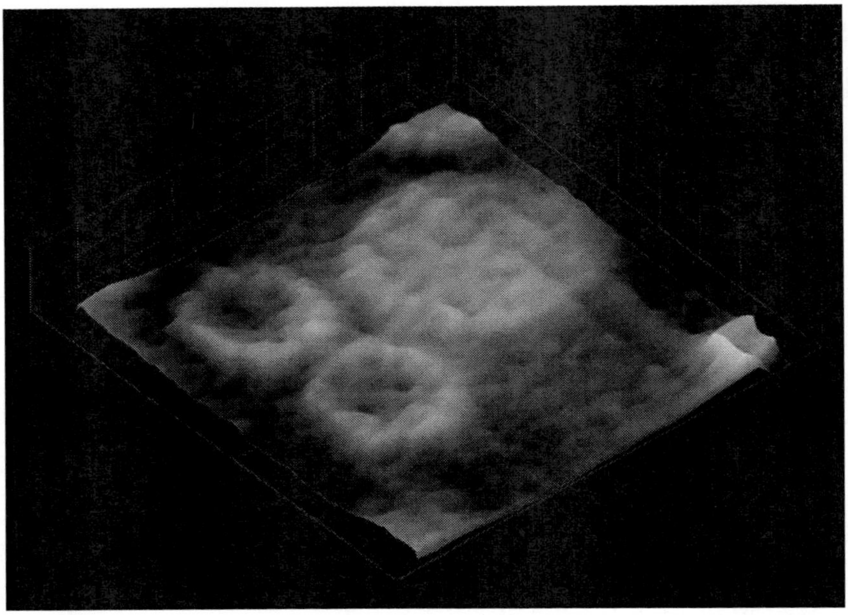

Figure 10. 3D image of the fragment of the human blood smear with a leukocyte and two erythrocytes.

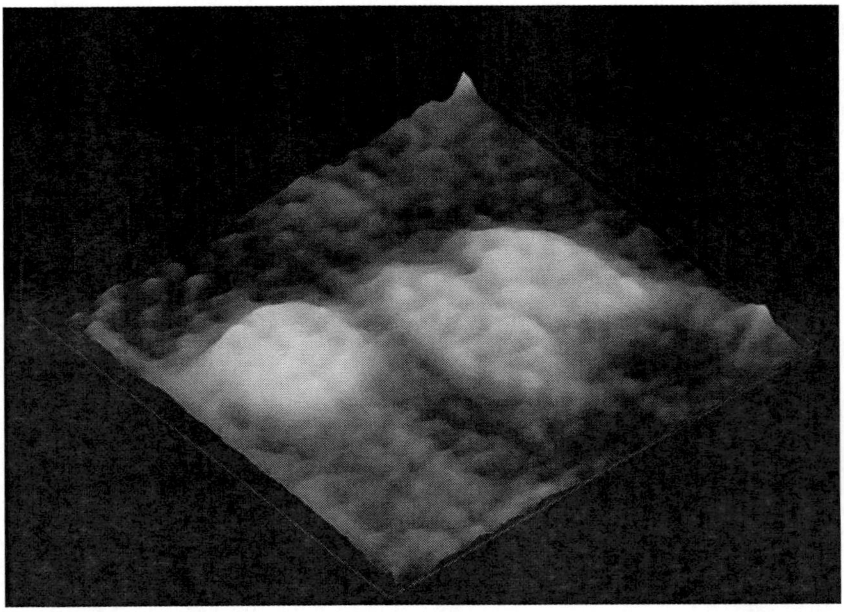

Figure 11. 3D image of the fragment of the rabbit blood smear with pathological erythrocytes.

2. APPLICATION OF THE DIGITAL HOLOGRAPHIC MICROSCOPY FOR PHASE MICROOBJECTS STUDY

In this chapter we present our pioneer results of DHIM application for experimental study of the 3D morphology of biological and technical phase microscopic objects. They are human blood erythrocytes and thin films.

2.1 DHIM Study of The 3D Morphology of Blood Erythrocytes

The study of the interaction of a living organism with the environment at a cellular level is of great scientific interest. A cell is a unit of a living organism that reflects and determines the status and functioning of the biological system as a whole. A number of papers have appeared in recent years in which it was established that the main target of the action of various physical and chemical factors of the environment, as well as internal pathologies and even of the mental states are the cellular plasmatic membranes. The variation of the elastic properties of the cellular membranes under the action of various effects must unavoidably shows up in a change in shape of the cells. The blood cells are of special interest. Blood unites the operation and functioning of all organs of the living organism. The red blood cells (erythrocytes) are the cells whose main function is the oxygen transport from lungs to tissues and the carbon dioxide transport to lungs. In addition, erythrocytes take part in the processes related to maintaining of the homeostasis at the organism level. Moreover, an erythrocyte is available for observation as a separate cell of a living organism. An erythrocyte is a cell without nucleus, and the content of protein hemoglobin in it is 98 %. For the optimal functioning, the functional activity of hemoglobin must be maintained and the optimal 3D shape of erythrocyte must be realized. The erythrocyte shape must correspond to maximum surface at the given volume and must ensure deformations providing the erythrocyte motion along thin capillaries. These conditions are satisfied for a biconcave disk shape, which is considered as the medical normal shape. The first image of erythrocyte as a biconcave disk was obtained using electron microscopy in [25]. Then, this result has been confirmed. It is commonly accepted that the fraction of the biconcave erythrocytes in the blood of healthy patients ranges from 60 to 97 %. It is knows that in the case of hematological diseases the modifications of erythrocytes shapes are observed. The results of electron microscopy show that, in addition to hematological diseases, the diseases of various genesis can be the reason for modifications of the 3D shape of erythrocytes [26]. This made it possible to formulate the concept of the erythrocyte pathomorphosis. However, this concept was under question, since the morphological modifications observed using electron microscopy can be caused by various effects related to the sample preparation.

Red blood cells, like other cells of a living organism, are phase microobjects. Therefore, the problem of studying the morphology of erythrocytes for purposes of medical diagnosis involves the problem of 3D visualization of phase microobjects and measuring their morphological parameters.

Human erythrocytes are microobjects with a size 7-8 μm and a maximum thickness of about 2 μm. Each one is a microobject with a low optical density and homogeneous refractive-index distribution, transparent for radiation from a He-Ne laser. The optical homogeneity of the erythrocytes makes it possible to use equation (27) to compute the thickness of the erythrocytes in different points and reconstruct their 3D images. Equation (27) includes the quantity Δn, which equals the refractive-index difference of the microobject and ambient medium. It is known that erythrocytes do not change their shape after drying. That makes it possible to use dry untreated blood smears on glass slides that are normally used in medical practice for study of 3D morphology of blood erythrocytes. Then Δn is the difference of the refractive indices of the erythrocytes and air. The refractive index of blood was measured by means of Abbe refractometer using a He-Ne laser and equals 1.352. This value was taken as refractive index of the erythrocytes. The refractive index of air equals 1. So, Δn is equal 0.352. This value was used in equation (27) under computer processing the interferograms of erythrocytes for their 3D imaging and measuring their morphological parameters.

Figure 12 shows the reconstructed 3D image of a fragment of the blood smear of a healthy donor. One can see the direction of blood smearing.

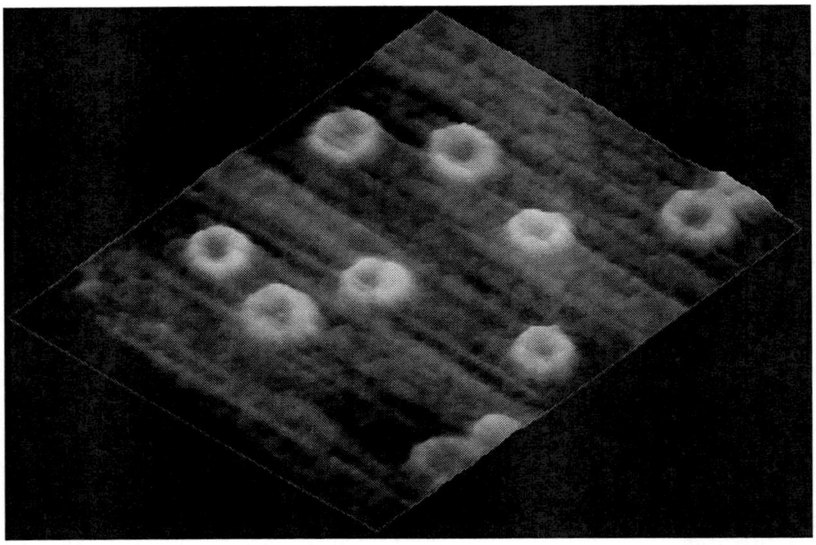

Figure 12. 3D image of the fragment of the blood smear.

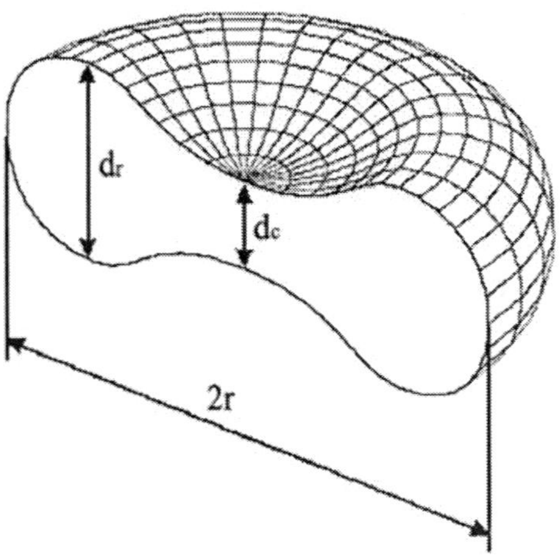

Figure 13. Determination of the sphericity coefficient *k*. d_c - thickness at the center; d_r - thickness at a half of radius.

In our experiments we have determined three main morphological types of erythrocytes: biconcave disk, flat disk, and spherocytes [27-29]. To characterize the morphological type, a sphericity coefficient *k* is introduced as a ratio of the erythrocyte thickness at the center to the thickness at half radius (Figure 13). For the biconcave erythrocytes, flat disks, and spherocytes, the sphericity coefficient is less than unity, about unity, and greater than unity, respectively. The sphericity coefficient is measured upon the computer processing of the DHIM erythrocyte interferograms.

Figure 14 demonstrated the 3D images of the three main morphological types and their sphericity coefficients.

The biconcave erythrocytes correspond to the medical norm; the functional possibilities of such erythrocytes are maximal. Functional possibilities of flat and spherical erythrocytes are reduced. These main morphological shapes of erythrocytes and their different variants were detected in the native blood smears of donors and patients with different diseases; but contain of these types of erythrocytes was quite different.

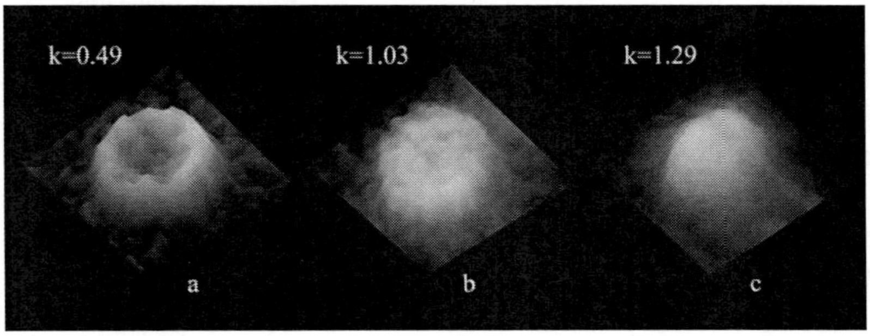

Figure 14. 3D images of the three main morphological types of erythrocytes: biconcave (a), flat (b), and spherical (c) and their sphericity coefficients

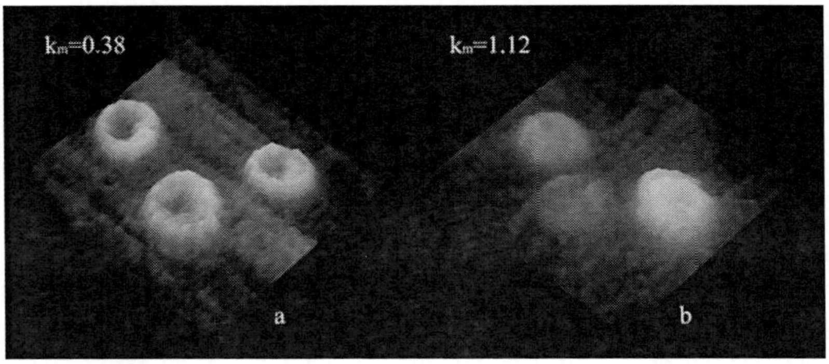

Figure 15. 3D images of the fragments of blood smears and the mean sphericity coefficients: (a) health patient ($k_m = 0.35$) and (b) diseased patient ($k_m = 0.96$).

Figure 15 shows the fragments of the native smears of blood of a healthy man aged 56 (a) and a diseased woman (cavernous hemangioma) aged 23 (b). The mean sphericity coefficients of the fragments are presented. The mean sphericity coefficient is determined as arithmetical mean of the spericity coefficients of the separate erythrocytes of the fragment.It is seen that the biconcave erythrocytes dominate in the blood smear of the healthy donor (Figure 15a). The mean sphericity coefficient of his smear is equal to 0.35.The fragment of the blood smear of the woman (Figure 15b) contains flat disks and a spherocyte. The mean sphericity coefficient of the fragment of her blood smear is equal to 0.96. The difference of blood smears of the healthy donor and the diseased woman is obvious.

Patients with different diseases were examined in our experiments. The majority of the patients had the morphological variations of the erythrocytes, the tendency to the increase of the mean sphericity coefficient of blood smears. But any specific variations of erythrocytes morphology which are distinctive for one or other disease were not detected. The development of a disease is always connected with functional disturbance of some sells of an organism. From the other hand, functional disturbance of some cells may cause the development of a disease. The question, what is the reason of the observed morphological variations of blood erythrocytes, is open and needs further investigations.

All observed morphological variations of erythrocytes are nonspecific and show the increase in their sphericity coefficients. The increase of the sphericity coefficient corresponds to the decrease of the surface square of the erythrocyte under its given volume. The morphological modifications related to a decrease in the erythrocyte surface area cause a decrease in the functionality with respect to the oxygen supply of tissues and organs.

3D model of erythrocyte was considered to quantitatively estimate the effect of morphological modifications of blood erythrocytes on their functionality with respect to the oxygen transfer [30]. As it is known, the sphere has the minimum surface under the given volume. On the assumption that the erythrocyte functionality with respect to the oxygen transport is linearly related to the surface area, we can introduce the functionality factor of the erythrocyte ϑ which is the ratio of the erythrocyte surface area to the surface area of the spherocyte with the same volume:

$$\vartheta = \frac{S}{S_0},$$

where $S_0 = 4\pi r_0^2$ (the surface area of the sphere). For a spherocyte we have $\vartheta = 1$, and, for any other shape we have $\vartheta > 1$.Our calculations show that increase in the sphericity coefficient k (transformation of the biconcave erythrocyte to the spherocyte) leads to a significant decrease in the surface area. For example, at $k = 0,4$ (biconcave erythrocyte), the functionality factor of the erythrocyte $\vartheta = 1.7$; at $k = 1.0$ (flat disk) the functionality factor of the erythrocyte $\vartheta = 1.2$. So, the functional factor of the biconcave erythrocytes greater than the functional factor of flat disks erythrocytes by the factor of 1.4. In this case the surface area of the biconcave disk is greater than the surface area of the flat disk by the factor 1.4, and greater than the surface area of the spherocyte by a factor 1.7. The total surface area of all the blood erythrocytes S_g is equal to the product of the number of erythrocytes in blood N and the surface area of a single erythrocyte S:

$$S_g = NS.$$

This quantity determines the oxygen capacity of blood. Evidently, the oxygen capacity depends on both the number of erythrocytes in blood and the erythrocytes surface area. A variation in the erythrocyte morphology in the direction of the increase of the sphericity coefficient (the transformation of medically normal biconcave disks to flat disks, figures 14, 15) leads to a decrease in the total surface area of the erythrocytes in blood by a factor of about 1.4; that is equivalent to the corresponding decrease of the oxygen capacity of the blood; and, to the corresponding decrease in the number of normal (biconcave) erythrocytes in blood.

A decrease in the oxygen capacity of blood causes hypoxia (the state that emerges upon the insufficient oxygen supply of the organism organs and tissues). In the medical literature, the blood hypoxia is only related to a decrease in the erythrocyte mass (the number of erythrocytes) and the effect of the erythrocyte morphological modifications on hypoxia is not considered. Apparently, this is due to the absence of the technical means for corresponding measurement. The above quantitative estimates prove that the modifications of the erythrocyte shapes detected in the blood smears of investigated patients with different diseases(even though the number and volume of erythrocytes and hemoglobin content correspond to the norm) is equivalent to a loss of one third of blood erythrocytes (moderate hemorrhage).

The hypoxia caused by various reasons (including a perturbation of the erythrocyte morphology) induces reactions aimed at maintaining homeostatic. If the adaptive response of an organism is insufficient, functional damages and structural changes are initiated.

Our investigations of blood erythrocytes morphology are pioneer. They put a lot of questions. The mechanism and reasons of the observed erythrocytes modifications have to be studied. But the necessity of 3D erythrocyte morphology examination under general medical investigation of the patients is out of doubt.

Investigation of ozone therapy influence on 3D morphology of blood erythrocytes

Lately ozone therapy is used in medical practice for normalization of supplying organs and tissues of an organism with oxygen. In our case ozone therapy is used for patient with neurosensor hardness of hearing [31-33]. The vitality of the problem is determined by its social importance, low efficiency of the existing methods of treatment. Hardness of hearing belongs to the diseases which are caused by negative influence of civilization. As to the data of the International Health Organization more than 450 millions people (that is about 7 % of the population of our planet) are suffering with different hearing pathologies.

According to the modern understanding of the problem, the main reason of the neurosensor hardness of hearing is deficiency of oxygen on any level of hearing sensors with posterior negative influence on the functions of the hearing system.

60 patients (men and women) with neurosensor hardness of hearing of different genesis were investigated. The ages of patients were from 18 to 67. All patients took the course of mono ozone therapy. The course of treatment consisted of 5 intravenous injections of 200 ml of ozonized physiological solution. Concentration of ozone in the solution was 0.48 mg/liter. Ozonizing of the physiological solution was performed using the device of the Russian firm "Medozone". Untreated blood smears of the patients were prepared before and just after injections of ozonized physiological solution.

All patients passed the audio testing after the course of ozone therapy. In all cases the positive medical effect was achieved.

Figure 16 shows images of blood smears of a patient before and after the injection of the ozonized physiological solution obtained using the classical optical microscope. It is seen that some changes in erythrocytes morphology happened; but 2D images does not allow seeing the character of these changes.

Figure 17 shows 3D images of the blood smears of the patient obtained using the DHIM.

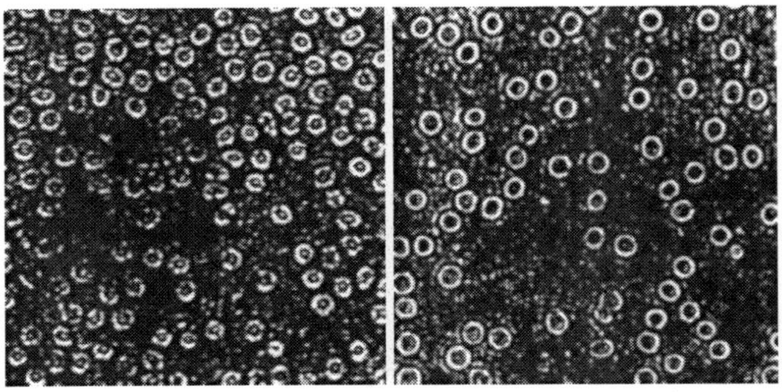

a b

Figure 16. Images of blood smears of a patient before (a) and after the injection of the ozonized physiological solution

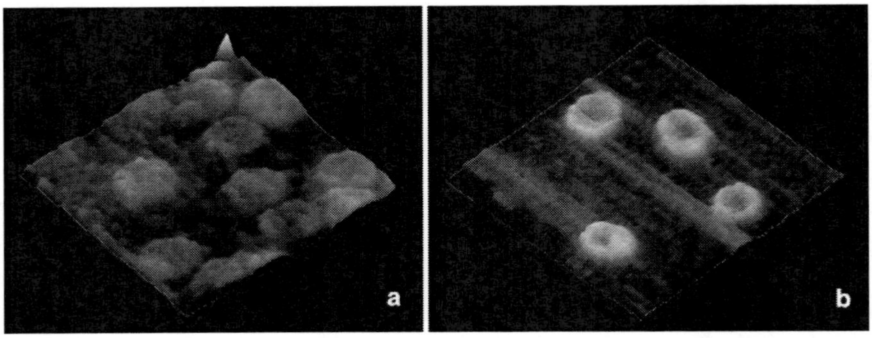

Figure 17. 3D images of fragments of blood smears of a patient before (a) and just after (b) injection of ozonized physiological solution.

Such results were obtained for all patients. It is seen that erythrocytes of the patients before the treatment have flat disk shapes (Figure 17a). After the injections of the ozonized physiological solution the shapes of the erythrocytes are changed. The erythrocytes have the shapes of biconcave disks (Figure 17b). It is apparent that flat disk shape of blood erythrocytes which does not corresponds to the norm is the main reason of oxygen deficiency, which causes neurosensor hardness of hearing. Injections of ozonized physiological solution result in normalization of erythrocyte morphology, in increasing their functional possibilities, and, consequently, in the positive medical effect.

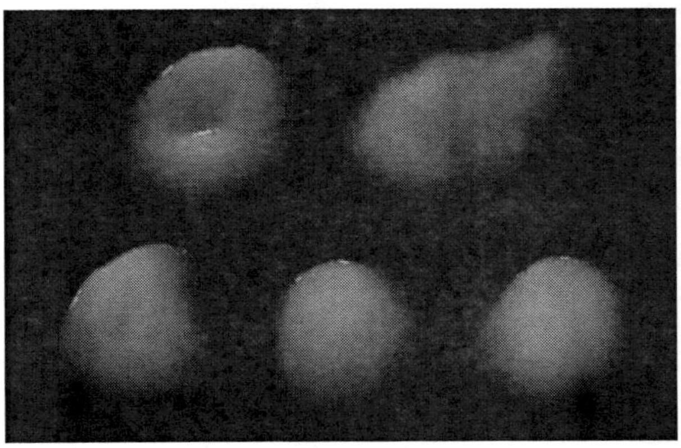

Figure 18. Variations of erythrocytes morphology of a patient in hemolytic anemia.

Of course, the lack of oxygen in tissues caused by erythrocytes modifications affect negatively a whole organism and can be the reason of different pathologies. It is necessary to investigate the reason of such morphological modifications and the way of the treatment.

Investigation of 3D morphology of blood erythrocytes in hematological diseases

A lot of degenerative shapes of erythrocytes were detected in blood smears of patients in hemolytic diseases. They resist classification (Figure 18).

Interesting results were obtained in the case of investigation of a patient in hereditary blood disease such as sickle-cell disease [34].

Figure 19 shows the dynamic of erythrocytes transformation of the patient in the conditions of decreasing oxygen content in blood (the local hypoxia was created by clamping the patient's finger).It was found that the transformation of erythrocyte shapes took place for 5 minutes.

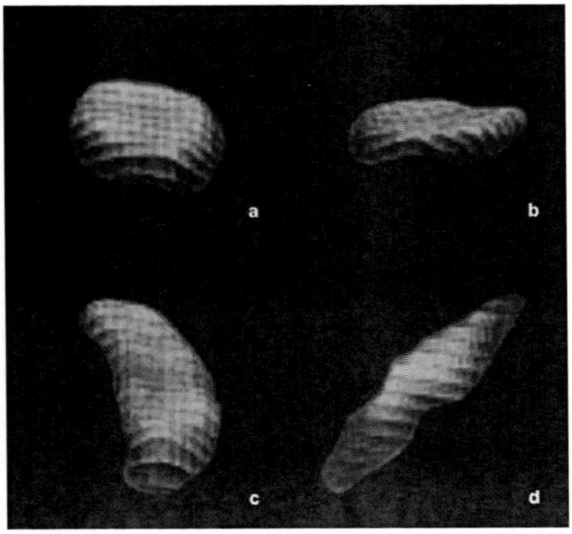

Figure 19. Change of shape of erythrocytes of the patient in sickle-cell disease under decreasing oxygen content in blood (a, b, c, d).

DHIM investigation of blood erythrocytes 3D morphology of pregnant women in diabetes mellitus and newborn infants

The most frequent reason of neonatal mortality and of different pathologies of newborns is prenatal hypoxia. Hypoxia is not a disease but the result of different pathologies of mother's and fetus's organisms. Enough supply of a fetus with oxygen is provided by uterine and placental blood circulation intensity, placental barrier penetration and functionality properties of mother's and fetus's erythrocytes. As it was shown above, different diseases can influence blood erythrocytes morphology, and the morphological changes can be the reason of different hypoxia pathologies of a mother and a child.

Diabetes mellitus is a widespread chronic disease. Progressive increase in the sickness rate put diabetes mellitus on the level of the leading problem of medicine which needs all round study. Deficiency of insulin is responsible for the disease. This results in the disorder of the carbohydrate and protein metabolism. Protein synthesis decreases; glucose content in blood increases. Glucose damages tissues and cells of an organism, and, thus, erythrocytes.

Morphological changes of blood erythrocytes of a mother in diabetes mellitus can be the reason of the fetal hypoxia. This made us carry out the investigation of 3D morphology of pregnant women (recently confined) without hematological pathology and their newborn infants [35, 36].

Blood smears were prepared in maternal hospital specializing in diabetes mellitus. 54 persons (41 women and 13 newborn infants) were investigated. The group of investigated women consisted of pregnant women suffering from carbohydrates metabolic derangement (without hematological pathology; aged from 19 to 36). The control group consisted of pregnant women in norm (10 persons) and healthy non-pregnant women (10 persons).New born infants born by the women with carbohydrates metabolic derangement and by the healthy women were investigated in an hour and in the third day after deliveries. Untreated blood smears of peripheral blood on glass slides, prepared according to the standard procedure, were used in our experiments.

It was detected that only 5 from 41 women had biconcave erythrocytes which correspond to the medical norm. Flat disk erythrocytes dominated in blood smears of other 36 women. Specific changes of 3D erythrocytes morphology of patients in diabetes metabolic derangement have not been detected. But the results have turned to be rather unexpected. It has been found that erythrocytes of majority of pregnant women with and without the pathology, and, of woman from the control group do not correspond to a medical norm. Such morphological changes of erythrocytes can be the reason of different hypoxia pathologies which decrease functional possibility of a human organism.

Correlation between erythrocytes shapes of a mother and her child has not been detected in our experiments. Erythrocytes of all investigated neonatal patients had flat disk shapes.

Figure 20 shows a fragment of blood smear of a neonatal patient.

Taking into consideration that erythrocytes of neonatal patients have some specific features (presence of nuclei, increased content of hemoglobin), it is possible to suppose that flat disk shape is the morphological feature of erythrocytes of newborn infants.

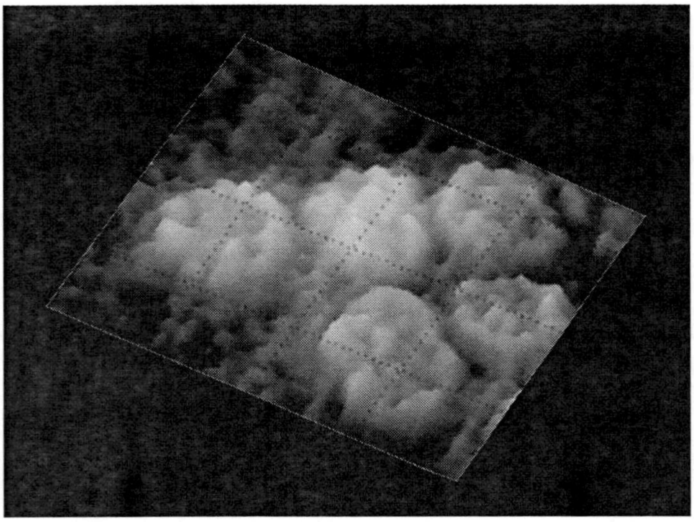

Figure 20. The fragment of the blood smear of a neonatal patient.

Gamma-radiation influence on 3D morphology of blood erythrocytes

Now in conditions of aggravating environment much attention are paid to investigation of different damaging factors influence on a human organism. In accordance with the modern scientific data, the main targets of different damaging factors influence are plasmatic cell membranes, in particular, membranes of red blood cells. Changes of the elastic properties of the cells membranes must result in morphology changes of erythrocytes. It made us study the influence of gamma-radiation on blood erythrocytes of a rat in vivo [37, 38]. The animal was exposed to irradiation from the gamma source (60 C); the doze of irradiation was lethal (200 Gr). The results of the experiments have confirmed the gamma- radiation sensitivity of the blood erythrocytes.

Figure 21 shows the results of the experiments. As one can see, biconcave erythrocytes dominate in the smear of arterial blood of the rat before irradiation (Figure 21a). The mean sphericity coefficient of the smear is equal to 0.2. The blood erythrocytes preserved their biconcave shape in an hour after irradiation (Figure 21c), but the mean sphericity coefficient of the erythrocytes has increase to 0.5. So, radiation caused morphological transformation of erythrocytes in the direction of the sphericity coefficient increase.

In addition, investigation of the morphological features of blood erythrocytes of arterial and venous blood of the rat was carried out. The erythrocytes of arterial blood are biconcave (Figure 21a), whereas the flat disc erythrocytes dominate in venous blood (Figure 21b). This indicates the fact of erythrocytes transformation in the process of gas exchange.

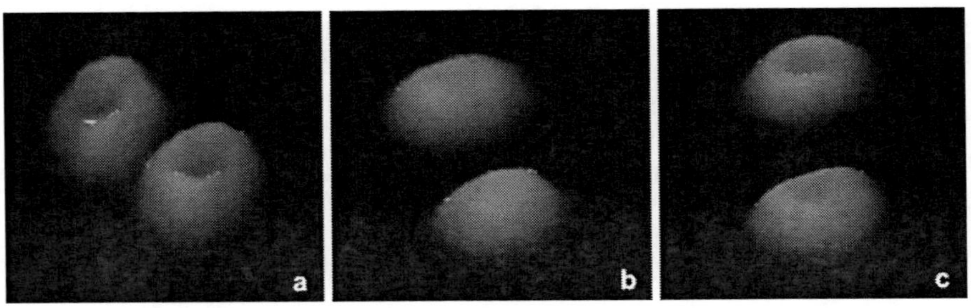

Figure 21. Erythrocytes of arterial (a) and venous (b) blood of a rat. Erythrocytes of arterial blood of the rat after irradiation by gamma-radiation in the dose 200 Gr *in vivo* (c).

Ionizing radiation (radiation therapy) is used in medical practice as part of cancer treatment. Figure 22 shows the results of investigation of influence of the radiation therapy on blood erythrocytes of a patient in breast cancer (woman, 53 years old). The course of radiation therapy involved 25 session of irradiation; the total doze was equal 70 Gr.

It is seen that biconcave erythrocytes dominate in blood smear of the patient before the course of radiation therapy (Figure 22a). The mean sphericity coefficient of the blood smear is equal 0.35. The considerable changes of erythrocytes morphology are observed after the course of the radiation therapy. Flat disk erythrocytes dominate in the smear after the radiation therapy; the mean sphericity coefficient of the smear is equal 0.9 (Figure 22b). So the radiation causes the morphological changes of blood erythrocytes. Such modifications can be the reason of hypoxia which is one more damaging factor for a human organism under radiation therapy.

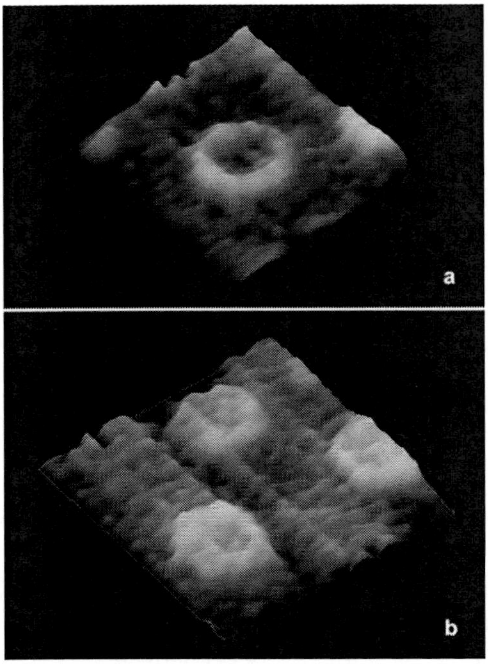

Figure 22. Fragments of the blood smears of a patient in breast cancer before (a) and after (b) the course of radiation therapy. The doze of radiation equal 70 Gr.

Conclusion

The DHIM experimental study of the 3D morphology of human blood erythrocytes have proved that, in addition to hematological diseases, the diseases of various genesis and external factors serve as the reason for the morphological modification of blood erythrocytes. It is detected that the morphologic modifications are nonspecific. These unspecific modifications correspond to an increase in the erythrocyte sphericity coefficient. It is proved that erythrocyte

3D morphology reflects the state of a living organism and the level of its biological response on different external factors influence. It is demonstrated that the observed morphological modifications of erythrocytes lead to a significant decrease in the blood oxygen capacity and can serve as a reason for hypoxia and, hence, functional and structural changes of organism.

2.2 DHIM Study of Thin Transparent Films

Lately the scientific and technical industry connected with thin film production is extensively developing. In the process of thin film deposition there is the necessity of the thin films morphology visual investigation and measurement of films thicknesses. For such investigation optical microscopes are widely used. But they allow only 2D imaging, quantitative measurements are impossible. Application of microinterferometers has some advantages due to the possibility of films thickness measurements. High accuracy of thickness measurement has been achieved for optically nontransparent coatings. But the known optical microinterferometers do not make it possible to obtain good results for transparent thin films (0.1-0.5 μm) on transparent substrates. Till now the electron microscopy method was the single method for thin film morphology investigation. But this method does not make it possible to carry out quantitative measurements. So, the problem of thin transparent films investigation has not been solved.

Thin films are phase microscopic objects. That makes it possible to use the DHIM for thin films investigation. In this chapter we present our pioneer results of application the DHIM for investigation of thin films morphology.

Now polymers are widely used. Lenses made of such materials, along with well known advantages, have shortcomings such as hyper plasticity, and a low value of hardness. Moreover, polymers lose its optical properties under influence of environment, especially solar radiation. Different transparent coatings are used for protection of plastic optical material. High transparence in the optical range, high firmness and chemical inertness makes AlN the perspective chemical compound for use on the polymer goods which are used for operation in the conditions of environment influence, especially under ultraviolet radiation influence. The technology of deposition of AlN coating on acryl substrates by vacuum-arc method is working out in the National Scientific Center "Kharkov Institute of Physics and Technology". Such thin AlN coatings on acrylic substrates were used as the objects under study in our experiments [40-42]. The influence of external damaging factors on the acryl goods with the protective coatings was also studied.

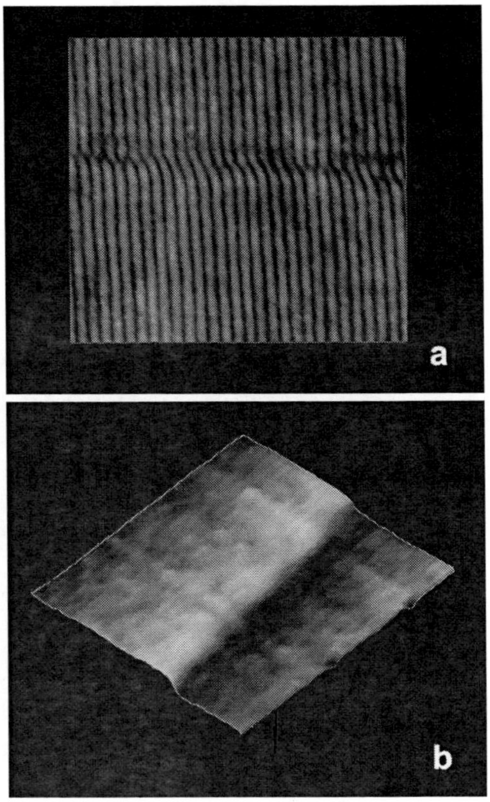

Figure 23. The fragment of the interferogram of the AlN film edge (a) and 3D image of the fragment (b). The thickness of the film is about 0.58 μm.

Figure 23 shows a fragment of an interferogram of the edge of AlN film on the acrylic substrate (a) and the reconstructed 3D image of the fragment. The thickness of the film is about 0.58 *μm.*

Figure 24 shows the fragments of the surface of AlN thin film deposited on acryl substrate with a deposition effect. The thickness of the film is about 0.1 μm.

Figure 25 shows the fragment of the surface of AlN thin film deposited on acryl substrate with the artificially created scratch.

DHIM application makes it possible to determine the character of the defects (convex upwards or concave downward) and to measure the sizes of the defects. So the maximum height of the surface defect (Figure 24) is about 0.7 μm. The width of the scratch is about 2 μm and the depth is about 0.1 μm (Figure 25). The obtained images show that film surface (except the places of the defects localization) is plane and homogeneous.

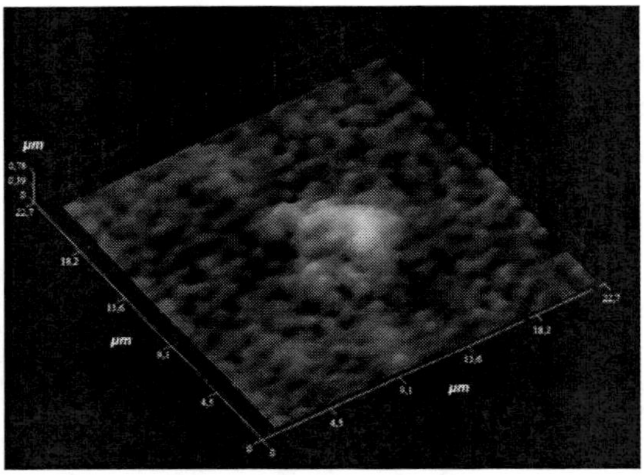

Figure 24. The fragment of the surface of AlN thin films deposited on acryl substrate with the deposition defect.

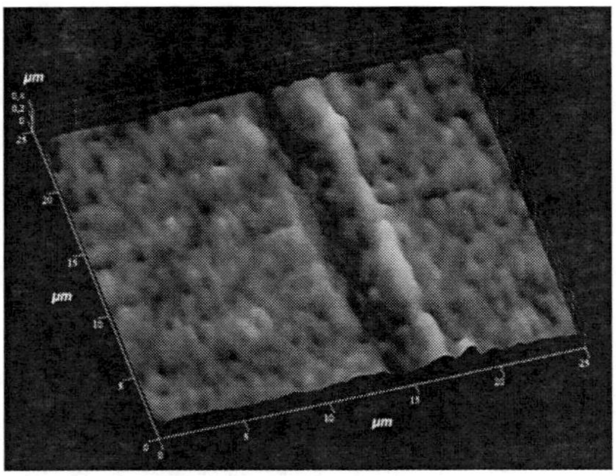

Figure 25. The fragment of the surface of AlN thin film deposited on acryl substrate with the artificially created scratch.

Figure 26 shows the fragment of the surface of AlN film on acryl substrates after UV-radiation influence.

Acryl without the protective coating loses its transparence .under the influence of UV-radiation The AlN coating protects acryl against damage; but when the critical doze of irradiation is achieved, coating cracks, detachments, and, wrinkles are observed. It is seen that cracks have formed after UV-radiation influence. The depth of the crack (Figure 26) is about 0.8 μm. This means that the crack is formed not only in the coating but in the substrate too. So, in this case the coating failed to protect the acryl good against UV-radiation influence. It is also seen that the whole surface of the film is damaged; it is wrinkled and uneven.

Figure 27 shows the surface of the AlN film on the acryl substrate after thermal damage.

So, the DHIM can be successfully used for transparent thin films morphology investigation. It combines the possibility of 3D imaging with the possibility of the measurement of the geometrical parameters of the films (thickness, sizes of defects, roughness).

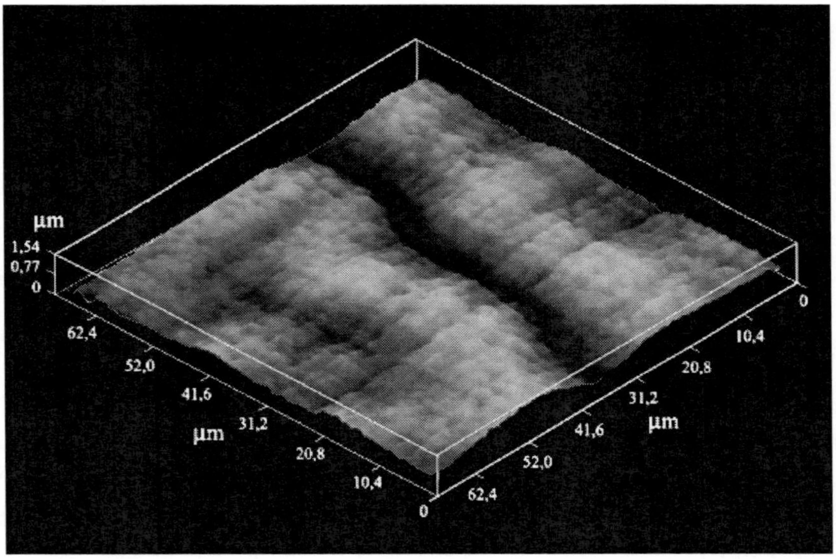

Figure 26. Fragment of the surface of AlN thin films deposited on acryl substrate damaged after UV-radiation influence.

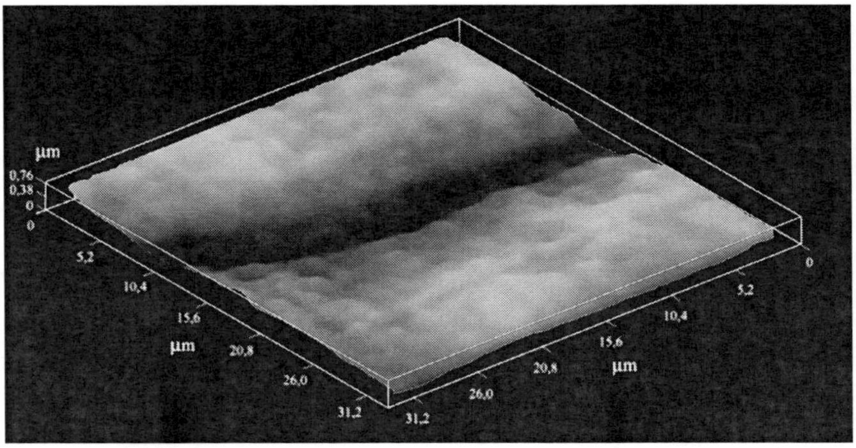

Figure 27. Fragment of the surface of AlN thin films deposited on acryl substrate damaged after thermal damage.

Conclusion

Combining the holographic methods with the methods for digital image processing has solved the problem of 3D visualization of phase microscopic objects. Creation of the digital holographic microscope allowing 3D real time imaging of phase microscopic objects and measurement of their morphological parameters has led to a new stage in light microscopy. For the first time 3D imaging of untreated microscopic objects has become possible. We presented pioneer results of DHIM application for investigation of medical and technical phase microobjects. These results obviously testify that 3D imaging allows obtaining new and very important information on the microobjects under study. So, the digital holographic microscopes can find application in medicine, biology and technique.

References

[1] Franson M. *Phase-Contrast and Interference Microscope.* Gosizdat, Fiz.-Mat. Lit., Moscow, Ru, 1960.
[2] D. Gabor. *J. Nature*. 1948, vol. 161, 777.
[3] Safronov G. S and Tishko T. V. *Ukrainsk. Fizich. Zh.* 1985, vol. 30, 333-337.
[4] Safronov G. S. and Tishko T. V. *Ukrainsk. Fizich. Zh.* 1985, vol. 30, 994-997.
[5] Safronov G. S. and Tishko T. V. *Prib. Tech. Eksp*. 1987, vol. 2, 249.
[6] Tishko T. V., Titar V. P. and Tishko D. N. *Opt. J.* 2005, vol. 72, № 2, 48-55.
[7] Tishko T. V., Titar V. P. and Tishko D. N. *J .Opt. Technol.* 2005, vol. 72, № 2, 203-209.
[8] Tishko T. V., Titar V. P., Panfilov D. A. and Tishko D. N. *Biol. Vestnik*. 1998, vol. 2, № 1, 107-111.
[9] P. Marquet, B. Rappaz and P. Magistretti. *J. et al. Opt. Lett.* 2005, vol. 30, 468-472.
[10] G. Popescu, T. Ikeda and C. A. Best. *J. Biomed. Opt.* 2005, vol. 10, 503-508.
[11] Born M. and Wolf E. *Principles of Optics*. Nauka, Moscow, Ru, 1973.
[12] Leith E. N., Upatnieks J. J. *Opt. Soc. Am*. 1962, vol. 52, 1123.
[13] Denisiuk Yu. N. *Dokl. of Acad. of Scien. of the USSA*. 1962, vol. 144, 1275.
[14] Ginzburg V. M. and Stepanov B. M. *Holographic measurements*. Radio I Svyaz. Moscow, Ru, 1961.
[15] R. J. Collier, C. B. Burckhardt and L. N. Lin. *Optical holography*. Academic press. N.Y. 1971.
[16] H. J. Caulfield. *Handbook of Optical holography*. Academic press. N.Y. 1979.
[17] R. F. van Lighten and G. Ostenberg. *Nature*. 211, 282, 1966.
[18] Lantzberg G. S. *Optics.* Fizmatlit. Moscow, Ru, 2003.
[19] G. W. Ellis. *Science*. 1966, vol. 154, 1195.
[20] Ostrovsky Ju. I., Butusov M. M., Ostrovskaya G. V. *Holographic interferometry.* Nauka. Moscow, Ru, 1977.
[21] Tishko T. V. and Titar V. P. *In Materials of the Third International Workshop "Laser and Fiber-Optiocal Network Modelling* (LFNM'2001)". Kharkov, 2001, 162-167.

[22] Tishko T. V. and Titar V. P. *Vestn. Khark. Nats. Univ.* Ser. Radiofiz. Electron. 2002, vol. 544, 56-61.

[23] Novitsky V. V., Ryazantzeva N. V., Stepovaya E. A., Shevtzova N. M., Miller A. A., Zaitzev B. N., Tishko T. V., Titar V. P. and Tishko D. N. *Theory and practice of erythrocyte microscopy*. Pechat. Manufact. Tomsk, Ru, 2008.

[24] Tishko T. V., Titar V. P. and Tishko D. N. *In Materials of the Sixth International Conference on Laser and Fiber-Optical Networks Modeling* (LFNM'2004). Kharkov, 2004.

[25] A. J. Salsbury and J. J. Clarke. *Clin. Pathol.* 1967, vol. 20, 603.

[26] Novitsky V. V., Ryazantseva N. V. et al. Atlas. *Clinical Erythrocyte Pathomorphosis*. St. Petersburg Univ. St. Petersburg, Ru, 2003.

[27] Tishko T. V., Titar V. P. and Tishko D. N. *In Materials of the Second international Conference on Advanced Optoelectronics and Lasers.* Yalta, 2005, vol. 1, 284-287.

[28] Tishko T. V., Titar V. P. and Tishko D. N. *Vestn. Khark .Nats. Univ.* Ser. Radiofiz. Electron. 2006, vol. 712, 52-56.

[29] Tishko T. V., Titar V. P., Tishko D. N. *Proc. of SPIE.* 2008, vol. 7006, 70060O-70060O-9.

[30] Tishko T. V., Titar V. P, Tishko D. N. and Nosov K. V. *Laser Physics*. 2008, vol. 18, № 4, 1-5.

[31] Tishko T. V., Titar V. P., Barchotkina T. M., et al. *Vestn. Khark. Nats. Univ.* Ser. Boifiz. Vestnik. 2000, vol. 497, 103-107.

[32] Tishko T. V., Titar V. P., Barchotkina T. M. and Tishko D. N. *In Materials of the First International Conference on Advanced Optoelectronics and Optics.* Alushta, 2003, vol. 2, 6-8.

[33] Tishko T. V., Titar V. P., Barchotkina T. M. and Tishko D. N. *Proc. of SPIE*. 2004, vol. 5582, 119-123.

[34] Tishko T. V., Titar V. P., Nekrasov V. I. and Shpachenko O. V. *In Materials of the Fourteenth International Scientific and Practical Conference on the Use of Laswers inMedicine and Biology*. Kharkov, 2000, 16.

[35] Tishko T. V., Titar V. P., Tishko D. N., et al. *Vestn. Khark. Nats. Univ.* Ser. Biolog. 2006, vol.729, 281-285.

[36] Tishko T. V., Titar V. P., Tishko D. N., et al. *In Materials of the Fourth International Conference on Advanced Optoelectronics and Lasers* (CAOL 2008). Alushta, 2008, 171-173.

[37] Tishko T. V., Titar V. P. *In Materials of The Fourth International Workshop on Laser and Fiber-Optical Network Modeling*. 2002, 266-268.

[38] Paranich A. V., Tishko T. V., Titar V. P., et al. *Vestn. Khark .Nats. Univ.* Ser. Radiofiz. Electron. 2002, vol. 544, 40-45.

[39] Tishko D. N., Tishko T. V., Titar V. P., et al. *Vestn. Khark. Nats. Univ.* Ser. Radiofiz. Electron. 2008, vol.806, 99-102.

[40] Tishko T. V., Tishko D. N. and Titar V. P. *Proceedings of 4-th European Microscopy Congress*. Aachen, Germany, 2008, vol. 1, 285-286.

[41] Tishko D. N., Tishko T. V. and Titar V. P. *J. Opt. Technol.* 2009, vol. 76, № 3, 147-149.
[42] Tishko D. N., Tishko T. V. and Titar V. P. *Opt. J.* 2009, vol. 76, № 3, 40-43.

In: 3D Imaging: Theory, Technology … ISBN: 978-1-60876-885-1
Editors: E. H. Duke and S. R. Aguirre, pp.93- 109

Chapter 3

ELECTRON MICROSCOPE TOMOGRAPHY IN STRUCTURAL BIOLOGY

J. J. Fernandez [1,2] ***and J. R. Bilbao-Castro*** [1,2]
[1]Dept. Computer Architecture and Electronics., University of Almeria, Almeria, Spain
[2]National Centre for Biotechnology (CSIC), Cantoblanco, Madrid. Spain

ABSTRACT

Electron microscope tomography (EMT) has emerged as the leading technique for three-dimensional (3D) structural analysis of unique complex biological specimens. EMT makes it possible to directly visualize the molecular architectures of organelles, cells and complex viruses at close-to-molecular resolution. EMT has been crucial to reveal some of the major breakthroughs in life sciences in the last few years. EMT combines electron microscopy with the power of 3D imaging to derive the 3D structure of complex specimens. A number of computational stages are involved in a typical structural study by EMT, which range from the image acquisition with the microscope to the 3D reconstruction by means of tomographic reconstruction algorithms. Afterwards, a number of computational steps are necessary to facilitate the interpretation of the 3D data: noise reduction, segmentation and analysis of subvolumes. As the computational demands are huge in some of the stages, high performance computing (HPC) techniques are also used to make the problem affordable in reasonable time. This chapter reviews the different computational stages involved in EMT, from image acquisition to interpretation of the 3D reconstruction. The HPC techniques normally used to cope with the computational demands are also briefly described.

INTRODUCTION

Electron microscope tomography (EMT) has emerged as the leading technique for three-dimensional (3D) structural analysis of unique complex biological specimens (McIntosh et al. 2005; Lucic et al., 2005). The great technological advances in the last decade have made it feasible to directly visualize the molecular architectures of organelles, cells and complex viruses as well as *in vivo* cellular dynamic events at close-to-molecular resolution (Medalia et al. 2002; He et al. 2003; Grunewald et al., 2003; Beck et al., 2004; Kurner et al., 2005; Nicastro et al., 2006; Al-Amoudi et al., 2007; He et al., 2008). The resolution attained by EMT is rapidly approaching the molecular level (better than 2nm), which allows the study of the 3D organization of the structural components at a detail sufficient for the identification of macromolecular complexes, the analysis of their spatial distribution and their interactions in the native cellular context (Nickell et al., 2006). A recent breakthrough in this area has been the 3D organization of polysomes (clusters of ribosomes simultaneously reading one strand of messenger RNA and synthesizing different occurrences of the same protein) in bacteria revealed by EMT (Brandt et al., 2009).

Electron tomography has got a unique potential to bridge the gap between Cellular and Molecular biology as it acts as a link between low resolution imaging techniques (light microscopy, X-ray tomography) and the high-resolution structural techniques (X-ray crystallography, nuclear magnetic resonance, electron crystallography, single particle electron microscopy). Therefore, EMT has the power to allow the integration of the structural information derived by the different techniques and gathered at multiple levels of the biological complexity so as to provide a comprehensive description of the cellular function in molecular and even pseudo-atomic detail (Sali et al., 2003; Robinson et al., 2007).

EMT involves essential computational stages to derive and interpret the 3D structure of the complex biological specimens being studied: data acquisition, image alignment, image restoration, 3D reconstruction, post-processing of the 3D volume and, finally, interpretation. However, prior to these computational stages, there is an important stage related to specimen preparation. Due to the vacuum conditions in the microscope, the sensitivity of the biological material and the limited penetrating power of the electrons, the specimen has to be specially prepared before being imaged in the electron microscope. For an in-depth description of specimen preparation techniques, the reader is referred to important reviews in the field (Frank, 2006; McIntosh, 2007, Leis et al., 2009; Hoenger and McIntosh, 2009).

This chapter is devoted to review the different computational stages and technologies involved to determine and analyse the 3D structure of complex biological specimens by EMT. The chapter is structured as follows. First, the procedures to acquire datasets from the electron microscope are briefly described. Next, the steps to align the acquired images and to determine and restore the effects of the transfer function of the microscope are presented. The essential step of the 3D reconstruction from the projection images is the core of the next section. To end up with the computational stages, the procedures for noise filtering, segmentation and pattern recognition are reviewed. Afterwards, these computational concepts are put into practice in the illustrative study of one of the most complex viruses. Next, some of the high performance computing techniques and technologies used to cope with the large computational demands in EMT are briefly mentioned. Finally, the most common software tools available for the EMT scientific community are surveyed.

Data Acquisition

The transmission electron microscope, whose optical principles are similar to the widely known light microscope, provides projection images of the specimen being imaged. A beam of electrons is shot towards the specimen, and scattered and unscattered electrons emerging from the specimen are then collected by magnetic lenses and focused to form an interference pattern, which constitutes the projection image (Frank, 2006). These projection images are thus formed by the integration of the 3D information of the specimen along the direction of the electron beam. In other words, the images look like "radiographs" of the sample. The images are then recorded on a CCD (charge-coupled device) camera.

The principle of EMT is the 3D reconstruction of a specimen from a series of projection images taken with a transmission electron microscope. This principle is commonly found in disciplines of science and engineering since late sixties and early seventies (DeRosier and Klug, 1968; Klug and Crowther, 1972). In EMT, a single individual biological sample is introduced in the electron microscope and a series of images (so-called tilt series) is recorded by tilting the sample around a single-tilt axis at different angles, typically over a tilt range of +/- 60 or 70 degrees and at small increments of 1-2 degrees (Figure 1). Sometimes, for better angular coverage, another tilt series is taken with the specimen rotated by 90 degrees (the double-axis tilting geometry) (Penczek, 1995; Mastronarde, 1997). Typical EMT data sets then range from 60 to 280 images. Due to the resolution requirements, the image size typically is 1024 x 1024, 2048 x 2048 or even 4096 x 4096 pixels.

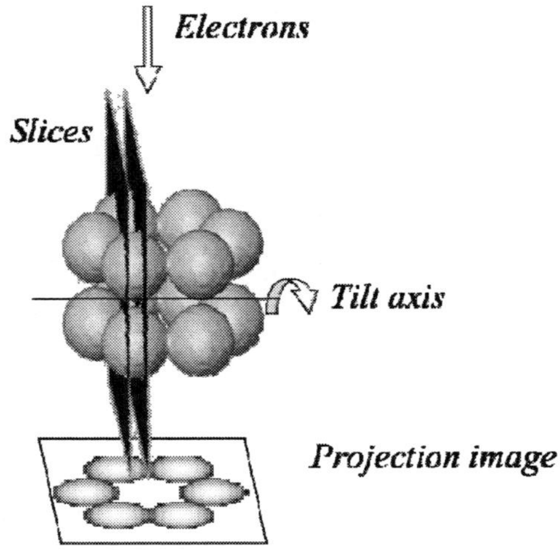

Figure 1. Single-tilt axis data acquisition geometry. The specimen is imaged in the microscope by tilting it over a range typically +/- 60 or 70 degrees in small tilt increments. As a result, a set of projection images (so-called tilt series) needed to structure determination is collected.

The computation of a distortion-free 3D reconstruction from a tilt series would require that a data set from the full tilt range (+/- 90 degrees) be available. Due to physical limitations of microscopes, the angular tilt range is limited and, as a result, tomographic tilt series have a wedge of missing data corresponding to the uncovered angular range. This limitation, which is not present in other disciplines such as medical tomography, causes distortions in 3D reconstructions, as described below.

Computer-automated data collection has been crucial for the advent of EMT as a structural technique in cellular biology (Dierksen et al., 1992; Koster et al., 1992; Dierksen et al., 1993). It allows automated tracking, focusing and recording of images under low electron-dose conditions by dividing the maximum tolerable dose over the total number of images, which preserves the specimen from radiation damage. But, as a consequence, the images exhibit a poor signal-to-noise ratio (SNR) around 0.1. During acquisition, the imperfections of the mechanical tilt system and the electron optics produce shifts in the images. The larger component of these shifts is compensated by the automated tracking procedure. However, a more accurate alignment of the images is needed afterwards by computational procedures.

PRE-PROCESSING: ALIGNMENT AND RESTORATION

The computational alignment is intended to mutually set the images to a common coordinate system by correction for the shifts and possible rotations and magnification changes. The standard procedure for the alignment starts at the preparation stage, where colloidal gold particles are included in the biological sample to be used as electron-dense fiducial markers. Once the tilt series is acquired, the coordinates of those markers are determined manually or semi-automatically throughout the images of the tilt series. Using the coordinates of those markers, the images are then mutually aligned by means of a least squares procedure aiming at minimizing the alignment error as a function of the shifts, rotations and other parameters included in the alignment model (Frank, 2006). An alternative automated procedure that does not require the use of fiducial markers is based on cross-correlation (Sorzano et al., 2009), however its sensitivity to noise limits its application to particular high-contrast EMT studies.

The electron microscope leaves an imprint in the acquired images as a result of its transfer function (so-called CTF, which stands for Contrast Transfer Function). The CTF arises from the aberrations of the lenses and from the defocus used in imaging. The artefacts of the CTF consist in oscillations that produce the attenuation of structural details and, even worse, in contrast reversals at certain spatial resolution ranges. The contrast reversal is especially harmful as the structural details at some resolution ranges are presented as white density over a black background whereas at other resolution ranges they appear as black over white. Correction for the CTF effects is essential for any image to faithfully represent a projection of the specimen at high resolution. So far there have not been urgent needs for that in electron tomography due to the relatively low-resolution limits. However, as the technique improves and the attainable resolution is pushed forward, the need for CTF correction is getting importance.

The first issue related to this restoration problem is the determination of the CTF as the low SNR hampers visualization of the oscillatory component of the CTF in the Fourier spectrum. An approach that is getting increasing interest in the field is based on the assumption that the tilt-series is eucentric (i.e. the defocus at the tilt axis is constant during acquisition) (Fernandez et al., 2006). The images of the tilt-series are split into tiles and the spectra of tiles at the same defocus, taken from the images throughout the tilt-series, are averaged. This yields an average spectrum with the CTF oscillations visible and highlighted, and hence an accurate fitting with the theoretical CTF model can be carried out. From this average CTF, the CTF at any point of any image in the tilt series can be easily determined by simple geometry.

The major problem of CTF correction in EMT is the gradient of the defocus along the direction perpendicular to the tilt axis in tilted images. This turns the restoration problem into a spatially variant one. Currently there are two approaches for CTF determination and correction that succeed in dealing with this CTF gradient in tilted images. The first approach is specially suited for high contrast studies and models the spatially variant restoration problem as an inverse problem (Winkler and Taylor, 2003). The second approach decomposes the global restoration problem into multiple local spatially invariant problems confined to strips parallel to the tilt axis (Fernandez et al., 2006). In both approaches the CTF correction is applied to the aligned tilt series prior to the tomographic reconstruction.

TOMOGRAPHIC RECONSTRUCTION

The reconstruction problem in EMT is to obtain the 3D structure of the specimen from the set of aligned, and possibly CTF-corrected, images in the tilt series. This is a very well known problem that arises in a myriad of scientific and engineering disciplines (Herman, 1980; Kak and Slaney; 2001). The mathematical principles of tomographic reconstruction are based upon the central section theorem, which states that the Fourier transform (FT) of a 2D projection of a 3D object is a central section of the 3D FT of the object (Frank, 2006). Therefore, the 3D FT of the specimen can be computed by assembling the 2D FTs of the images in the tilt series, which yields the 3D structure of the specimen by an inverse FT. One problem of this approach is related to the interpolation in Fourier space.

The standard method for tomographic reconstruction is Weighted Backprojection (WBP), which essentially is equivalent to the Fourier approach just described but working in real space (Frank, 2006). WBP assumes that the projection images represent the amount of mass density encountered by imaging rays. The method simply distributes the known specimen mass present in projection images evenly over computed backprojection rays. This way, the specimen mass is projected back into a reconstruction volume (i.e., backprojected). When this process is repeated for all the projection images in the tilt series, backprojection rays from the different images intersect and reinforce each other at the points where mass is found in the original structure. Therefore, the 3D mass of the specimen is reconstructed from a series of 2D projection images. The backprojection process involves an implicit low-pass filtering that makes reconstructed volumes strongly blurred. In practice, in order to compensate the transfer function of the backprojection process, a previous high-pass filter (i.e., weighting) is applied to the projection images, hence the term ``weighted backprojection''. This weighting is necessary to properly represent the high frequency information in the reconstruction. Figure 2 shows a sketch of the backprojection process to 3D reconstruction from projections. For a detailed description of the method, refer to (Frank, 2006).

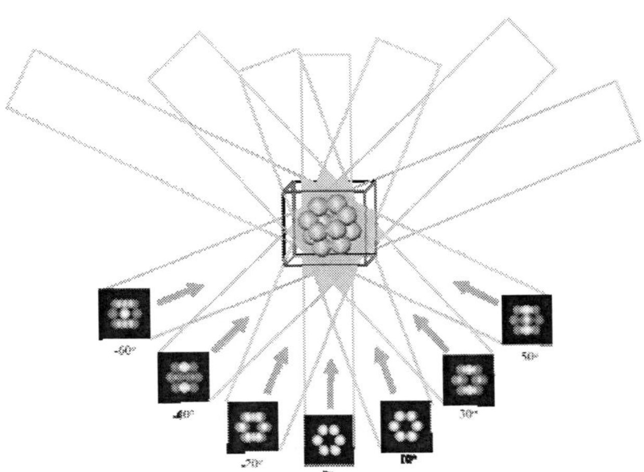

Figure 2. Three-dimensional reconstruction from projections by backprojection. The projection images in the tilt-series are projected back into the volume to be reconstructed.

The relevance of WBP in EMT mainly stems from the linearity and the computational simplicity of the method. The main disadvantages of WBP are that (i) the results may be strongly affected by limited tilt angle data obtained with the microscope, and (ii) WBP does not implicitly take into account the transfer function of the microscope or the noise conditions. As a consequence of the latter, *a posteriori* regularization techniques (such as low-pass filtering) may be needed to attenuate the effects of the noise.

There exist alternative real-space reconstruction algorithms that formulate the 3D reconstruction problem as a large system of linear equations to be solved by iterative methods (Gilbert, 1972; Fernandez et al., 2002). These methods are characterized by an inherent regularization nature that makes them robust to face the particularities of EMT: limited angle data and noisy conditions. In essence, these methods aim at minimizing the error between the experimental projection images and the equivalent projections calculated from the reconstructed volume. Conceptually, iterative methods proceed in the following way (Figure 3): First, they start from an initial model (either a null model, a constant model, or even the result of a previous reconstruction method, e.g. WBP), and the model is progressively refined as iterations evolve. In every iteration, (1) projections are computed from the current model; (2) the error between the experimental projections and those computed from the model is calculated; (3) the model is refined so that the error is minimized (which is known as ``error backprojection"). Among the iterative methods, SIRT (Simultaneous Iterative Reconstruction Technique) (Gilbert, 1972) and ART (Algebraic Reconstruction Technique) (Gordon et al., 1970) are probably the most known.

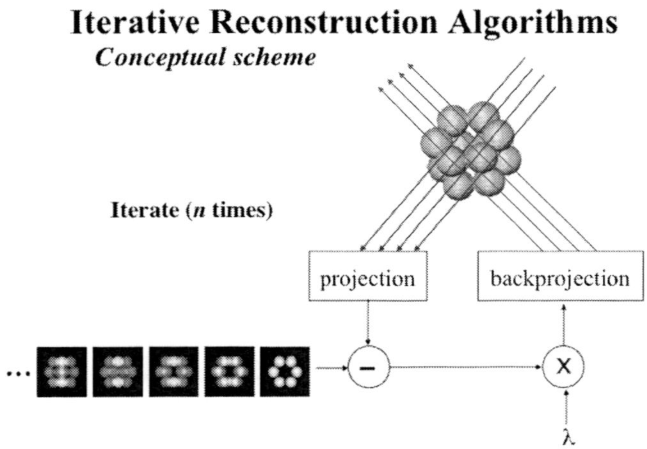

Figure 3. Three-dimensional reconstruction by iterative methods. The tomographic reconstruction is progressively refined by minimizing the error between the experimental and calculated projections.

These alternative iterative algorithms are getting increasing interest in the field because their robustness against the experimental conditions found in EMT (Lucic et al., 2005; Leis et al., 2006). These methods have not been used extensively in this field so far because of their computational demands. However, high performance computing and the advent of modern computing platforms such as multi-core computers or GPUs (graphics processors) are making them viable alternatives to WBP (Fernandez, 2008).

The limited tilt range in EMT results in a region empty of information in the Fourier space of the 3D reconstruction (so-called "missing wedge"). The resolution of the reconstruction is thus anisotropic (i.e., direction-dependent). In real space, it produces artefacts as blurring of the spatial features in the beam direction, making some features appear as elongated in that direction (i.e. there is a significant loss of resolution in the Z-direction), features oriented perpendicular to the tilt axis tend to fade from view, and others are not resolved at all. A +/- 70 tilt range involves that 22% of the information is missing. The use of double-tilt axis acquisition geometry significantly reduces the missing information (down to 7% in the case of +/- 70 tilt range). The angular sampling, that is, the interval between successive tilt images, is another point affecting the resolution of the reconstruction. The more projection images, the better the angular sampling, and as a consequence the better the resolution.

Post-Processing and Interpretation of Tomograms

Although tomographic reconstructions (also know as tomograms in the field) contain a wealth of information, their interpretation is complicated due to a number of factors: the artefacts due to the missing wedge, the low SNR and the inherent biological complexity. Significant efforts are spent to facilitate the interpretation by several stages of post-processing of the tomograms: noise reduction, segmentation, analysis of macromolecular complexes and resolution assessment.

Tomograms are significantly corrupted by noise, which precludes their visualization and analysis. Standard linear filtering techniques based on local averages, Gaussian kernels or low pass Fourier filtering succeed in reducing the noise, but at the expense of blurring edges and features. This has led to the development of more sophisticated noise reduction techniques that preserve the structural features of interest. Iterative median filtering (van der Heide et al., 2007) is a nonlinear technique that succeeds in preserving the structures by, for some rounds, substituting a voxel by the median of its neighbours. It is well suited for high contrast tomograms. The Beltrami flow (Fernandez, 2009) is another nonlinear method that considers the 3D volume as a 3-manifold embedded into a 4D space, with the latest dimension being the density. This method manages to tune the strength of the filtering according to an edge indicator based on geometry operators, hence preserving structures of interest. Bilateral filtering (Jiang et al., 2003) is an anisotropic nonlinear technique that filters noise by applying Gaussian kernels on the spatial domain and on the density domain. Here a voxel is substituted by the weighted mean of the neighbours with a weight reflecting the similarity in terms of density and the spatial relationships. Anisotropic nonlinear diffusion is by far the standard noise reduction algorithm in the field (Frangakis and Hegerl, 2001; Fernandez and Li, 2003). It achieves feature preservation and enhancement as the strength and direction of the smoothing are adaptively tuned to the local structures around each voxel. The performance of this technique has been quantitatively assessed and it outperforms the other methods (Narasimha et al., 2008). Figure 4 sketches the fundamentals of some nonlinear and anisotropic filtering procedures.

Segmentation intends to decompose the tomogram into its structural components by identifying the sets of voxels that constitute them. Though tedious, manual segmentation is the simplest and the most common approach, which consists in that the user assigns the structural features using visualization tools (e.g. He et al., 2008). Several automatic or semi-automatic approaches have been proposed in the field. There exist methods based on simple density thresholds (McIntosh, 2007) or more sophisticated optimal thresholding (Cyrklaff et al., 2005), the Watershed transform extended to 3D (Volkmann, 2002), eigenvector analysis of an affinity matrix (Frangakis and Hegerl, 2002), oriented filters (Sandberg and Brega, 2007), fuzzy logic (Garduno et al., 2008). In addition, template matching with simple 3D geometric templates has been proposed for high contrast tomograms (Lebbink et al., 2007). However, none of these methods has stood out as a general applicable method yet. Most of them are sensitive to noise, though their success is greatly improved if combined with the noise reduction methods discussed above, and the results should be supervised in any case (McIntosh, 2007; Pruggnaller et al., 2008; Salvi et al., 2008).

Electron tomograms of the cell environment are crowded of macromolecular complexes. The high-resolution structure of many of these complexes are usually available from techniques such as X-ray crystallography or single particle electron microscopy. The current resolution levels in EMT allow detection of these complexes in the *in situ* cell environment using these available structures as search-templates against the tomogram. This allows the analysis of the spatial distribution of these macromolecular complexes and their interactions in the native cellular context, an approach that is referred to as 'visual proteomics' (Nickell et al., 2006). Detection is carried out by a template-matching procedure based on cross-correlation function (CCF) on the three coordinates and the three orientation parameters of the putative occurrences in the tomogram. In order to account for the limited tilt conditions, the missing wedge is taken into account during the CCF computation (Frangakis et al., 2002). The numerous false positives have to be discarded by visual inspection or statistics (Ortiz et al., 2006). The putative complexes are then extracted from the tomogram, mutually aligned and averaged, with consideration of the missing wedge (Schmid and Booth, 2008). Finally, once the location and the orientation of the positive complexes are known, it is then possible to locate them back in the tomogram space with the proper orientation, thereby creating a macromolecular atlas of the cell that allows the analysis of their 3D distribution and their interactions.

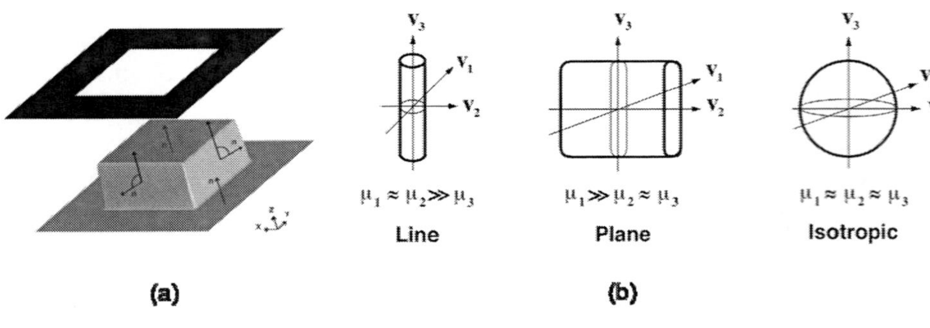

Figure 4. Approaches for noise filtering. (a) The Beltrami flow considers a 3D volume as a 3-manifold embedded into a 4D space. This sketch shows the 2D case, where an image with a white square over black background (top) is viewed as a surface in a 3D space (bottom). The edges are seen as cliffs in the Z direction. At each point of the surface, the projection of the normal (arrows in blue) to the Z direction (arrows in black) acts as an edge indicator, yielding little value at sharp edges where the smoothing should be attenuated or cancelled out. (b) In anisotropic nonlinear filtering, the local structure around each voxel is determined based on an eigen-analysis that provides three orthogonal eigenvectors (**v**) and their corresponding eigenvalues (μ). This analysis allows identification of basic geometric figures, as shown, and the strength and direction of the smoothing are adaptively tuned so that the edges of these structures are preserved and enhanced.

Resolution estimation aims to find out the level of detail that is undoubtedly present and reliable in the tomogram. An approach that is getting interest in the field is inspired in the Fourier Shell Correlation (FSC) commonly used in other electron microscopy modalities like single particle electron microscopy (Fernandez et al., 2006). This approach, known as FSCe/o, splits the tilt series into two halves (containing the even and odd projection images, respectively). From these half tilt series, two independent tomograms are computed that are then compared in Fourier space to find out the maximum spatial resolution up to which both are mutually consistent (Cardone et al., 2005). Another approach, more time-consuming, is known as noise-compensated leave one out (NLOO). Here, for each projection image, a tomogram is computed from the whole tilt series except that projection image. Then, a projection is calculated from the tomogram at the direction of the missing projection, and a comparison in Fourier space (according to the 2D version of the FSC) between the calculated and the missing projection is carried out (Cardone et al., 2005). Therefore, this method estimates the quality of the tomogram as the resolution up to which it is possible to predict a missing projection. For small tilt intervals (1 degree) FSCe/o and NLOO yield similar results, otherwise NLOO is more reliable. On the other hand, in cases where averaging of substructures or macromolecular complexes is involved, the resolution is estimated from the FSC of two independent averages computed from half-sets of substructures.

An Illustrative Example: EMT of Vaccinia Virus

Vaccinia virus is one of the largest (around 360 nm) and most complex viruses whose 3D structure at 5 nm resolution was elucidated for the first time in 2005 by EMT (Cyrklaff et al., 2005). Vaccinia virus is well known because it was successfully used for vaccination against the smallpox disease, which led to its eradication. In this section, the steps that led to the determination of the structure of this virus by EMT are reviewed.

The data acquisition stage yielded the tilt series, which consisted of 61 images taken from the specimen in the angular range [-60°,60°] at an interval of 2°. The pixel size of the images was 1.64 nm. Figure 5 shows two projection images (at 0° and 40°) of the tilt series. Five virions can be identified. Figure 6 shows three projection images (at -60°, 0° and 40°) of a specific virion. After tomographic reconstruction with the standard method, WBP, the tomogram was obtained, as shown in Figure 7. Note the loss of resolution in the direction of axis Z due to the missing wedge produced by the limited tilt range. Also note the low SNR of the projection images, which in turn makes the tomogram extremely noisy as well.

Noise reduction with the standard method, anisotropic nonlinear diffusion, produced data well suited for interpretation and visual inspection. Figure 8 shows the result of the denoising when applied to one of the subtomograms containing a virion. The different membranes and components of the virus become visible and are highlighted over the background. This much cleaner data allows visualization in 3D, as shown on the right panel in Figure 8.

Segmentation was then carried out based on optimal thresholding and manual tracing (Figure 9). This segmentation procedure revealed that the Vaccinia virus is a brick-shaped structure with fixed dimensions of 360 x 270 x 250 nm, composed by an outer membrane (yellow), and an inner core (blue) where the genetic material is located. A membrane that has a palisade of spikes surrounds the core. Systematic inspection of the denoised and segmented tomograms allowed discovery of pores through which the genetic material presumably can pass during infection. There also exist lateral densities (orange) behind the outer membrane and there is room to speculate that they may be special areas for the storage of viral components required for the infection process.

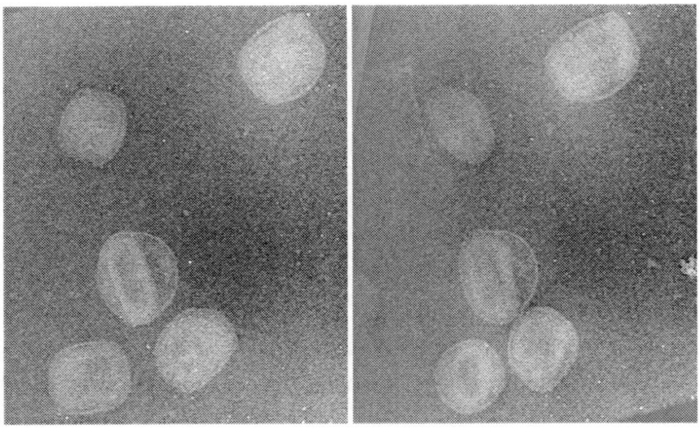

Figure 5. Acquisition of Vaccinia virus tilt-series. Two projection images of the tilt series, taken with the sample tilted at 0 ° and 40 °, are shown.

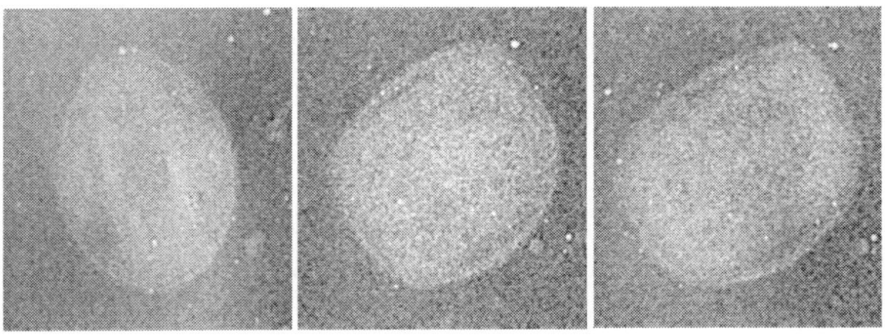

Figure 6. Projection images of a specific Vaccinia virion. Three projection images of a specific virion extracted from the tilt series (see the virion at the top of the panels in Figure 5), corresponding at -60°, 0 ° and 40 ° tilts are shown.

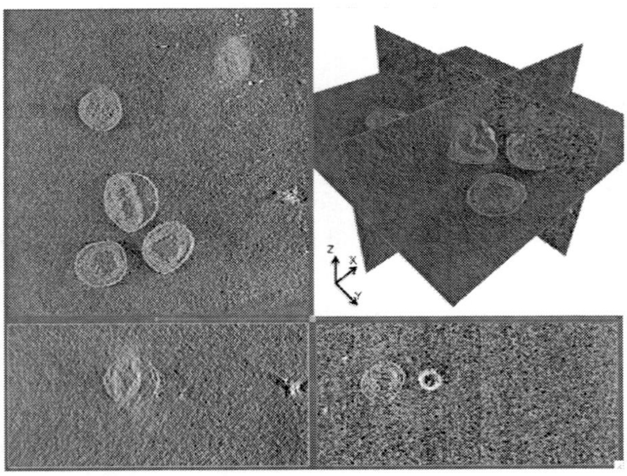

Figure 7. Tomogram computed from the tilt-series. Different slices at different orthogonal axes are shown.

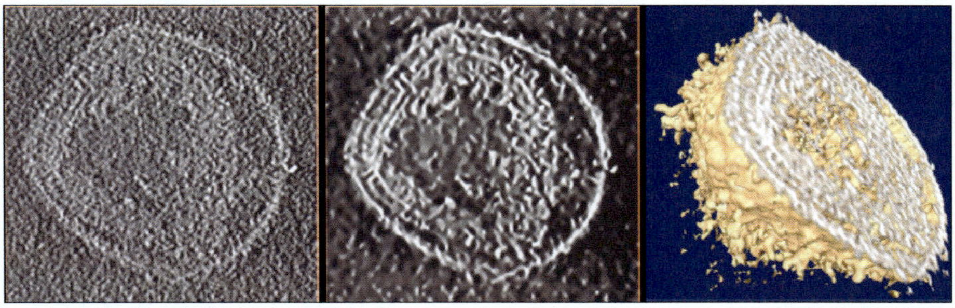

Figure 8. The effects of noise reduction over a subtomogram containing a Vaccinia virion. A slice of the original subtomogram and of the denoised one are shown on the left and middle. Visualization in 3D of the virion is now possible, as seen on the right.

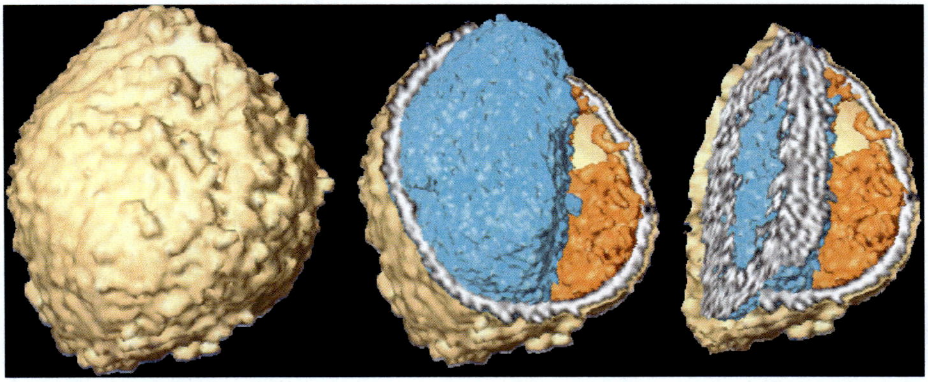

Figure 9. Segmentation of a Vaccinia virion by manual tracing and optimal thresholding. The virus comprises an outer membrane (yellow) that encloses a core (blue) where the genetic material is. The core has a membrane and a palisade of spikes. Lateral densities (orange) are speculated to be material to assist the infection process.

The procedure for pattern recognition was used to determine the arrangement of the spikes anchored in the membrane of the core. An area containing several spikes crystallites was extracted and used as a template for cross-correlation search. The results showed that the spikes formed hexagonal patches throughout the core's outer surface (Cyrklaff et al., 2005). In this study, the resolution could be assessed by the crystal order of the patches that showed information up to 5 nm resolution.

High Performance Computing in EMT

There are a number of stages in EMT characterized by huge computational demands deriving from the data size along with the algorithmic complexity of the methods (e.g. 3D reconstruction, denoising, segmentation, template matching, etc). High performance computing (HPC) has been traditionally applied to address the computationally demanding problems in EMT and using the different computational platforms and paradigms at the time (Fernandez, 2008).

The single-tilt axis geometry typically used in EMT allows decomposition of the 3D reconstruction problem into multiple independent reconstructions of slabs of slices orthogonal to the tilt axis (Fernandez, 2008). This has been applied for WBP or for iterative methods, traditionally using supercomputers (Perkins et al., 1997), clusters of workstations (Fernandez et al., 2002; 2004; 2008), and recently on modern multicore platforms (Bilbao-Castro et al., 2009). These HPC implementations have provided linear speed-up factors, i.e. the effective reduction of computation time is proportional to the number of processors used. In the last decade, computational grids have emerged as powerful large-scale high-performance distributed computing infrastructures where computation and storage can be spread across a myriad of geographically dispersed machines. Decomposition of the tomographic problem into independent slabs has turned out to be well suited for grid computing and it has thus been possible to obtain excellent acceleration factors (Peltier et al., 2003; Fernandez et al., 2007). However, strategies to deal with the stability issues have been necessary to fully exploit the potential of the grid (Bilbao-Castro et al., 2007). Recently, the advent of graphics processors (GPUs) for general-purpose computing has made it possible to obtain outstanding speed-up factors (60x) in reconstruction (Castano-Diez et al., 2007; 2008).

Anisotropic nonlinear diffusion, the standard denoising method in EMT, is extremely demanding, and parallel implementations for clusters and modern multicore computers have been developed to reduce the computation time with linear acceleration factors (Tabik et al., 2007). Essentially, the volume is decomposed into overlapping subvolumes to be filtered and, at each iteration, the overlap areas are updated with data from neighbour processors or nodes. Simpler filtering techniques, such as the median or bilateral, have been implemented for GPUs, obtaining exceptional acceleration factors, around 70x (Castano-Diez et al., 2008). Segmentation has also been carried out in parallel by splitting the volume into several subvolumes to be processed in parallel using a master-worker paradigm (Garduno and Herman, 2008).

Template matching allows automated identification of macromolecules in tomograms as well as objective annotation of cellular structures. The tomogram is scanned in search of structures matching templates of the macromolecules or the features of interest. The searches for the templates at different orientations can be run in parallel and, at the end, the results are joined so as to obtain the matching parameters, This strategy has been implemented for supercomputers (Bohm et al., 2000), clusters of workstations (Ortiz et al., 2006) or grids (Lebbink et al., 2007). Recently, GPUs have been applied as well, achieving a reduction factor of the computation time around 22x (Castano-Diez et al., 2008).

Software Tools for EMT

A number of software packages for EMT in biology are freely available for the scientific community. Most of them are accessible through the wikipedia "Software Tools For Molecular Microscopy":
http://en.wikibooks.org/wiki/Software_Tools_For_Molecular_Microscopy.
A list of these packages and their main features follows.

General packages: They contain a comprehensive set of tools for the different computational stages in the EMT workflow.

Bsoft: http://lsrbr.niams.nih.gov/bsoft/

EM3D: http://em3d.stanford.edu/
IMOD: http://bio3d.colorado.edu/imod/
Priism/IVE: http://www.msg.ucsf.edu/IVE/
Protomo: http://www.electrontomography.org/
Spider: http://www.wadsworth.org/spider_doc/spider/docs/spider.html
TOM: http://www.biochem.mpg.de/en/rd/baumeister/tom_e/
TOMOJ: http://u759.curie.u-psud.fr/softwaresu759.html

Specific packages: They contain tools for specific stages of the EMT workflow.

AV3: Alignment and averaging of macromolecules detected in tomograms. http://www.biochem.mpg.de/en/rd/baumeister/research/ContentFrido/Content_Software/index.html
EMPackage: Filtering and segmentation tools. http://www.embl-heidelberg.de/frangakis/
MOLMATCH: Detection of macromolecules in tomograms. http://www.biochem.mpg.de/en/rd/baumeister/research/ContentFrido/Content_Software/index.html
Leginon: Automated acquisition of tilt series. http://leginon.org
PEET: Alignment and averaging of particles in volumes extracted from tomograms. ftp://bio3d.colorado.edu/pub/PEET/
RAPTOR: Alignment of tilt series. http://www-vlsi.stanford.edu/TEM/software.htm
Shape: Automated segmentation of membranes. ftp://bio3d.colorado.edu/pub/Shape/
SerialEM: Automated acquisition of tilt series. http://bio3d.colorado.edu/SerialEM/
TOMOAND: Anisotropic nonlinear noise reduction. http://www.ual.es/~jjfdez/SW/tomoand.html
TOMOBFLOW: Nolinear noise reduction with Beltrami flow. http://www.ual.es/~jjfdez/SW/tomobflow.html
TOMOCTF: Determination and correction of the transfer function. http://www.ual.es/~jjfdez/SW/ tomoctf.html
UCSF Tomography: Automated acquisition and real-time reconstruction. http://www.msg.ucsf.edu/ em/EMNEW2/ tomography_page.html

Some of these packages are already provided with HPC solutions to reduce the computation time: Bsoft, IMOD, MOLMATCH, Priism/IVE, Spider, UCSF Tomography. In these packages, the HPC techniques are mainly applied to tomographic reconstruction, denoising and template matching.

Conclusion

Electron microscope tomography has matured as a structural technique in biology, making it possible to visualize the molecular architectures of organelles, cells and complex viruses at near molecular resolution. EMT has got a unique potential to bridge the gap between cellular and molecular biology, allowing the integration of the multi-resolution structural information derived by the different structural techniques and thus a comprehensive description of the cellular function. EMT combines electron microscopy with the power of 3D imaging and relies on essential computational image processing stages to derive and interpret the 3D structure of the complex biological specimens: data acquisition, image alignment, image restoration, 3D reconstruction, post-processing and interpretation of the structure. In this chapter, the computational methods and technologies involved in experimental EMT studies have been reviewed. These methods are expected to play a key role to help EMT scientists explore untrodden paths in cell biology and at a level of detail ever imagined.

Acknowledgments

The authors thank the support of the grants MCI-TIN2008-01117 and JA-P06-TIC-01428. J.R. Bilbao-Castro is a fellow of the Spanish "Juan de la Cierva" postdoctoral contracts program, co-financed by the European Social Fund.

References

Al-Amoudi, A., Diez, D. C., Betts, M. J. and Frangakis, A. S. (2007). The molecular architecture of cadherins in native epidermal desmosomes. *Nature*, 450, 832-837.

Beck, M., Forster, F., Ecke, M., Plitzko, J. M., Melchior, F., Gerisch, G., Baumeister, W. and Medalia, O. (2004). Nuclear pore complex structure and dynamics revealed by cryoelectron tomography. *Science*, 306, 1387-1390.

Bilbao-Castro, J. R., Garcia, I. and Fernandez, J. J. (2007). EGEETomo: A user-friendly, fault-tolerant and grid-enabled application for 3D reconstruction in electron tomography. *Bioinformatics*, 23, 3391-3393.

Bilbao-Castro, J. R., Marabini, R., Sorzano, C. O. S., Garcia, I., Carazo, J. M. and Fernandez, J. J. (2009). Exploiting desktop supercomputing for three-dimensional electron microscopy reconstructions using ART with blobs. *Journal of Structural Biology, 165*, 19-26.

Bohm, J., Frangakis, A. S., Hegerl, R., Nickell, S., Typke, D. and Baumeister, W. (2000). Toward detecting and identifying macromolecules in a cellular context: template matching applied to electron tomograms. *Proceedings of the National Academy of Sciences of USA*, 97, 14245-14250.

Brandt, F., Etchells, S. A., Ortiz, J. O., Elcock, A. H., Hartl, F. U. and Baumeister, W. (2009). The native 3D organization of bacterial polysomes. *Cell*, 136, 261-271.

Cardone, G., Grunewald, K. and Steven, A. C. (2005). A resolution criterion for electron tomography based on cross-validation. *Journal of Structural Biology*, 151, 117-129.

Castaño-Díez, D., Mueller, H. and Frangakis, A. S. (2007). Implementation and performance evaluation of reconstruction algorithms on graphics processors. *Journal of Structural Biology*, 157, 288-295.

Castaño-Díez, D., Moser, D., Schoenegger, A., Pruggnaller, S. and Frangakis, A. S. (2008). Performance evaluation of image processing algorithms on the GPU. *Journal of Structural Biology*, 164, 153-160.

Cyrklaff, M., Risco, C., Fernandez, J. J., Jimenez, M. A., Esteban, M., Baumeister, W. and Carrascosa J. L. (2005). Cryo-electron tomography of Vaccinia virus. *Proceedings of the National Academy of Sciences of USA*, 102, 2772-2777.

DeRosier, D. J. and Klug, A. (1968). Reconstruction of 3 dimensional structures from electron micrographs. *Nature*, 217, 130-134.

Dierksen, K., Typke, D., Hegerl, R., Koster, A. J. and Baumeister, W. (1992). Towards automatic electron tomography. *Ultramicroscopy*, 40, 71-87.

Dierksen, K., Typke, D., Hegerl, R. and Baumeister, W. (1993). Towards automatic electron tomography II. Implementation of autofocus and low-dose procedures. *Ultramicroscopy*, 49, 109-120.

Fernandez, J. J. (2008). High performance computing in structural determination by electron cryomicroscopy. *Journal of Structural Biology*, *164*, 1-6.

Fernandez, J. J. (2009). TOMOBFLOW: feature-preserving noise filtering for electron tomography. *BMC Bioinformatics*, 10, 178.

Fernandez, J. J., Lawrence, A. F., Roca, J., Garcia, I., Ellisman, M. H. and Carazo, J. M. (2002). High-performance electron tomography of complex biological specimens. *Journal of Structural Biology*, 138, 6-20.

Fernandez, J. J. and Li, S. (2003). An improved algorithm for anisotropic nonlinear diffusion for denoising cryo-tomograms. *Journal of Structural Biology*, 144, 152-161.

Fernandez, J. J., Carazo, J. M. and Garcia, I. (2004). Three-dimensional reconstruction of cellular structures by electron microscope tomography and parallel computing. *Journal of Parallel and Distributed Computing*, 64, 285-300.

Fernandez, J. J., Li, S. and Crowther, R. A. (2006). CTF determination and correction in electron cryotomography. *Ultramicroscopy*, 106, 587-596.

Fernandez, J. J., Garcia, I., Carazo, J. M. and Marabini, R. (2007). Electron tomography of complex biological specimens on the Grid. *Future Generation Computer Systems*, 23, 435-446.

Fernandez, J. J., Gordon, D. and Gordon, R. (2008). Efficient parallel implementation of iterative reconstruction algorithms for electron tomography. *Journal of Parallel and Distributed Computing*, 68, 626-640.

Frangakis, A. S. and Hegerl, R. (2001). Noise reduction in electron tomographic reconstructions using nonlinear anisotropic diffusion. *Journal of Structural Biology*, 135, 239-250.

Frangakis, A. S. and Hegerl, R. (2002). Segmentation of two- and three-dimensional data from electron microscopy using eigenvector analysis. *Journal of Structural Biology*, 138, 105-113.

Frangakis, A. S., Bohm, J., Forster, F., Nickell, S., Nicastro, D., Typke, D., Hegerl, R. and Baumeister, W. (2002). Identification of macromolecular complexes in cryoelectron tomograms of phantom cells, *Proceedings of the National Academy of Sciences of USA*, 99, 14153-14158.

Frank, J. (Editor) *Electron Tomography: Methods for Three-Dimensional Visualization of Structures in the Cell.* Berlin, Springer; 2006.

Garduno, E., Wong-Barnum, M., Volkmann, N. and Ellisman, M. H. (2008). Segmentation of electron tomographic data sets using fuzzy set theory principles. *Journal of Structural Biology*, 162, 368-379.

Garduno, E. and Herman, G. T. (2008). Parallel Fuzzy Segmentation of Multiple Objects. *International Journal of Imaging Systems and Technology*, 18, 336-344.

Gilbert, P. (1972). Iterative methods for the reconstruction of three dimensional objects from their projections, *Journal of Theoretical Biology*, 36, 105-117.

Gordon, R., Bender, R. and Herman, G. T. (1970). Algebraic reconstruction techniques (ART) for three-dimensional electron microscopy and x-ray photography. *Journal of Theoretical Biology*, 29, 471-481.

Grunewald, K., Desai, P., Winkler, D. C., Heymann, J. B., Belnap, D. M., Baumeister, W. and Steven, A. C. (2003). Three-dimensional structure of herpes simplex virus from cryo-electron tomography. *Science*, 302, 1396-1398.

He, W., Cowin, P. and Stokes, D. L. (2003). Untangling desmosomal knots with electron tomography. *Science*, 302, 109-113.

He, W., Ladinsky, M. S., Huey-Tubman, K. E., Jensen, G. J., McIntosh, J. R. and Bjorkman, P. J. (2008). FcRn-mediated antibody transport across epithelial cells revealed by electron tomography. *Nature*, 455, 542-546.

Herman, G. T. (1980). *Image Reconstruction from Projections*. Academic-Press, New York.

Hoenger, A. and McIntosh, J. R. (2009). Probing the macromolecular organization of cells by electron tomography Current Opinion in Cell *Biolology*, 21, 89-96.

Jiang, W., Baker, M. L., Wu, Q., Bajaj, C. and Chiu, W. (2003). Applications of a bilateral denoising filter in biological electron microscopy. *Journal of Structural Biology*, 144, 114-122.

Kak, A. C. and Slaney, M. Principles of Computerized Tomographic Imaging, *Society of Industrial and Applied Mathematics*, Philadelphia, 2001.

Klug, A. and Crowther, R. A. (1972). Three-dimensional image reconstruction from the viewpoint of information theory. *Nature*, 238, 435-440.

Koster, A. J., Chen, H., Sedat, J. W. and Agard, D. A. (1992). Automated microscopy for electron tomography. *Ultramicroscopy*, *46*, 207-227.

Kurner, J., Frangakis, A. S. and Baumeister, W. (2005). Cryo-electron tomography reveals the cytoskeletal structure of Spiroplasma melliferum. *Science*, 307, 436-438.

Lebbink, M. N., Geerts, W. J. C., van der Krift, T. P., Bouwhuis, M., Hertzberger, L. O., Verkleij, A. J. and Koster, A. J. (2007). Template matching as a tool for annotation of tomograms of stained biological structures. *Journal of Structural Biology*, 158, 327-335.

Leis, A. P., Beck, M., Gruska, M., Best, C., Hegerl, R., Baumeister, W. and Leis, J. W. (2006). Cryo-electron tomography of biological specimens. *IEEE Signal Processing Magazine*, 23(3), 95- 103.

Leis, A., Rockel, B., Andrees, L. and Baumeister, W. (2009). Visualizing cells at the nanoscale, *Trends in biochemical sciences*, 34, 60-70.

Lučić, V., Förster, F. and Baumeister, W. (2005). Structural studies by electron tomography: from cells to molecules. *Annual Review of Biochemistry*, 74, 833-865.

Mastronarde, D. N. (1997). Dual-Axis Tomography: An Approach with Alignment Methods that preserve Resolution. *Journal of Structural Biology*, 120, 343-352.

McIntosh, R., Nicastro, D. and Mastronarde, D. (2005) New views of cells in 3D: An introduction to electron tomography. *Trends in Cell Biology*, 15, 43-51.

McIntosh, R. (Editor) *Cellular Electron Microscopy*, Volume 79 of Methods in Cell Biology. Academic press, New York, 2007.

Medalia, O., Weber, I., Frangakis, A. S., Nicastro, D., Gerisch, G. and Baumeister, W. (2002). Macromolecular architecture in eukaryotic cells visualized by cryoelectron tomography. *Science*, 298, 1209-1213.

Narasimha, R., Aganj, I., Bennett, A. E., Borgnia, M. J., Zabransky, D., Sapiro, G., McLaughlin, S. W., Milne, J. L. S. and Subramaniam, S. (2008). Evaluation of denoising algorithms for biological electron tomography. *Journal of Structural Biology*, 164, 7-17.

Nicastro, D., Schwartz, C., Pierson, J., Gaudette, R., Porter, M.E. and McIntosh, J.R. (2006) The molecular architecture of axonemes revealed by cryoelectron tomography. *Science*, 313, 944-948.

Nickell, S., Kofler, C., Leis, A. P. and Baumeister, W. (2006) A visual approach to proteomics. *Nature Reviews Molecular Cell Biology,* 7, 225-230.

Ortiz, J. O., Forster, F., Kurner, J., Linaroudis, A. A. and Baumeister, W. (2006) Mapping 70S ribosomes in intact cells by cryoelectron tomography and pattern recognition. *Journal of Structural Biology,* 156, 334-341.

Penczek, P., Marko, M., Buttle, K. and Frank, J. (1995) Double-Tilt Electron Tomography. *Ultramicroscopy*, 60, 393-410.

Peltier, S. T., Lin, A.W., Lee, D., Mock, S., Lamont, S., Molina, T.,Wong, M., Dai, L., Martone, M.E. and Ellisman, M. H. (2003) The Telescience portal for tomography applications. *Journal of Parallel and Distributed Computing,* 63, 539–550.

Perkins, G. A., Renken, C. W., Song, J. Y., Frey, T. G., Young, S. J., Lamont, S., Martone, M. E., Lindsey, S. and Ellisman,M. H. (1997) Electron tomography of large, multicomponent biological structures. . *Journal of Structural Biology*, 120, 219–227.

Pruggnaller, S., Mayr, M. and Frangakis, A.S. (2008) A visualization and segmentation toolbox for electron microscopy. *Journal of Structural Biology,* 164, 161-165.

Robinson, C. V., Sali, A. and Baumeister, W. (2007) The molecular sociology of the cell. *Nature,* 450, 973-982.

Sali, A., Glaeser, R., Earnest, T. and Baumeister, W. (2003) From words to literature in structural proteomics. *Nature*, 422, 216-225.

Salvi, E., Cantele, F., Zampighi, L., Fain, N., Pigino, G., Zampighi, G., and Lanzavecchia, S. (2008) JUST (Java User Segmentation Tool) for semi-automatic segmentation of tomographic maps. *Journal of Structural Biology,* 161, 287-297.

Sandberg, K. and Brega, M. (2007) Segmentation of thin structures in electron micrographs using orientation fields. *Journal of Structural Biology*, 157, 403–415.

Schmid, M. F. and Booth, C. R. (2008) Methods for aligning and for averaging 3D volumes with missing data. *Journal of Structural Biology*, 161, 243-248.

Sorzano, C. O. S., Messaoudi, C., Eibauer, M., Bilbao-Castro, J.R., Hegerl, R., Nickell, S., Marco, S. and Carazo, J.M. (2009) Marker-free image registration of electron tomography tilt-series. *BMC Bioinformatics*, 10, 124.

Tabik, S., Garzon, E. M., Garcia, I. and Fernandez, J. J. (2007) High performance noise reduction for biomedical multidimensional data. *Digital Signal Processing*, 17, 724-736.

van der Heide, P., Xu, X. P., Marsh, B. J., Hanein, D. and Volkmann, N. (2007) Efficient automatic noise reduction of electron tomographic reconstructions based on iterative median filtering. *Journal of Structural Biology,* 158, 196-204.

Volkmann, N. (2002) A novel three-dimensional variant of the watershed transform for segmentation of electron density maps, *Journal of Structural Biology,* 138, 123–129.

Winkler, H. and Taylor, K. A. (2003) Focus gradient correction applied to tilt series image data used in electron tomography. *Journal of Structural Biology,* 143, 24-32.

In: 3D Imaging: Theory, Technology … ISBN: 978-1-60876-885-1
Editors: E. H. Duke and S. R. Aguirre, pp.111- 137

Chapter 4

THREE-DIMENSIONAL IMAGING AND PROCESSING

Tsutomi Gomi
Kitasato University, Sagamihara, Kanagawa, Japan

ABSTRACT

The purpose of this chapter is to provide a tutorial overview on the subject of three-dimensional (3D) imaging and processing. We expect the chapter to the useful for practicing engineers, medical scientists for gaining an understanding of what can and cannot be done with theory, technology, and reconstruction algorithm. Toward this end, we have tried to strike a balance among purely algorithmic issues, topics (tomosynthesis imaging etc.) dealing with how to generate data for reconstruction in different domains, and artifacts inherent to different data collection strategies.

This chapter is structured to cover the basics of computed tomography (CT) from x-ray modern cone-beam CT. However, the main focus of the chapter is concerned with detailed derivations of reconstruction algorithms in 2D and modern 3D CBCT systems. Since the impact of CBCT will undeniably increase in the future, 3D reconstruction algorithms are illustrated and derived in detail. A thorough analysis of CT artifacts and a discussion of practical issues, such as dose considerations, provide further insight into modern CT systems. The chapter is addressed to a wide interdisciplinary readership in an effort to explain both the fundamentals and applications of tomography. Consequently, the focus is on physics and technology, whereas radiological aspects are addressed only marginally. There is no requirement for special prior knowledge. With respect to detail problems or questions, relevant literature is referenced.

1. INTRODUCTION

About 30 years have passed since Dr. Hounsfield developed a practicable CT system. The arrival of CT devices in the field of medical diagnosis has resulted in a revolution equivalent to the discovery of X-ray by Dr. Roentgen. Since then, most researchers aiming for a higher quality in medical diagnosis have worked toward the functional improvement of CT devices leading to the development of fan-beam CT devices, helical scan CT devices, multislice CT devices, cone-beam CT devices. The time needed for image reconstruction has been reduced with these new devices and the image quality has improved dramatically. With the increasing demand for better technology, development research of high performance CT devices is being carried out.

Current image reconstruction methods using helical scanning with a multislice CT generates cone-beam and helical artifacts [3,5,12]. These methods require a 32-mm detector and a 30-s breath-hold time when regions such as the chest and abdomen are being scanned with a scanning range of 20 mm. This results in large interscan variations, while slices have to be thin to reduce the helical pitch. However, appropriate scan parameters can yield high-resolution reconstructed images.

For cone-beam CT scanning systems, volume reconstruction algorithms have been developed and applied in various studies in order to show their full potential for use in future applications. As is true for standard medical CT systems with one-dimensional detectors, because the basic system geometry is unchanged for cone-beam CT scanners, two different scanning modes are of particular interest: circular and helical modes. These are of special interest for applications such as medical imaging and nondestructive testing. The problem of cone-beam reconstruction for helical source–detector trajectories is a topic of ongoing discussion [1–9]. The method developed by Feldkamp et al. [10] seems to be the most used technique for circular trajectories.

The approximate reconstruction method, which was developed as a straightforward adaptation of two-deimansional (2D) filtered backprojection (FBP) to cone-beam geometry, has several advantages. Apart from its easy implementation, it is exact for scanning objects in the central plane containing the circular source trajectory and those that are homogeneous in the direction parallel to the rotation axis. Since the method was reported, it has been most widely used for three-dimensional (3D) cone-beam reconstruction. The inexactness of the Feldkamp algorithm is a consequence of the missing data problem. The 3D Radon transform cannot be determined completely when projection data are acquired along a circular source–detector trajectory [11,12]. Nevertheless, circular trajectories may be used in future cone-beam CT systems because artifacts are produced in Radon space due to missing small cone angles.

In the biomedical field, the most popular method for cone-beam imaging reconstruction is the 3D FBP, which uses a circular scanning locus and reconstructs images well in the case of a small cone angle [10]. However, the Feldkamp algorithm produces significant image artifacts, such as a dropping away of intensity from the mid-plane in the case of a moderate to large cone angle. Consequently, several variants of the Feldkamp algorithm were developed for practical applications that involve larger cone angles [13–16,27,29].

Recently, medical CT began a transition from fan-beam to cone-beam geometry with the introduction of multislice CT systems [17–19]. These systems allow the scanning of regions requiring a broad scanning range, such as the chest and abdomen, because they use a multislice CT employing a large number of channels (i.e., 128 and 256 rows etc). Use of a wide-range cone-beam CT with a wide angle results in reconstruction with low image quality accompanied by cone-beam artifacts in the reconstruction planes away from the mid-plane in the longitudinal direction. A cone-beam CT with a wide-angle lens, which reduces cone-beam artifacts and generates high-quality reconstruction images with a wide exposure range, would thus be clinically very useful.

The advent of flat-panel detectors has opened a new avenue of imaging technology research, including the experimental use of such detectors for CT. Therefore, in parallel with the development of multislice CT systems with a constantly increasing number of detector rows, CT imaging with flat-panel detectors has been considered mainly because of the high spatial resolution achievable. Various experimental and clinically useful systems have been developed. Clinically established products include the use of X-ray intensifiers with rotating C-arm systems, enabling high-resolution 3D angiographic images, which are used, for example, in interventional neuroradiology [21] and orthopedic surgery [22,23].

Clinical reports have indicated the usefulness of cone-beam CT in an angiography system and image-guided radiation therapy in a current medical service system [23–34]. However, cone-beam artifact and scatter measures are problems affecting the image quality of the reconstruction image. Many researchers suggest that computer simulation methods may improve control over the cone-beam artifact. Other reports indicate that it can reduce scatter X-ray measure by bow-tie filtering and image processing.

Interest in tomosynthesis and its clinical applications has been revived by recent advances in digital X-ray detector technology. Conventional tomography technology provides planar information of an object from its projection images. In tomography, an X-ray tube and an X-ray film receptor are positioned on either side of the object. The relative motion of the tube and film is predetermined based on the location of the in-focus plane [30]. A single image plane is generated by a scan, and multislice CT scans are required to provide a sufficient number of planes to cover the selected structure in the object. Tomosynthesis acquires only one set of discrete X-ray projections that can be used to reconstruct any plane of the object retrospectively [31]. The technique has been investigated in angiography and imaging of chest, hand joints, lungs, teeth, and breasts [32–37]. A review of tomosynthesis has been given by Dobbins et al. [38]. Tomosynthesis was shown to outperform planar imaging to a statistically significant extent. Various types of tomosynthesis reconstruction methods have been explored.

2. Current Status and Problem

Because the human body is a 3D object aligned in a longitudinal direction, it is not easy to obtain projection data from all directions. Multislice CT has the benefit of multidetector channels, and improvement is being sought in the spatial resolution in the longitudinal direction and examination efficiency. However, multislice CT has the problem of short acquisition time of projection data, and improvement of spatial resolution in the longitudinal direction is required. Methods adopting cone-beam CT for improving resolution are regarded as the solution for short acquisition time, which is a problem of multislice CT, and there is an increasing interest in this technical development trend. In addition, a cone-beam CT can generate a high-resolution 3D image because the spatial resolution in the longitudinal direction is determined by the size of the search element consisting of 2D detectors. Image intensifiers were used as detectors before flat-panel detector (FPD) came to be used in cone-beam CT systems [26]. The dynamic range (linearity) of a signal is inadequate for 16–18 bit demand and it is only 10 bit in a CT detector with this image intensifiers. For this reason, a cone-beam CT that uses an image intensifiers as a detector is useful for acquiring a volume of data from subjects with a high contrast, such as lungs, bone, contrasting blood vessels, but the extraction of data from a low-contrast subject for CT is difficult. Use of the FPD algorithm enables the digital acquisition of X-ray images, and the dynamic range is wider than that of an image intensifiers (12–14 bits). Therefore, for using FPD as a detector for cone-beam CT, the low-contrast resolution and methods to use image intensifiers, need to improve. Consequently, research and development of FPD is flourishing. However, there are some problems as well. First, FPD can generate a reconstruction (central plane) in the neighborhood of the center of rotation as an exact image. However, it is difficult to generate an accurate image if there is a rearrangement away from center of rotation. In such instances, a cone-beam artifact arises distorting the appearance of the object and an exact reconstruction cannot be obtained. Second, removal of X-ray scatter is difficult and gives a bad influence to a reconstruction image using detectors in two dimensions. Third, it is data velocity collection of FPD at 30–60 frames/second and it compares it with 900–1800 frames/seconds used in CT as far late. Consequently, it seems that it is difficult to obtain a dynamic scan in a short time. For dynamic acquisition, the utility of four-dimensional (4D) CT using a 256-channel detector has been reported [27–28].

Analogous to geometric tomography, the most basic reconstruction method for tomosynthesis is simple backprojection. Backprojection alone, however, leads to significant contrast-reducing tomographic blur from distant structures, which is imposed upon the reconstructed plane of interest. More sophisticated tomosynthesis reconstruction methods including FBP [39–46], iterative deblurring [47–51], and iterative reconstruction [51–53], attempt to correct the overlying tomographic blur and/or poor depth resolution. Wu et al. [54] recently evaluated the performance of a tomosynthesis method by a maximum likelihood (ML) algorithm for artifact reduction in digital breast tomosynthesis.

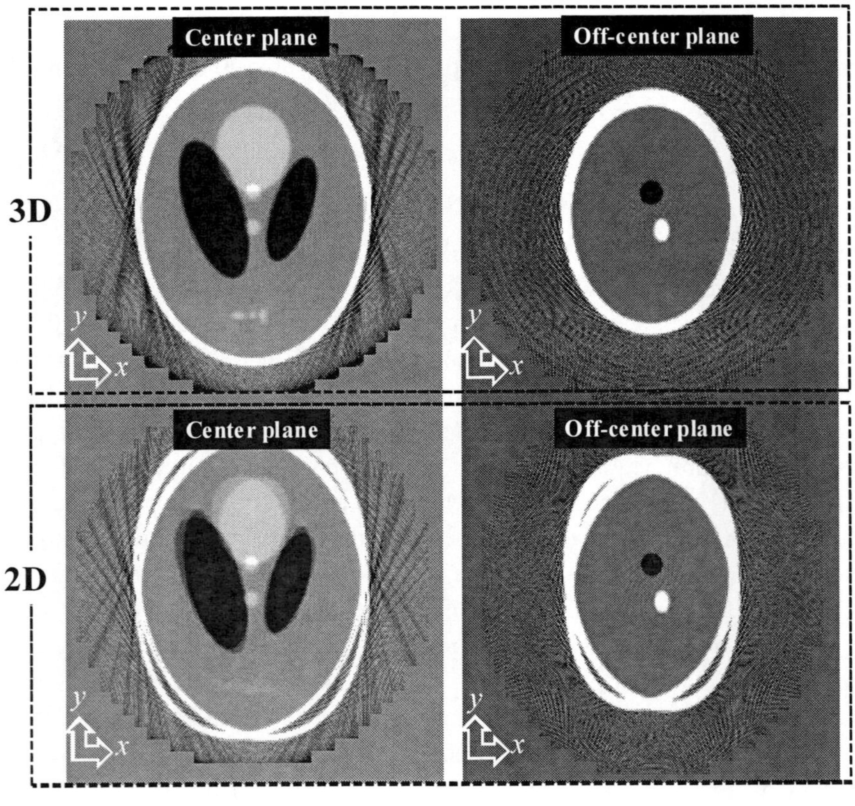

Figure 1. Comparison of 3D FBP algorithm reconstruction images with images obtained from 3D FBP reconstruction, 2D FBP reconstruction of the different slice plane (use of 3D Shepp-Logan phantom at z=-0.25).

Ideally, structures in a given plane of interest should be clearly displayed in the corresponding tomosynthesis reconstruction plane, whereas structures located outside the plane should not be visible. Practically, the limited angular range of the tomosynthesis image acquisition geometry dictates that the spatial resolution is limited in the dimension perpendicular to the detector plane. Consequently, out-of-plane structures cannot be totally removed from the reconstruction plane. Out-of-plane structures are present in every reconstruction plane, but most of them are not conspicuous because the various low-amplitude structures from various projections overlap with each other in the reconstruction plane and are therefore blurred. However, out-of-plane structures with high-attenuation features are not blurred. They appear as multiple replicates of the particular feature in every reconstruction plane except the one in which the actual high-attenuation feature is located. At a projection angle, these ghosting features are distributed along the line made by the X-ray source and the actual feature.

3. 3D Reconstruction Algorithm

3.1 Cone-beam CT System

Figure 1 shows the simulation results obtained by the 2D and 3D FBP methods for an object having 3D information (the 3D Shepp–Logan phantom was used). The 2D filter backprojection method was not reproducible and it was difficult to regard a geometric variation of an image, but the 3D FBP method could reproduce the 3D information from the phantom. From these results, it appears necessary to use the 3D FBP method in reconstruction using cone-beam CT. We refer to the 3D reconstruction algorithm of a circular orbit system in the main manuscript.

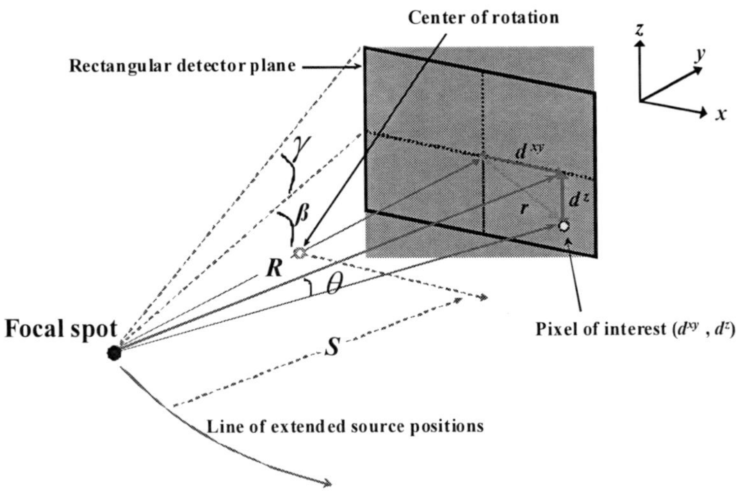

Figure 2. Schematic view of the projection geometry for a rectangular detector plane the corresponding extended source. The geometric relations necessary for the calculation of the projection angle weighted theory can be derived.

3.1.1 Feldkamp algorithm [10]

By analogy with 2D FBP, cone-beam data were acquired along a circular source–detector trajectory (Figure 2). For a given 2D detector, the cone-beam produced by a source illuminating a focus detector can be described as follows. Let $\vec{R}$ be the vector from the center of the detector of the scanning system to the source and $\vec{D}$ the vector from the center of rotation to the center of the detector. For a scanning system moving along a circular trajectory, the position of the source and detector results in:

$$\vec{R} = R\begin{pmatrix} \cos\alpha \\ \sin\alpha \\ 0 \end{pmatrix} \qquad \vec{D} = \begin{pmatrix} -\cos\alpha \\ -\sin\alpha \\ 0 \end{pmatrix} \tag{1}$$

The set of 2D projection data $p^f(\alpha,\beta,\gamma)$ on a focus detector measured along a circular focus–detector trajectory is parameterized by the angular focus position on the circular trajectory $\alpha \in \left[0,\ 2\pi\right]$, the fan angle $\beta \in \left[-\beta_{\max},\ +\beta_{\max}\right]$, and the cone angle $\gamma \in \left[-\gamma_{\max},\ +\gamma_{\max}\right]$. To obtain the projection data in a rectangular detector plane to be used in 3D cone-beam reconstruction, resampling to Cartesian coordinates in the column direction is applied. The projection data on the resulting rectangular detector are parameterized in the following by $p^{uv}(\alpha,d^{xy},d^z)$, with $(\cos\alpha,\sin\alpha,0)$ being the vector normal to the rectangular plane. d^{xy} and d^z are the two Cartesian coordinates within the new rectangular detector plane, where $d^x\left(d^{xy}\right)$ marks the direction in the detector plane orthogonal to the plane of rotation:

$$p^f(\alpha,\beta,\gamma) \rightarrow p^{uv}\left(\alpha,d^{xy},d^z\right) \tag{2}$$

The two Cartesian coordinates have a range of $d^{xy} \in \left[-d^{xy}_{\max},\ +d^{xy}_{\max}\right]$ and $d^z \in \left[-d^z_{\max},\ +d^z_{\max}\right]$. The maximum values are calculated as follows:

$$d^{xy}_{max} = R\,tan(\beta_{max}) \tag{3}$$

and

$$d^{z}_{max} = R\,tan(\gamma_{max}) \tag{4}$$

This rectangular plane is the largest that fits completely into the convex area. The data contained in the outer area do not need to be measured in the original focus–detector plane if the proposed method is used. Therefore, the use of a suitable collimator reduces the dose applied to the patient or object.

Consequently, a simplified 3D FBP method can be applied to the rebinned data lacking the distance weighting factor $\left(\frac{R}{r}\right)^2$, which is well known from the Feldkamp algorithm approach. While R is the length of the vector R from the source to the center of the detector of rotation, r describes the length of the vector from the source to a voxel under consideration projected onto $\vec{R}$ within the original method.

The resulting Feldkamp algorithm thus has reduced computational complexity and can be expressed in the following manner:

$$g_1 = p^f(‡, \%\alpha,)\cdot{}^{-}(\%\alpha,) \tag{5}$$

$$g_2 = g_1(\alpha, \beta, \gamma) * h(\beta) \tag{6}$$

$$f\left(\vec{x}\right) = \frac{1}{2¶}\int_0^{2¶}\left(\frac{R}{r}\right)^2 g_2(‡, \%\alpha,)\ d‡ \tag{7}$$

where equation (5) and (6) is pre processing, equation (7) is the reconstruction image from the 2D projection data. The pre-weighting factor $\omega(\beta,\gamma)$ is geometrically interpreted as the angle between the ray and central ray of the projection.The one-dimensional ramp filter $h(\%)$ is applied along the lines to the plane of rotation in the detector plane (d^{xy} direction).

3.1.2 Variations of the Feldkamp algorithm

3.1.2 (a) The P-FDK method [14]

The Turbell is proposed as a rebinning of the projection data into a geometry that removes this factor from the backprojection formula. The resulting beam geometry is parallel in the fan direction but divergent in the cone direction and the algorithm exploiting this geometry is named parallel FDK (P-FDK).

Let φ be a projection angle of the system on the circular source–detector trajectory from which a parallel-beam projection has to be calculated. Then, from the available cone-beam projections, the data are transformed as

$$p^f(\alpha, \%\delta\gamma) \rightarrow p^p(\square, \%\alpha,) \tag{8}$$

The reconstruction algorithm P-FDK for the cylindrical detector case proceeds with pre-weighting and filtering of the rebinned data according to

$$g_1 = p^P(\varphi, \beta, \gamma) \cdot \omega^P(\beta, \gamma) \tag{9}$$

$$g_2 = g_1(\square, \%\alpha,) * h(\%\alpha) \tag{10}$$

The backprojection formula is written as

$$f\left(\vec{x}\right) = \frac{1}{2¶} \int_0^{2\pi} g_2(\square, \%\alpha,)\ d\square \tag{11}$$

where equation (9) and (10) is pre processing, equation (11) is the reconstruction image from the 2D projection data. The pre-weighting factor $\omega^P(\beta, \gamma)$ is geometrically interpreted as the angle between the ray and central ray of the projection.The one-dimensional ramp filter $h(\%\alpha)$ is applied along the lines to the plane of rotation in the detector plane (d^{xy} direction).

3.1.2 (b) The T-FDK method [13]

By modifying the filtering directions of P-FDK, Grass, Kohler, and Proksa have formulated an algorithm, T-FDK, with attractive geometrical properties as well as seemingly improved image quality.

Let φ be a projection angle of the system on the circular source–detector trajectory from which a parallel-beam projection has to be calculated. Then, from the available cone-beam projections, the data are transformed as

$$p^f(\alpha, \%\sigma\gamma) \rightarrow p^P(\square, \%\alpha,) \tag{12}$$

The projection data on the resulting virtual rectangular detector are parameterized in the following by $p^{uv}(\varphi, d^{xy}, d^z)$, with $(\cos\varphi, \sin\varphi, 0)$ being the vector normal to the rectangular plane. φ still describes the projection angle of a scanning system with an extended source. d^{xy} and d^z are the two Cartesian coordinates within the new rectangular detector plane, where $d^z(d^{xy})$ marks the direction in the detector plane that is orthogonal (parallel) to the plane of rotation:

$$p^P(\varphi, \beta, \gamma) \rightarrow p^{uv}(\varphi, d^{xy}, d^z) \tag{13}$$

The reconstruction algorithm P-FDK for the cylindrical detector case proceeds with pre-weighting and filtering of the rebinned data according to

$$g_1 = p^{uv}(\varphi, d^{xy}, d^z) \cdot \omega^T(d^{xy}, d^z) \tag{14}$$

$$g_2 = g_1(\square d^{xy}, d^z) * h(d^{xy}) \tag{15}$$

The backprojection formula lacks is written as

$$f\left(\vec{x}\right) = \frac{1}{2\pi}\int_{0}^{2\pi} g_2\left(\square, d^{xy}, d^{z}\right) d\square \tag{16}$$

where equation (14) and (15) is pre processing, equation (16) is the reconstruction image from the 2D projection data. The pre-weighting factor $\omega^T\left(d^{xy}, d^{z}\right)$ is geometrically interpreted as the angle between the ray and central ray of the projection.The one-dimensional ramp filter $h\left(d^{xy}\right)$ is applied along the lines to the plane of rotation in the detector plane (d^{xy} direction).

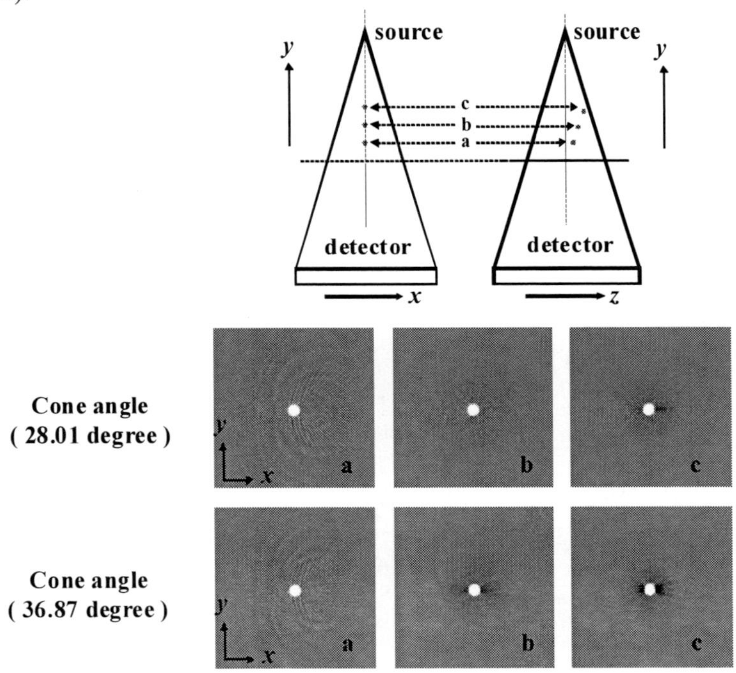

Figure 3. Comparison of 3D FBP algorithm (Feldkamp algorithm) reconstruction images with images obtained from con-angle at 28.01 degree, cone-angle at 36.87 degree of the different microsphere phantom position. The cone-beam artifact of a reconstruction image tends to become large cone-angle and away from the mid-plane.

3.1.2 (c) The nonlinear weighted hybrid method [29]

The cone-beam artifact has a large cone angle and becomes greater at greater distances in the longitudinal direction (Figure 3). In addition, it was confirmed that when there are large amounts of artifacts, the trajectory of the projected data is larger. Considering these results, we suggest a method of correction by changing the weighting through the rotation angle while reconstructing objects at a long distance from the mid-plane position.

As shown in Figure 4a, b, the detector channel to which the microspheres-phantom is projected differs at each projection angle, and orbit displacement (L) increase as it moves away from the mid-plane in longitudinal direction. As shown in Fifure 4c, when a single scan is conducted at projection angles of 0 degree and 359 degree, and by plotting the relationship between the channel data, it is possible to confirm the phenomenon where the trajectory is following a constant cycle.

Because the number of occurrences of cone-beam artifacts increases with larger trajectories, multiplication of each projection angle by a correction coefficient, which is inversely proportional to the size of the orbit displacement, will reduce the cone-beam artifact (Figure 4). It is possible to reduce the cone-beam artifact by creating and using a correction coefficient that will reduce weighting of the projection data at around 180° at which the displacement of the trajectory is at its maximum. The correction coefficient can be found by finding the inverse function ($\omega^s(\alpha)$) and cosine function.

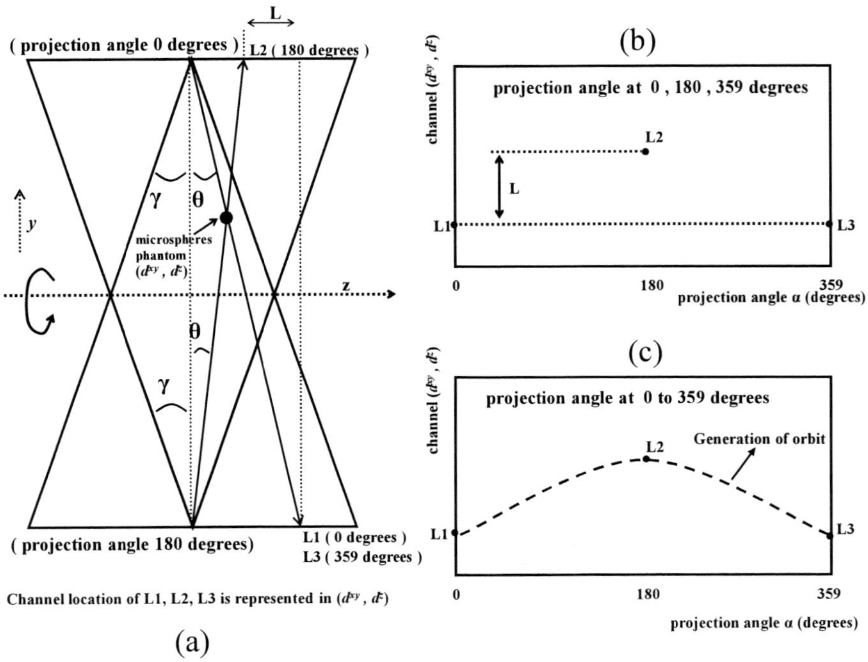

Figure 4. Figurative representation of theory to analyze factors generating cone-beam artifact.

The inverse function is shown in equation (17).

$$\omega^s(\alpha) = [\Gamma(\alpha)]^{-1} \tag{17}$$

$$\Gamma(\alpha) = \left(\frac{Rd^z}{S - \cos(\ddagger - ,\,)}\right)^{-1}$$

The correction coefficient $\omega^T(\alpha, d^{xy}, d^z)$ is

$$\omega^T(\alpha, d^{xy}, d^z) = \omega^s(\alpha) \cdot \cos(\theta(d^{xy}, d^z)) \tag{18}$$

$$\cos(\theta(d^{xy}, d^{z})) = \frac{l_s}{l_p}$$

and compensates for the different ray length through the volume. d^{xy} and d^{z} are the two Cartesian coordinates within the new rectangular detector plane. The height of the extended source position over the central line of the rectangular detector is described by $l_s = \sqrt{R^2 - d^{xy2}}$, since the extended source is positioned on the circular trajectory with radius R. The length of the ray from the extended source position to the pixel under consideration is then given by $l_p = \sqrt{l_s^{\,2} - d^{z2}}$. A schematic view of the geometry can be found in Figure 1.

Consequently, the resulting projection angle-weighted algorithm has reduced computational complexity and can be expressed in the following manner:

$$p^{f} = (t, \%\alpha) \rightarrow p^{uv}(t, d^{xy}, d^{z}) \tag{19}$$

$$g_1 = p^{uv}(t, d^{xy}, d^{z})^{-T}(t, d^{xy}, d^{z}) \tag{20}$$

$$g_2 = g_1(t, d^{xy}, d^{z}) * h(d^{xy}) \tag{21}$$

$$f(\vec{x}) = \frac{1}{2\pi}\int_0^{2\pi} g_2(\varphi, d^{xy}, d^{z})\, d\alpha \tag{22}$$

The one-dimensional ramp filter $h(d^{xy})$ is applied along the lines to the plane of rotation in the detector plane (d^{xy} direction).

3.1.3 *Simulation study*

We performed computer simulation by using the 3D Shepp–Logan phantom to evaluate the Feldkamp algorithm, P-FDK, T-FDK, and the nonlinear weighted hybrid algorithm. The source-to-origin distance was set to 4.0. The number of detectors per cone-beam projection was 256 × 256 (rectangular plane). The size of the 2D detector plane was 2.0 × 2.0. The full-cone angle and fan-angle was 23.8 degree, respectively. The number of projections was 360. The numbers of radial and angular samples were 256 and 360, respectively. Each reconstructed image volume had dimensions of 2.0 × 2.0 × 2.0 and contained 256 × 256 × 256 voxels.

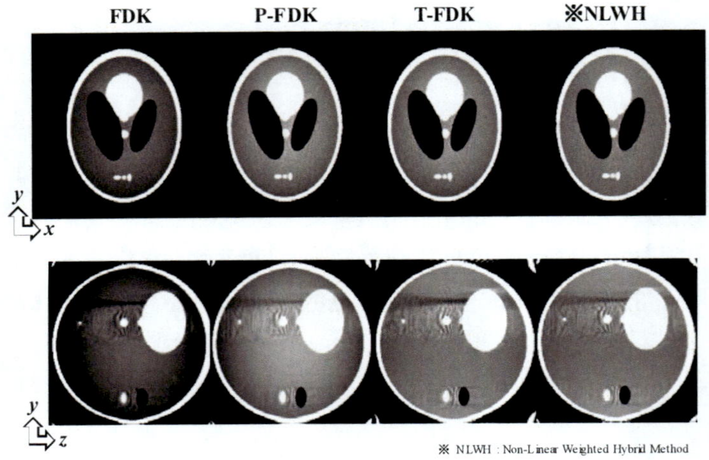

Figure 5. Ideal and reconstructed slices of the 3D Shepp-Logan phantom at z=-0.25 with Feldkamp, P-FDK, T-FDK and non-linear weighted hybrid (NLWH) reconstruction method.

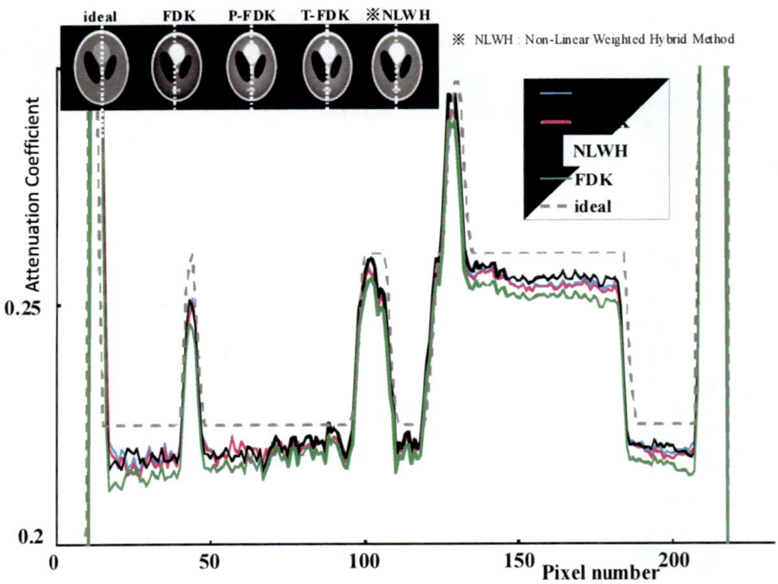

Figure 6. Intensity profiles (The central vertical line in the selected slice of the 3D Shepp-Logan phantom).

In the numerical simulation, 3D Shepp–Logan phantoms were used to evaluate the nonlinear weighted hybrid algorithm against existing Feldkamp, P-FDK, and T-FDK algorithms. Representative reconstruction results are presented in Figure 5. This figure shows that the traditional Feldkamp, P-FDK, and T-FDK algorithm reconstructions suffered from a significant drop in intensity away from the mid-plane, which is a well-known drawback of the Feldkamp algorithm (Figure 6). On the other hand, the nonlinear weighted hybrid algorithm improved the image quality remarkably, giving a better image quality than the Feldkamp, P-FDK, and T-FDK algorithms. Specifically, the nonlinear weighted hybrid algorithm suppressed artifacts very well, even for a fairly large cone angle that was several times larger than that with the traditional Feldkamp, P-FDK, and T-FDK reconstructions for similar image quality.

3.1.4 *Effectiveness of reduced X-ray scatter methods*

The effect of scatter from a 3D object which is incident on two dimensions of a detector with a large field cannot be ignored. We confirmed that a capping phenomenon that decreases the pixel value of a rearranged image results when the scatter of the content increases in the center of the subject. We used a bow-tie filter to correct this capping and could suppress the capping for intensity distribution so that direct X-ray intensity after subject transmission becomes same (Figure 7). When a pixel value of a rearrangement image does not use a bow-tie filter, there is a tendency to decrease large in image edge regions, but can confirm what is improved when bow-tie filter is used (Figure 8).

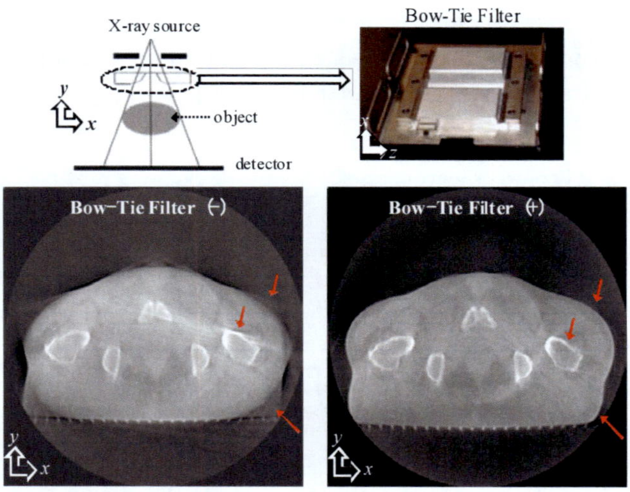

Figure 7. Real and slices of the human pelvis (prostate) at axial direction with bow-tie filtering and non bow-tie filtering processing, respectively.

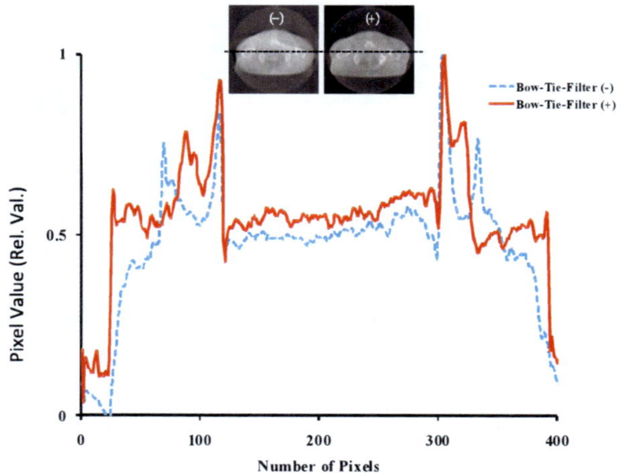

Figure 8. Intensity profiles (The central horizontal line in the selected slice of the human pelvic image).

3.2 Tomosynthesis System

Existing tomosynthesis algorithms can be divided into three categories: backprojection algorithms, FBP algorithms, and iterative algorithms. The conventional tomosynthesis reconstruction algorithm is called “shift-and-add” (SAA), whereby projection images taken at different angles are electronically shifted and added to generate an image plane focused at a certain depth below the surface. The projection shift is adjusted so that the visibility of features in the selected plane is enhanced while those in other planes are blurred. Using a digital detector, image planes at all depths can be retrospectively reconstructed from one set of projections. The SAA algorithm is valid only if the motion of the X-ray focal spot is parallel to the detector. FBP algorithms are widely used in CT in which many projections (typically a few hundred to about one thousand) acquired over 360 degree are used to reconstruct cross-sectional images. The X-ray tube and detector are rotated during CT acquisition. The Fourier central slice theorem has a fundamental role in FBP theory. In 2D CT imaging, a projection of an object corresponds to sampling the object along the direction perpendicular to the X-ray beam in the Fourier space [57].

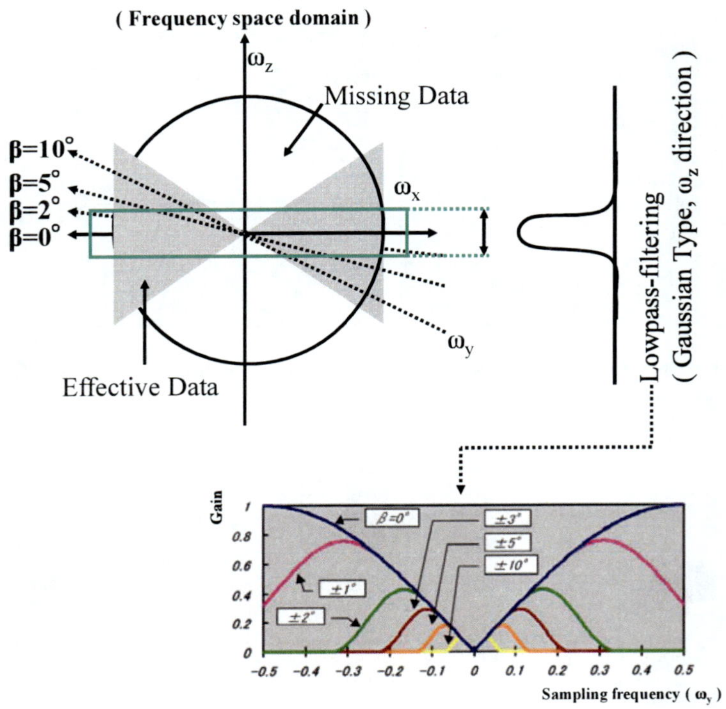

Figure 9. Illustration of the effective area and defect area in tomosynthesis.The Fourier space data having undergone three-dimensional Fourier transform have missing cones centred on the ω_z -axis, with the vertices, meeting at the origin of the Fourier space coordinates. Thus, Fourier space low-pass filtering is characterized by applying a low-pass filter in the direction of the sectional axis to lessen the influence of the missing cone data.

For many projections, information about the object is well sampled and the object can be restored by combining the information from all projections. In 3D cone-beam imaging, the information about the object in Fourier space is related to the Radon transform of the object. The relation between the Radon transform and the cone-beam projections has been well studied and solutions to the cone-beam reconstruction have been provided [58–59]. An iterative algorithm performs the reconstruction in a recursive fashion [60–61], unlike the one-step operation in the backprojection and FBP algorithms. During iterative reconstruction, a 3D object model is repeatedly updated until the model converges to the solution that optimizes an objective function. The objective function defines the criteria of the reconstruction solution. The maximum likelihood (ML) algorithm, a widely used iterative algorithm, was the comparison study in this manuscript. The objective function in the ML algorithm is the likelihood function, which is the probability of getting the measured projections in a given object model. The solution of the ML algorithm is an object model that maximizes the probability of getting the measured projections.

3.2.1 Reconstruction algorithm

A modified FBP algorithm has been reported that provides a description of filtering that can used in combination with backprojection to yield tomosynthesis slice images with desired properties [62]. The following description of the generalized 3D impulse function is adapted from this previous work [44]. The 3D version of the Fourier slice theorem states that when a 2D image of an object is acquired at some particular orientation to that object, the 2D Fourier transform of that projection image yields a plane through the 3D Fourier space of the object. Characteristics are estimated in the modified FBP by low-pass filtering processing. The Fourier space low-pass filtering unit applies a low-pass filter in the direction along the sectional axis of the Fourier space data that have undergone a 3D Fourier transform (Figure 9). This process is effective in reducing artifacts in the 3D volume data generated by a 3D back Fourier transform of the Fourier space data after low-pass filtering. The 3D Fourier transform of the 3D volume data generated by the backprojection is based on the following equation (23):

$$F(\omega_x,\omega_y,\omega_z) = \iiint f(x,y,z)\cdot \exp\{-j(\omega_x\cdot x+\omega_y\cdot y+\omega_z\cdot z)\}dx\cdot dy\cdot dz \qquad (23)$$

where $f(x,y,z)$ is the simple backprojection intermediate image, and x, y, and z are real numbers. The meaning of the filtering process performed in 3D Fourier space is described below, and it is mathematically expressed by the following equation (24):

$$FM(\omega_x,\omega_y,\omega_z) = F(\omega_x,\omega_y,\omega_z)\cdot M(\omega_x,\omega_y,\omega_z) \qquad (24)$$

where $FM(\omega_x,\omega_y,\omega_z)$ is the filtered 3D Fourier distribution image, and $M(\omega_x,\omega_y,\omega_z)$ is a function representing filter characteristics. The filtering process carried out in 3D Fourier space is to weight the 3D Fourier distribution image of complex data with the real-valued filter function M dependent on the respective frequency values. The weighting function M is compressed in the ω_z direction. $M(\omega_x,\omega_y,\omega_z)$ is expressed by the following equation (25) as a product of three functions representing the filter characteristic:

$$M(\omega_x, \omega_y, \omega_z) = H_{prof}(\omega_z) \cdot H_{spec}(\omega_r) \cdot H_{inverse}(\omega R) \tag{25}$$

A typical example of each filter function system shown in equation (3) is described next. $H_{prof}(\omega_z)$ has a low-pass filter characteristic, i.e., a Gaussian characteristic, which is expressed by the following equation (26):

$$H_{prof}(\omega_z) = \exp\left(-0.693 \left[\frac{\omega_z}{CFD} \right]^2 \right) \tag{26}$$

where CFD is the frequency with the Gaussian attenuation halved.

$H_{spec}(\omega_r)$ has a filter characteristic which is expressed by the following equation (27):

$$\begin{cases} H_{spec}(\omega_r) = 1 & \left(case \quad \omega_r < \frac{CFR - WFR}{2} \right) \\ H_{spec}(\omega_r) = \frac{1 - \sin(\omega_r - CFR) \cdot \pi / WFR}{2} & \left(case \quad \frac{CFR - WFR}{2} < \omega_r < \frac{CFR + WFR}{2} \right). \\ H_{spec}(\omega_r) = 0 & \left(case \quad \frac{CFR + WFR}{2} < \omega_r \right) \end{cases} \tag{27}$$

However, $\omega_r = \sqrt{\omega_x^{\ 2} + \omega_y^{\ 2} + \omega_z^{\ 2}}$. The function has a sine wave form with high-frequency components smoothly attenuated. CFR is the cut-off frequency, and WFR is the total transition frequency width of the filter strength. $\frac{CFR + WFR}{2}$ is the Nyquist frequency and $\frac{CFR - WFR}{2}$ is the no-processing region frequency. This $H_{spec}(\omega_r)$ removes high-frequency components from the origin of the 3D Fourier space. $H_{inverse}(\omega R)$ has a filter characteristic which is expressed by the following equation (28):

$$H_{inverse}(\omega R) = |\omega R| \qquad , \qquad \omega R = \sqrt{\omega_x^{\ 2} + \omega_y^{\ 2}} \tag{28}$$

The 3D back Fourier transforms the Fourier space data back to 3D volume data, having undergone Fourier space low-pass filtering. The 3D back Fourier transform is expressed by the following equation (29):

$$fm(x, y, z) = \frac{1}{8}\pi^3 \iiint FM(\omega_x, \omega_y, \omega_z) \cdot \exp\{j(\omega_x\ x + \omega_y\ y + \omega_z\ z)\} d\omega_x d\omega_y d\omega_z \tag{29}$$

where equation (29) is the transformation from the frequency domain to the space domain. It is the inverse of the relation described by equation (23).

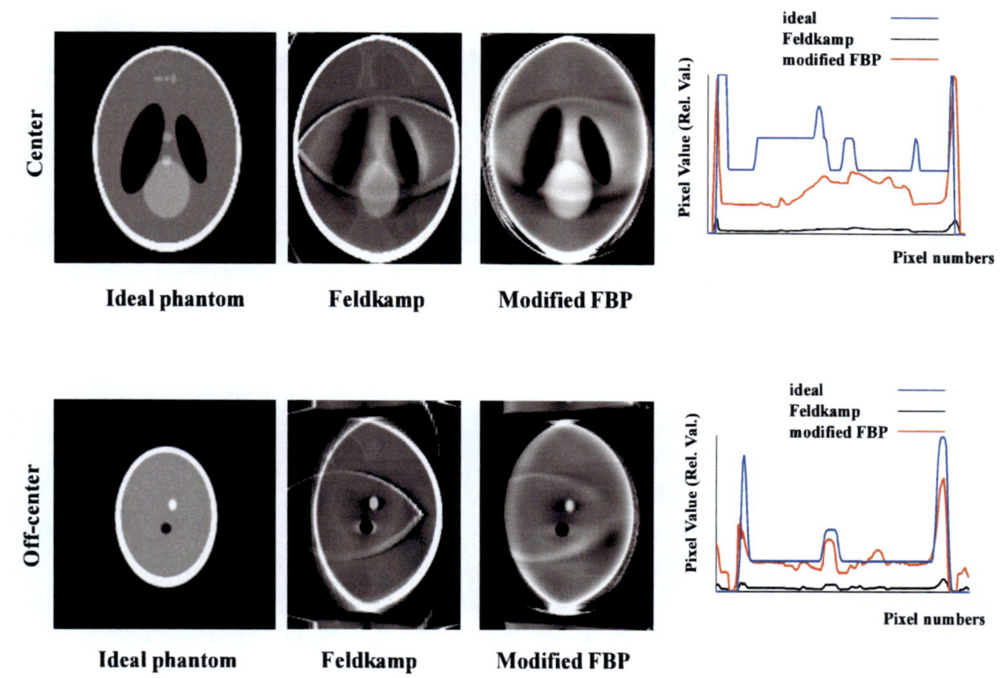

Figure 10. Reconstruction simulation images of the 3D Shepp-Logan phantom at different heights. In addition, comparison of axial profile plots through the reconstructed 3D image function in comparison with discretization of the 3D Shepp-Logan phantom.

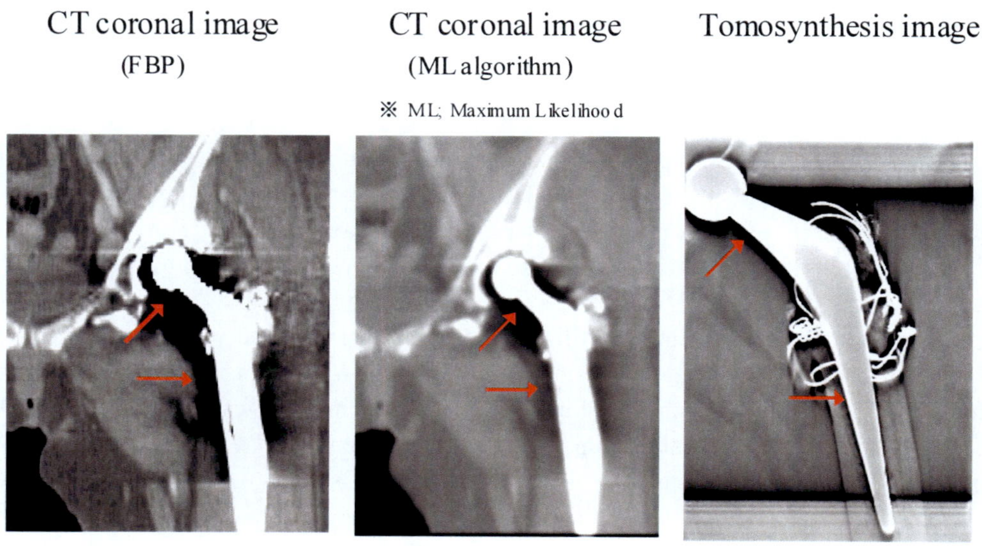

Figure 11. Tomosynthesis and CT (FBP and ML algorithm) images of the hip prostheses at same heights. (soft-tissue information)

3.2.1 (a) Conventional FBP vs. modified FBP

The simulation requires the program to be fed with data concerning the geometrical layout (detector, source, and trajectories) and the virtual object (phantom), and it is necessary to specify which physical effects (beam hardening, partial occlusion) should be simulated. Projections of a 3D Shepp–Logan phantom object, centered at the origin, were simulated with a tomographic angle of 40.8 degree. A dataset with 90 views was generated to examine the Feldkamp and modified FBP algorithms. This simulation was performed under the same conditions (tomographic angle, pixel size, and view number) as real scan examinations (Figure 10). The source-to-origin distance was set to 511 mm. The source-to-detector distance was set to 1024 mm. The detector type was a rectangular plane. The detector size was set to 512 × 512 pixels (216 × 216 mm^2). The reconstruction grid was set to 512 × 512 × 512 voxels. The detector was assumed to have a pixel size of 421 mm and the images were backprojected onto a 200 mm pixel grid.

3.2.1 (b) CT vs. modified FBP

X-ray CT has matured over the last three decades, and it is now a powerful tool in medical diagnostics. As a noninvasive imaging technique, CT has become essential, especially since the advent of spiral CT in the 1990s, which led to shorter scan times and improved 3D spatial resolution. CT provides high resolution in the tomographic plane but limited resolution in the axial direction. Therefore, the partial-volume effect may make it difficult to evaluate structures that are not oriented in the direction of the CT tomographic plane. However, the quality of images generated with a CT scanner can still be reduced by the presence of metal objects in the field of view. Imaging of patients with metal implants, such as marker pins, dental fillings, or hip prostheses, suffer from artifacts, generally in the form of bright and dark streaks, cupping and capping, etc (Figures 11-12). These artifacts are mostly due to quantum noise, scattered radiation, and beam hardening [55]. Metal artifacts influence image quality by reducing contrast and by obscuring details, thus impairing the detectability of structures of interest, which can make a diagnosis impossible. In addition, CT values are impaired, which can lead to errors in using these data, such as in attenuation correction in PET/CT [56]. The metallic components of arthroplasty devices are high-contrast objects, and as such generate artifacts when imaged using CT scans. These artifacts can make it extremely difficult or impossible to interpret images of these devices. These artifacts, along with the partial-volume effect, severely limit the potential for objective quantification of total joint replacements with CT.

Methods for reduction of metal artifacts aim to improve the quality of images affected by this type of artifact. In recent years, modified iterative [63–66] or wavelet reconstruction techniques [67] have produced promising results, but these methods cannot be combined with the fast and robust FBP algorithm, which is the standard reconstruction technique implemented in modern CT scanners.

3.2.1 (c) Metal artifact reduction processing [68]

Artifacts caused by high-attenuation features in hip prostheses were observed in digital linear tomosynthesis reconstruction as a result of the small number of projections and the narrow angular range typically employed in tomosynthesis imaging. We developed artifact reduction methods based on a modified Shepp–Logan reconstruction filter kernel, realized by taking into account additional weighting by direct current components in the frequency domain space. Processing leads to an increase in the ratio of low-frequency components in an image (Figure 13).

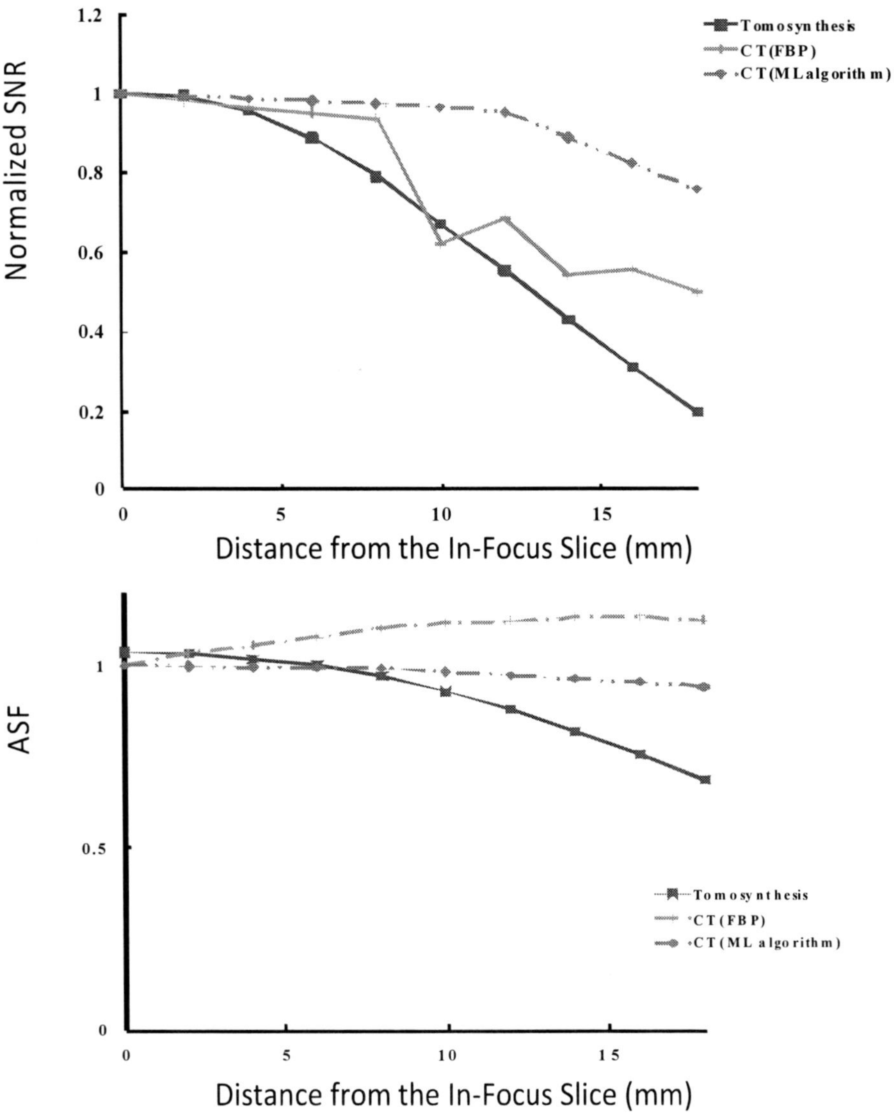

Figure 12. Artifact spread function (ASF) and signal-to-noise ratio (SNR) versus distance from the in-focus plane for each algorithm. (Wu et al. [54] proposed an ASF metric to quantify artifacts observed in planes outside the focus image plane. The SNR is defined as $(N_1\text{-}N_0) / \sigma_0$, where N_1 is the mean pixel value in the region of interest (ROI) within the normal bone object , N_0 is the mean pixel value in the ROI in a background area, and σ_0 is the standard deviation of pixel value in the background ROI)

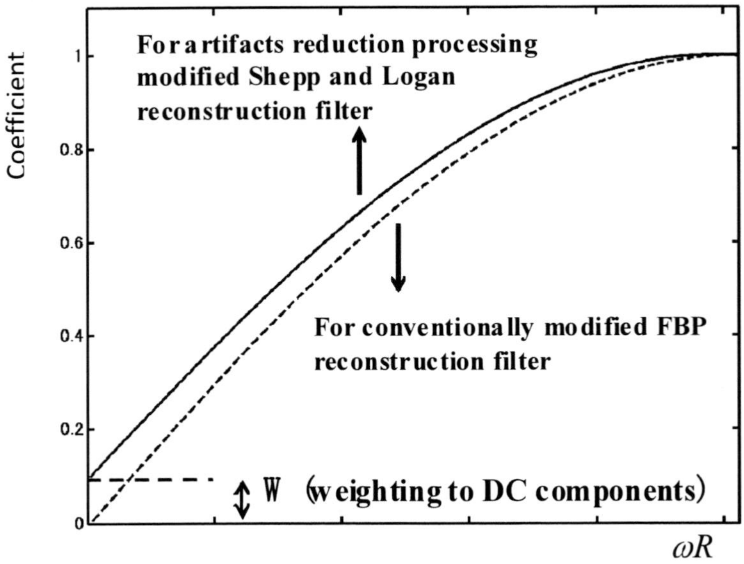

Figure 13. Concept of the new artifact reduction processing method. It can consider weighing by direct current (DC) components to be processed similar to the image that multiplied the different weight coefficient by and added to the shift image and the conventionally modified FBP image.

Artifact reduction processing was performed with a basic and modified FBP algorithm. Artifact reduction processing provides a method of filtering that can be used in combination with backprojection to yield tomosynthesis sliced images with desired properties (Figures 14-16).

$H_{inverse}(\omega R)$ has a filter characteristic expressed by the following equation (30):

$$\omega_{R\_temp} = W + \sqrt{\omega_x^{\ 2} + \omega_y^{\ 2}}$$

$$\omega_{R\_norm} = \frac{\omega_{R\_temp}}{\omega_{R\_\max}}$$

$$H_{inverse}(\omega R) = \left|\omega_{R\_norm}\right| \tag{30}$$

where W is the addition of a direct current component (Figure 13). $\omega_{R\_\max}$ is the maximum value of a ω_{R_temp} value. The characteristics in the negative direction along the horizontal axis are omitted because these are in linear symmetry about the vertical axis with the characteristics in the positive direction. $H_{spec}(\omega_r)\cdot H_{inverse}(\omega R)$ is expressed by the following equation (31):

$$\begin{cases} H_{spec}(\omega_r)\cdot H_{inverse}(\omega R) = \frac{2_{\rho H}}{\pi}\left|\left|\omega_{R\_norm}\right| + sin\left(\frac{\pi\rho}{2_{\rho H}}\right)\right| & (|\rho| \le \rho H) \\ \\ H_{spec}(\omega_r)\cdot H_{inverse}(\omega R) = 0 & (|\rho| > \rho H) \end{cases} \tag{31}$$

ρH is the Nyquist frequency $\left(\frac{CFR+WFR}{2}\right)$ and ρ is the no-processing region frequency $\left(\frac{CFR-WFR}{2}\right)$.

The 3D back Fourier transforms the Fourier space data back to 3D volume data, having undergone Fourier space low-pass filtering.

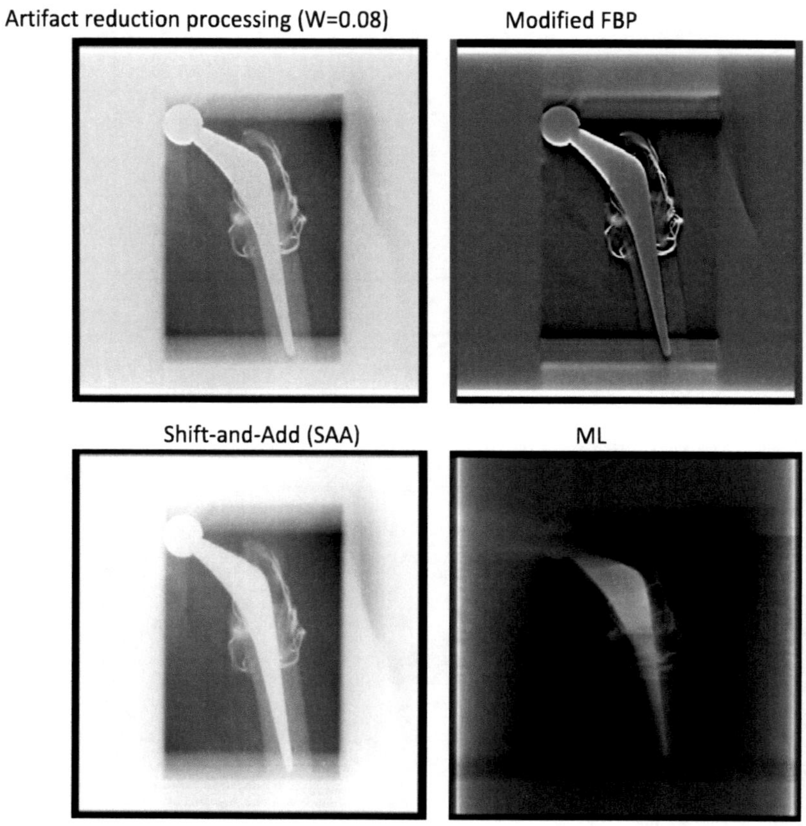

Figure 14. Comparison of artifact reduction processing images with images obtained from artifact reduction processing, conventionally modified FBP, shift-and-add (SAA) and ML algorithms of the in-focus plane. Artifact reduction processing provided better visualization of the hip prosthesis by eliminating blurring and reducing above and below visualized planes.

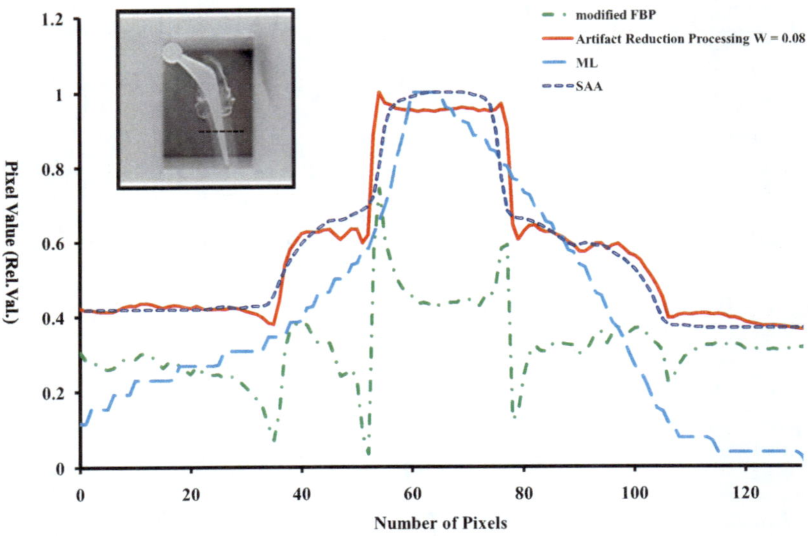

Figure 15. Comparison of line profiles using artifact reduction processing, modified FBP, SAA, and ML algorithms in the in-focus plane. Artifacts (part of undershooting) are reduced by artifact reduction processing.

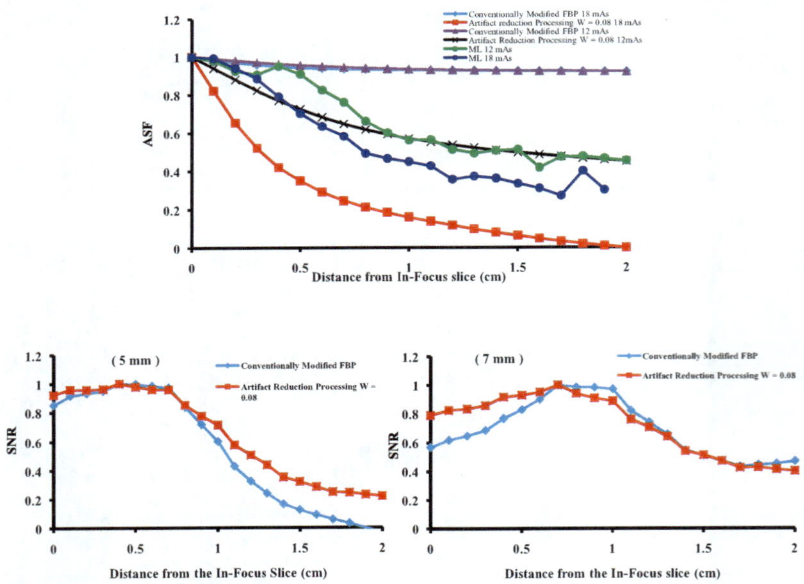

Figure 16. top column; Comparison of an ASF and conventionally modified FBP and ML algorithms using the same weighting coefficients of DC components (70 kVp, W=0.08) in the distance from the in-focus plane. Artifacts are reduced by artifact reduction processing. ASF realizes is improved by radiation dose increase. bottom column; Comparison of the SNR using different signal size (5 and 7 mm φ) of DC components and conventionally modified FBP algorithm in the distance from the in-focus plane. The SNR improves with artifact reduction processing.

4. Future Directions

4.1 Cone-Beam CT

In the reconstruction of cone-beam CT, when a wide imaging range is required, FBP processing that takes account of the cone angle is needed. This reproduces subject information as faithfully as possible, and ideally, 3D FBP processing should be used in such a manner as to prevent deterioration of image artifacts. One of the image quality improvement problems of cone-beam CT is to develop a reconstruction method to reduce the cone-beam artifact. Another problem in image quality improvement is the effect of x-ray scatter. In the trial that used bow-tie filter, image processing disappeared. According to the manufacturer, owing to the use of the cone-shaped X-ray beam and the "smart beam technology," the absorbed dose from a cone-beam CT scan is approximately equivalent to two to five panoramic exposures; however, this claim needs further investigation.

Clinical reports have indicated the usefulness of cone-beam CT in an angiography system and image-guided radiation therapy in a current medical service system. However, cone-beam artifact and scatter measures are problems affecting the image quality of the reconstruction image. Many researchers suggest that computer simulation methods may improve control over the cone-beam artifact. Other reports indicate that it can reduce scatter X-ray measure by bow-tie filtering and image processing.

4.2 Tomosynthesis

The digital tomosynthesis images in this study were acquired using linear motion of the X-ray tube and detector. The type of motion used during data acquisition dictates the type of blurring of off-focal-plane objects in the image. Linear motion blurs objects in one dimension only, which leads to linear streak artifacts caused by high-contrast off-focal-plane objects. On the other hand, 3D reconstruction schemes (tomosynthesis and CT) require complete knowledge of the X-ray source projection geometry prior to exposure. This limitation precludes much of the potential task-dependent flexibility. The optical analog would be a photographer limited to a camera with no provision for adjusting its f-stop. This limitation also precludes accurate reconstruction from projections acquired from a patient who moves unpredictably between exposures because this is geometrically equivalent to not knowing the projection geometry.

Image reconstruction schemes may be selected by taking the metric outcome into consideration. It seems that the number of projections, the total exposure dose, and the pixel size of the detector are better than with tomosynthesis. Ideally, the number of X-ray quanta for the reconstruction of this voxel equals that from a single projection acquired with the same amount of total exposure. The effect of projection angle, which decreases photon transmission and reduces the effective detector pixel size, also reduces the SNR further.

Artifact reduction processing showed an adequate overall performance, but its effectiveness strongly depended on the image region. Digital linear tomosynthesis images gave good results independently of the type of metal present in the patient and showed good results for the removal of noise artifacts (particularly at greater distances from metal objects). The application of digital linear tomosynthesis to the imaging of hip prostheses appears promising. The 3D visualization of hip joints on images with artifact reduction processing is far superior to that on images processed with conventionally modified FBP and ML algorithms. Flexibility in the choice of imaging parameters in artifact reduction processing based on the desired final images and realistic imaging conditions may be beneficial.

REFERENCES

[1] Grangeat, P; Sire, P; Guillemaud, R; La, V. *Computational Imaging and Vision: Three-Dimensional Image Reconstruction in Radiology and Nuclear Medicine* (Kluwer, Dordrecht), 1996.

[2] Grangeat, P; Sire, P; Guillemaud, R; La, V. *Contemporary Perspectives in Three-Dimensional Biomedical Imaging: Indirect Cone-beam Three-Dimensional Image Reconstruction* (IOP Press), 1997.

[3] PMB, "1997 International Meeting on Fully Three-Dimensional Image Reconstruction in Radiology and Nuclear Medicine" *Phys. Med. Biol.*, 1998, 43.

[4] Carlsson, CA. "Imaging modalities in x-ray computerized tomography and in selected volume tomography," Phys. Med. Biol., 1999, 44, 23-56.

[5] Sliver, MD. "High Helical pitch cone-beam computed tomography," *Phys. Med. Biol.*, 1998, 43, 847-856.

[6] Tam, KC; Samarasekera, S; Sauer, F. "Exact cone-beam CT with a spiral scan," *Phys. Med. Biol.*, 1998, 43, 1015-1024.

[7] Taguchi, K; Aradate, H. "Algorithm for image reconstruction in multi-slice helical CT," *Med. Phys.*, 1998, 25, 550-561.

[8] Noo, F; Defrise, M; Clack, R. *"Single-slice rebinning method for helical cone-beam CT," Phys. Med. Biol.*, 1999, 44, 561-570.

[9] Kudo, H; Noo, F. *"Cone-beam filtered backprojection algorithm for truncated helical data," Phys. Med. Biol.*, 1998, 43, 2885-2909.

[10] Feldkamp, LA; Davis, LC; Kress, JW. "Practical cone-beam algorithm," *J. Opt. Soc.* Am. A, 1, 1984, 612-619.

[11] Tuy, HK. "An inversion formula for cone-beam reconstruction," *SIAM J. Appl. Math*, 1983, 43, 546-552.

[12] Smith, BD. "Image reconstruction from cone-beam projections: necessary and sufficient conditions and reconstruction methods," *IEEE Trans. Med. Imaging*, 1985, 4, 14-25.

[13] Grass, M; et al., "3D cone-beam CT reconstruction for circular trajectory," *Phys. Med. Biol.*, 2000, 45, 329-347.

[14] Turbell, H. 2001, *"Cone-beam reconstruction using filtered backprojection,"* Linkoping Studies in Science and Technology, Thesis No 672.

[15] Noo, F; Kudo, H; Defrise, M. "Approximate Short-scan Filtered backprojection for Helical CB Reconstruction," *IEEE Nuclear Science Symposium,* 1998, 3, 2073-2077.

[16] Flohr, T. "Clinical benefits of a multi row detector spiral CT system," *Radiology*, 1997, 205, 214-215.

[17] Hu, H. "Multi-slice helical CT: Scan and reconstruction," *Med. Phys.*, 1999, 26, 5-18.

[18] Wang, G; Vannier, MW. "Pitch analysis in multi-slice spiral/helical CT," *Med. Phys.*, 1999, 26, 2648-2653.

[19] Katsevich, A. "Theoretically exact filtered backprojection-type inversion algorithms for spiral CT," SIAM (Soc. Ind. Appl. Math) *J. Appl. Math*, 2002, 62, 2012-2026.
[20] Wang, G; Lin, TH; Cheng, PC; Shinozaki, DM. "A general cone-beam reconstruction algorithm," *IEEE Trans. Med. Imaging,* 1993, 17, 261-370.
[21] Anxionnat, R; Bracard, S; Macho, J; Da Costa, E; Vaillant, R; Launay, L; et al. 3D angiography. Clinical interest. First applications in interventional neroradiology. *J Neuroradiol*, 1998, 25(4), 251-262.
[22] EI Sheik; M; Heverhagen, JT; Alfke, H; Froelich, JJ; Hornegger, J; Brunner, T; et al. Multiplanar reconstructions and three-dimensional imaging (computed rotational osteography) of complex fractures by using a C-arm system:initial results. *Radiology,* 2001, 221(3), 843-849.
[23] Linsenmaier, U; Rock, C; Euler, E; Wirth, S; Brandl, R; Kotsianos, D; et al. Three-dimensional CT with a modified C-arm image intensifier: feasibility. *Radiology,* 2002, 224(1), 286-292.
[24] Letourneau, D; Wong, JW; Oldham, M; et al. Cone-beam-CT guided radiation therapy: technical implementation. *Radiother Oncol*, 2005, 75(3), 279-286.
[25] Nakagawa, K; Yamashita, H; Shiraishi, K et al. Verification of in-treatment tumor position using kilovoltage cone-beam computed tomography: a preliminary syudy. *Int J Radiation Oncology Biol Phys*., 2007, 69(4), 970-973.
[26] Baba, R; Konno, Y; Ueda, K; et al. Comparison of flat-panel detector and image-intensifier detector for cone-beam CT. *Computerized Medical Imaging and Graphics*, 2002, 26(3), 152-158.
[27] Mori, S; Endo, M; Komatsu, S; et al. A combination-weighted Feldkamp-based reconstruction algorithm for cone-beam CT. *Phys Med Biol.*, 2006, 51(16), 3953-3965.
[28] Mori, S; Endo, M; Tsunoo, T; et al. Physical performance evaluation of a 256-slice CT-scanner for four-dimensional imaging. *Med Phys.*, *2004*, 31(6), 1348-1356.
[29] Gomi, T; Koshida, K; Miyati, T. Development of a non-linear weighted hybrid cone-beam CT reconstruction for circular trajectories. *Computerized Medical Imaging and Graphics*, 2007, 31(7), 561-569.
[30] Ziedses des Plante, BG. Eine neue methode zur differenzierung in der roentgenographie (planigraphie). *Acta Radiol,* 1932, 13, 182-92.
[31] Grant, DG. omosynthesis. A three-dimensional radiographic imaging technique. *IEEE Trans Biomed*, 1972, 19, 20-8.
[32] Stiel, G; Stiel, LG; Klotz, E; Nienaber, CA. Digital flashing tomosynthesis: A promising technique for angiographic screening. *IEEE Trans Med Imaging*, 1993, 12, 314-21.
[33] Warp, RJ; Godfrey, DG; Dobbins, JT. Applications of matrix inverse tomosynthesis. *Proc SPIE*, 2000, 3977, 376-83.
[34] Duryea, J; Dobbins, JT; Lynch, JA. Digital tomosynthesis of hand joints for arthritis assessment. *Med Phys.*, 2003, 30, 325-33.
[35] Sone, S; Kasuga, T; Sakai, F; Kawai, T; Oguchi, K; Hirano, H; et al. Image processing in the digital tomosynthesis for pulmonary imaging. *Eur Radiol*, 1995, 5, 96-101.
[36] Badea, C; Kolitsi, Z; Pallikarakis, N. A 3D imaging system for dental imaging based on digital tomosynthesis and cone beam CT. *Proc Int Federation Med Biol Eng.*, 2001, 2, 739-41.

[37] Niklason, LT; Christian, BT; Niklason, LE; Kopans, DB; Castleberry, DE; Opsahl-Ong BH; et al. *Digital tomosynthesis in breast imaging. Radiology*, 1997, 205, 399-406.
[38] Dobbins 3rd, JT; Godfrey, DJ. Digital x-ray tomosynthesis: curent state of the art and clinical potential. *Phy Med Biol.*, 2003, 48, R65-106.
[39] Edholm, P; Granlund, G; Knutsson, H; Petersson, C. Ectomography-a new radiographic method for reproducing a selected slice of varying thickness. *Acta Radiol*, 1980, 21, 433-42.
[40] Knutsson, HE; Edholm, P; Granlund, GH; Petersson, CU. Ectomography-a new radiographic reconstruction method. 1.Theory and error estimates. *IEEE Trans Biomed Eng.*, 1980, 27, 640-8.
[41] Petersson, CU; Edholm, P; Granlund, GH; Knutsson, HE. Ectomography-a new radiographic reconstruction method. 2.Computer-simulated experiments. *IEEE Trans Biomed Eng.*, 1980, 27, 649-55.
[42] Matsuo, H; Iwata, A; Horiba, I; Suzumura, N. 3-Dimensional image reconstruction by digital tomo-synthesis using inverse filtering. *IEEE Trans Med Imaging*, 1993, 12, 307-13.
[43] Badea, C; Kolitsi, Z; Pallikarakis, N. Image quality in extend arc filtered digital tomosynthesis. *Acta Radiol*, 2001, 42, 244-8.
[44] Lauritsch, G; Harer, WH. A theoretical framework for filtered backprojection in tomosynthesis. *Proc SPIE*, 1998, 3338, 1127-37.
[45] Stevens, GM; Fahrig, R; Pelc, NJ. Filtered backprojection for modifying the impulse response of circular tomosynthesis. *Med Phys.*, 2001, 28, 372-80.
[46] Stevens, GM. Volumetric tomographic imaging. *Thesis,* 2001.
[47] Ruttimann, UE; Groenhuis, RAJ; Webber, RL. Restoration of digital multiple tomosynthesis by a constrained iteration method. *IEEE Trans Med Imaging*, 1984, 3, 141-8.
[48] van der Stelt, PF; Ruttimann, UE; Webber, RL. Enhancement of tomosynthesis images in dental radiology. *J Dent Res.*, 1986, 65, 967-73.
[49] Engelke, W; Ruttimann, UE Tsuchimochi, M; Bacher, JD. An experimental study of new diagnostic methods for the examination of osseous lesions in the temporomandibular joint. *Oral Surg Oral Med Oral Pathol*, 1992, 73, 348-59.
[50] Webber, RL; Underhill, HR; Freimanis, RL. A controlled evaluation of tuned-aperture computed tomography applied to digital spot mammography. *J Dig Imaging,* 2000, 13, 90-7.
[51] Suryanarayanan, S; Karellas, A; Vedantham, S; Glick, SJ; D'Orsi, CJ; Baker, SP; et al. Comparison of tomosynthesis methods used with digital mammography. *Acta Radiol*, 2000, 7, 1085-97.
[52] Bleuet, P; Guillemaud, R; Desbat, L; & Magnin, I. An adapted fan volume sampling scheme for 3-D algebraic reconstruction in linear tomosynthesis. *IEEE Trans Nucl Sci.*, 2002, 49, 2366-72.
[53] Wu, T; Stewart, A; Stanton, M; McCauley, T; Phillips, W; Kopans, DB; et al. Tomographic mammography using a limited number of low-dose cone-beam projection images. *Med Phys.*, 2003, 30, 365-80.
[54] Wu, T; Moore, RH; Kopans, DB. Voting strategy for artifact reduction in digital breast tomosynthesis. *Med Phys.*, 2006, 33, 2461-71.

[55] Hsieh, J. Image artifacts; causes; and correction. In: LW; Goleman, JB; Fowlkes, (Eds). *Medical CT and ultrasound; current technology and applications; Madison: Advanced Medical Publishing,* 1995, 487-518.

[56] Kamel, EM; Burger, C; Buck, A; von Schulthess, GK; Goerres, GW. Impact of metallic dental implants on CT-based attenuation correction in a combined PET/CT scanner. *Eur Radiol*, 2003, 13, 724-8.

[57] Kak, A; Slaney, M. Principles of computerized tomographic imaging. New York:*IEEE*, 1988.

[58] Smith, DB. Image reconstruction from cone-beam projections: necessary and sufficient conditions and reconstruction methods. *IEEE Trans Med Imaging*, 1985, M1-4, 14-25.

[59] Grangeat, P. Mathematical framework of cone-beam 3D reconstruction via the first derivative of the Radon transform. *Math Methods Tomogr*, 1991, 13, 66-97.

[60] Ruttimann, U; Groenhuis, R; Webber, R. Restoration of digital multilane tomosynthesis by a constrained iteration method. *IEEE Trans Med Imaging*, 1984, MI-3, 141-8.

[61] Bleuet, P; Guillemaud, R; Magin, I; Desbat, L. An adapted fan volume sampling scheme for 3D algebraic reconstruction in linear tomosynthesis. *IEEE Trans Nucl Sci.*, 2002, 49, 2366-72.

[62] Gomi, T; Hirano, H. Clinical potential of digital linear tomosynthesis imaging of total joint artroplasty. *J Digit Imaging*, 2008, 21(3), 312-22.

[63] Wang, G; Snyder, DL; O'Sullivan, JA; et al. Iterative debluring for metal artifacts reduction. *IEEE Trans. Med. Imaging*, 1996, 15, 657-664.

[64] Wang, G; Vannier, MW; Cheng, PC. X-ray cone-beam tomography for metal artifacts reduction and local region reconstruction. *Microsc Microanal*, 1999, 5, 58-65.

[65] Wang, G; Frei, T; Vannier, MW. A fast iterative algorithm for metal artifact reduction in x-ray CT. *Acad. Radiol,* 2000, 7, 607-614.

[66] Man B, De; Nuyts, J; Dupont, P; et al. Reduction of metal streak artifacts in x-ray computed tomography using a transmission maximum a posteriori algorithm. *IEEE Trans. Nucl. Sci.*, 2000, 47, 997-981.

[67] Robertson, DD; Yuan, J; Wang, G; Vannier, MW. Total hip prosthesis metal-artifact suppression using iterative deblurring reconstruction. *J. Comp. Assist. Tomog*, 1997, 21, 293-298.

[68] Gomi, T; Hirano, H; Umeda, T. Evaluation of the X-ray digital linear tomosynthesis reconstruction processing method for metal artifact reduction. *Computerized Medical Imaging and Graphics*, 2009, 33(7), 257-274.

In: 3D Imaging: Theory, Technology … ISBN: 978-1-60876-885-1
Editors: E. H. Duke and S. R. Aguirre, pp.139-157

Chapter 5

BIOLUMINESCENCE *IN VIVO* IMAGING OF ORTHOTOPICALLY IMPLANTED TUMOR CELLS IN THE PRECLINICAL DRUG DISCOVERY

Ralph Graeser and Norbert Esser
ProQinase GmbH, Freiburg, Germany

ABSTRACT

Since the 1970s, human tumor cell lines, subcutaneously implanted into immunodeficient mice, rapidly advanced to become the most important pre-clinical efficacy models. However, in recent years, doubts concerning their predictive value increased. A part of the problem may reside within the combination of tumor cell lines selected for fast growth through many rounds of passaging in 2D-petri dish cultures, with the artificial subcutaneous implantation site. Recent evidence pointed towards an important role of the stromal compartment for many aspects of tumorigenesis. Along with other groups, we therefore set out to implant tumor cell lines orthotopically, i.e. into the organ of their origin. This technique requires surgery, and, since the tumors don't grow visibly, a sensitive imaging system for the detection of the implanted cells. A variety of tools have been developed that provide the sensitivity required, some only applicable for experimental models, e.g. fluorescence (GFP, RFP...), and bioluminescence, others, e.g. PET/CT or MRI translatable to the clinic. Bioluminescence imaging (BLI) was our choice due to its cost-effectiveness compared to the latter, and the excellent signal to noise ratio. Tumor cells thus need to be transduced with luciferase before surgical implantation into the given organ. BLI may then be used to check implantation to the correct site, growth of the tumors, and randomization of the mice into treatment groups. Upon treatment start, the effect of the drug on primary tumor and metastases may be monitored via weekly BLI measurements. Upon termination of the experiment, organs may be investigated for metastatic tumor cells via BLI, or by homogenization followed by quantitative *in vitro* luciferase assays.

This set-up has been successfully applied to test novel treatments, or novel formulations of classical chemotherapy. It allows to distinguish between drug action against the primary tumor or metastases, yielding quantitative results.

INTRODUCTION

An efficient filter is required to select compounds that are effective not only *in vitro* or *in cellulo*, but also in a whole organism. Thus, pre-clinical development of novel compounds requires animal testing, which, for efficacy studies, mainly includes mouse studies. However, the predictivity of such models was questioned from the very beginning. Syngeneic mouse models, which became available for drug testing in the early 1950s, were criticized for their fast growth, and their murine origin. Indeed, mainly cytotoxic compounds active against fast growing tumors emerged from campaigns using these models (1). With the advent of the nude mouse in the beginning of the 1970s, the growth of human tumor cells in the mouse became possible. This solved both issues mentioned above. Not only could human tumor cell lines be used, but these cells also tended to grow somewhat slowlier than their murine counterparts. Even so, issues about the predictive value of mouse models in general prevail (2, 3). Reasons for the failure to correctly predict the clinical outcome of a test compound include tumor cell lines that may have lost many of their original characteristics through too many passages *in vitro*, and the very artificial subcutaneous implantation site. In the first section, we will discuss some of the reasons why we think that orthotopic tumor models are superior to their subcutaneous counterparts. In the following section we will then discuss sensitive imaging modalities used to detect orthotopically implanted tumor cells. Finally we will elaborate on experiences using bioluminescence for orthotopic tumor models, and their use in pre-clinical drug development.

Mouse models

Subcutaneous / ectopic implantation

Since the 1970s, growing human tumor cell lines subcutaneously in rodents has become the standard way to pre-clinically test novel compounds. Reasons are availability of a wide range of well-characterised, established cell lines and relative ease and reproducibility of tumor inoculation and growth measurement in nude mice. As mentioned in the above section, however, the quality of these models have recently become subject to serious controversy.

A part of the problem with human xenograft models may reside in the fact that repeated passaging of human tumor cell lines has selected for fast growing, undifferentiated and homogenous cell lines, which may have lost many of the features of the original tumor. Primary isolates passaged via continuous subcutaneous implantations seem to keep their original histiotype better (4-6).

Even using primary isolates, however, subcutaneously implanted tumor cells rarely metastasize. Amongst others, this may be due to a lack of organotypical stromal cell interactions and an aberrant vascularisation at the ectopic implantation sites. Since, in the human situation, many patients succumb to metastases rather than the primary tumor (which may often be surgically removed), the absence of metastases represents a major drawback of subcutaneous tumor models.

Orthotopic implantation

In contrast to subcutaneously engrafted cells, cells injected into the organ of their origin ('orthotopically') spread to metastatic sites in other organs, with specificities comparable to the human situation (7). Besides allowing the cells to spread, the organotypical stromal interaction that are allowed to occur in such orthotopic models may also affect the growth, differentiation, and drug sensitivity of the tumor cells.

The former two points were nicely shown in a study using three subtypes of a Dunning R3347 PCa syngenic rat prostate cancer cell line. When implanted either orthotopically or subcutaneously, differences between the subtypes became apparent with respect to their grade of differentiation, hormone-dependence, growth rate, vascularisation, as well as histiotype. Orthotopically implanted tumors tended to grow slower, preserved, in the case of the well differentiated subline, their differentiation, and had a higher microvessel density and more mature vessels than their subcutaneous implants (8).

Altered drug sensitivity, perhaps induced via tumor-stromal interactions at the orthotopic site could be shown using a CT-26 colon tumor cell line implanted into various sites in the mouse. When tested for their sensitivity towards doxorubicin or 5-FU, cells growing subcutaneously were most sensitive to doxorubicin, whereas their counterparts growing in the spleen and cecum were most sensitive to 5-FU. Tumors in the liver were highly resistant to both drugs, whereas experimental lung metastases were sensitive to 5-FU but resistant to doxorubicin (9). Moreover, in an approach aimed at predicting the most suitable treatment for patients suffering from pancreatic cancer, directly explanted tumor cells were implanted subcutaneously into nude mice. Samples from two patients were treated with Mitomycin C, and both tumors responded. However, when the drug was applied to the patients, only one showed progression free survival, the other patient progressed after one week. The same patient samples, implanted orthotopically, reflected this situation much better in that only the sample from the patient who benefited from the treatment was sensitive in the orthotopic implantation model, the other was not affected by the treatment (10).

The drawbacks of orthotopic tumor implantation include, on the one hand, the requirement of, sometimes, sophisticated surgery, and, on the other hand, the need for sensitive imaging, since the tumors do not grow visibly on the flank of the mouse. Whereas the former issue just complicates the tumor cell inoculation for such models, the latter requires careful consideration of available techniques and the minimal requirements of the experiments planned (unless funds are unlimited).

In vivo Imaging

Several imaging modalities for small animals have been developed in the recent years, some modified from the use in humans (e.g. PET/CT, MRI), others, like fluorescence and bioluminescence, are available almost exclusively to model animals. Working in an institution with limited funds, two imaging technologies appeared most appealing: eGFP/RFP mediated fluorescence, or bioluminescence generated by luciferase enzymes. Both modalities require genetically altered cells and are therefore not translatable to the clinic, but they offer sensitive, affordable means to detect tumor cells in the mouse. The next section will, therefore, be devoted to these two techniques, with, probably, a slight bias towards bioluminescence, which is the modality we finally selected for our purpose.

Fluorescent proteins (eGFP, RFP...)

The green fluorescent protein (GFP) from Aequoria victoria was discovered by Shimomura and co-workers as early as 1962 (11), but it was the isolation of its cDNA in 1992, which revolutionized biology (12), and resulted in the 2009 Nobel prize. For the first time, real time observations of cellular processes were possible, but the technique was also used to track cells in mice. Micrometastases, as well as single cells floating in blood vessels could be detected in fresh tissues from mice inoculated with GFP-marked tumor cells (13, 14). Miliary seeded GFP expressing B16F10 cells could be detected in liver, bone, brain and lymph nodes in the live animal. The detection limit of this cell line in relation to the tissue depth was established using isolated tissues at a depth of 0.5 mm for ca. 60 cells, and 2.2 mm for ca. 2000 cells (15, 16).

The tissue penetrance of visible light is limited by the strong absorption of hemoglobin between 400-600 nm. Beyond 900 nm, water absorption starts. Red-shifted fluorescence is therefore better suited for *in vivo* imaging purposes (for a review, see (17)), and the isolation of a red fluorescent protein (dsRed) helped to increase the sensitivity of fluorescence *in vivo* imaging (18, 19). Fluorescent protein expressing cells may be detected at a single cell level. A combination of a host mouse expressing GFP and RFP expressing tumor cells allowed to visualize tumor angiogenesis as well as host cell infiltration of the tumors in extracted tissue (20). Using a spinning disk confocal microscope, a mix of cells labeled with fluorescent proteins or fluorescent dyes with up to 4 colours could be monitored *in vivo* in a skin flap mouse breast cancer tumor model (21). Using FACS, circulating tumor cells could be isolated from the blood of orthotopically, but not subcutaneously, implanted eGFP expressing PC3 prostate tumor cells. When implanted as a mix with RFP-labeled parental cells, mainly eGFP marked tumor cells were found at metastatic sites, suggesting that circulating tumor cells represented a more metastatic subpopulation (22).

Cells expressing fluorescent proteins may be monitored *in vivo* and ex vivo when implanted orthotopically. Several tumor models had been developed that allow monitoring of drug effects on tumors and metastases *in vivo* (23-25). A good correlation of RFP fluorescence and MRI could be demonstrated (26).

However, high resolution detection of GFP/RFP-expressing tumor cells often requires a skin flap window or an excision of the tumors, complicating the use of such models in larger drug trials. Also, a very high expression level of the fluorescent proteins is generally required for the detection of the cells *in vivo*.

Bioluminescence

In 1985, the gene for firefly luciferase (FLuc) was cloned and expressed in E. coli as an active enzyme which uses luciferin and ATP as co-substrates to generate light (27). HeLa cells transfected with a luciferase expression construct could be detected in live animals. As few as 30 cells could be detected *in vitro*, and *in vivo* growth curves could be established from intraperitoneally (ip), intravenously (iv), and subcutaneously (sc) applied HeLa cells (28). Injected ip at increasing numbers showed a dose-dependent light emission, with 2500 cells being the detection limit. The signal increased proportionally over 4 logs. Therapy effects of SCID mice injected ip with HeLa cells expressing luciferase and treated with a variety of therapeutic agents could be monitored *in vivo*. 'Cured' mice with undetectable luciferase signals were subjected to PCR analysis, which confirmed the absence of the luciferase gene (29). The signal intensity correlated well with size as measured using MRI (30). Using subcutaneous injected luciferase marked tumor cell lines, calliper measurements were compared to intraperitoneal or intratumoral applied luciferin induced BLI signals in a high-throughput setting. A very good correlation was found, indicating that weekly single point luciferase measurements, affordable both in terms of time and cost, may be used to determine tumor burden in the mouse (31).

A second luciferase gene, which also depends on ATP, but uses coelenterazine as a substrate, was isolated from a soft coral, Renilla reniforma, in 1991 (RLuc; (32)). RLuc was also tested as a marker to trace tumor cells *in vivo*, and compared to FLuc. RLuc, as well as FLuc expressing cells were implanted sc into the same mouse. Both cells were readily detected, and there was no cross-reactivity between the two substrates. However, the kinetics of light generation upon simultaneous injection of both substrates (luciferine: 150 mg/kg; coelenterazine: 0.7 mg/kg) differed significantly. Whereas RLuc luminescence peaked one minute after injection and gradually decreased thereafter, FLuc luminescence increased until ca. 3-4 minutes after injection and stayed high for at least 10 minutes (33). Besides the kinetics, also the wavelength emitted differs between the two luciferases: RLuc peaks at 480 nm, whereas Fluc has an emission maximum at 560 nm (27, 33).

Luciferase marked tumor cells have been widely used to follow the growth and metastasation of orthotopic mouse models, and to test the effects of experimental and novel treatments. The good tissue penetrance of bioluminescence allows the detection of metastases in bones or the brain, or in deeper organs of the mouse.

A model for breast cancer mediated bone metastasation was generated using a luciferase expressing, bone seeking clone of MDA-MB-231, MDA-MB-231B. The diffuse BLI signal indicating distribution of the cells over most of the body immediately after injection was gone after 24 h, but reappeared 24 days later, focused to the hindlegs and maxillofacial region. After 38 days, the metastatic lesions in the femur could be visualised using radiography. Growth curves of individual metastases could be established (34). A bone metastasis model based on the injection of luciferase marked neuroblastoma cells into the femur of nude mice was developed by Mouchess and co-workers. Tumor cell growth in the femur, as well as spread to other organs could be followed via bioluminescence. The results could be confirmed using T2 weighted MRI analysis. Also, osteolytic activity of the tumor cells was monitored using x-ray and CT scans. The latter could be used to calculate the degree of bone resorption (35).

U87M cells marked with luciferase were injected into the brain to generate an orthotopic model of glioblastoma. The growth of the tumors was monitored using BLI and gadolinium-enhanced MRI, which allowed three-dimensional volumetric reconstruction. A very good correlation was observed between the two imaging modalities. Treatment effects of an adenovirus encoding soluble VEGFR could be followed using BLI (36).

Fluorescence or Bioluminescence ?

The use of eGFP-luciferase fusion proteins permits a direct comparison of fluorescence and bioluminescence *in vivo* imaging in mice. A set of studies using a triple fusion protein consisting of luciferase, thymidine kinase, and mRFP suggested that fluorescence was useful for imaging and sorting of individual cells *in vitro*, but had limited *in vivo* potential. Bioluminescence imaging, however, provided very sensitive small animal imaging (37, 38). Our own experiences using an eGFP-luciferase fusion protein confirmed these results (unpublished observations). Thus, due to the extremely good signal to background ratio and the less pronounced requirement for very high over-expression, we chose bioluminescence rather than fluorescence for our *in vivo* testing facility. The next section will focus on the authors' experience in using bioluminescence for orthotopic tumor models in a pre-clinical drug testing facility.

The Use of Luciferase Marked Orthotopic Metastasizing Mouse Models in Pre-Clinical Drug Testing

Generation of luciferase-expressing cell pools

A downside of using bioluminescence – or cells expressing fluorescent proteins – for *in vivo* imaging is the requirement to generate cells that stably express a transgene. This process usually involves cloning of cell lines, a process which may alter the characteristics of tumor

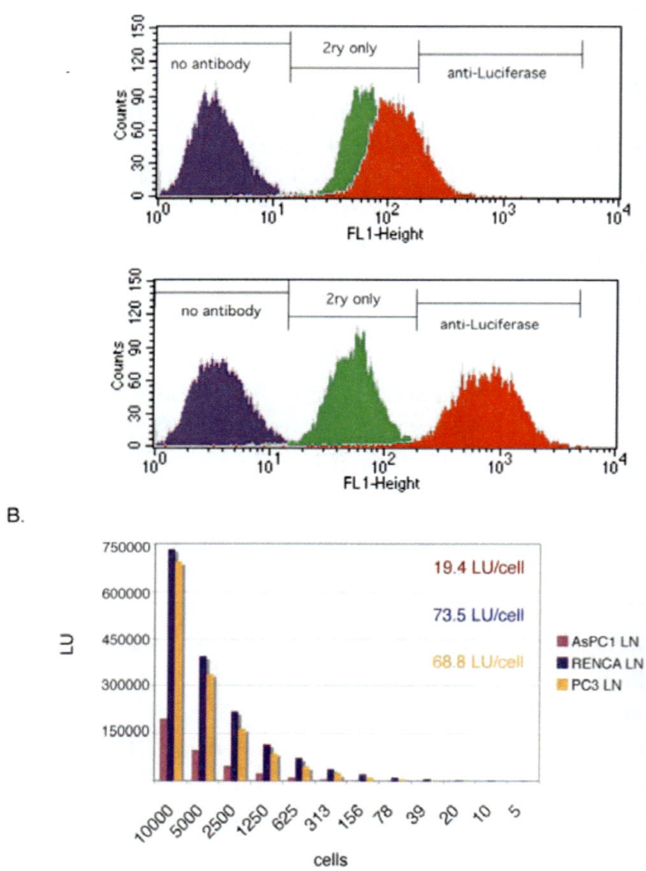

Figure 1. Characterization of luciferase expressing cell lines

A. FACS analysis. Blue, cells left unstained, green, cells stained with the FITC-labeled secondary only, and red with both, the anti-luciferase and a secondary FITC-labeled secondary antibody. The upper panel shows the parental cell line, the lower the corresponding luciferase-expressing cell pool.

B. *In vitro* luciferase assays.Luciferase expressing cell pools of AsPC1 LN (pancreatic carcinoma), RENCA LN (mouse renal carcinoma), and PC3 LN (prostate carcinoma) were lysed and serially diluted, starting at 10000 cells.

cell lines. Such cells should therefore be carefully checked whether they still represent the original disease (see (39)). Also, the expression of a transgene may affect cells - GFP expression induces oxidative stress and may alter drug sensitivity (40) whereas only very high levels of luciferase expression appeared to alter tumor growth behaviour (41).

Our approach to generate luciferase expressing cell lines makes use of a luciferase-neomycin-resistance fusion protein, transduced using a retroviral or lentiviral protocol. The use of a bi-functional protein that mediates both, G418 selection and luciferase activity eliminates the requirement to isolate cell clones, since the two markers cannot diverge. Furthermore, the very efficient retroviral gene transduction process reduces the selection time to about one week, keeping the stress to the cells at a minimum level. This protocol results in cell pools that express luciferase, albeit maybe not totally uniformly, but with the whole cell population being clearly shifted when analysed by FACS (Figure 1A). As a quality control, the mean luciferase activity per cell may be determined using an in vitro luciferase assay (Figure 1B). The expression, as detected in such an assay, remains stable, even in the absence of G418. This is essential, since it is not possible to select cells in the mouse. Some cells, however, appear to down-regulate viral promoters. In such cell lines, a construct with an additional EF1alpha promoter appears to enhance expression levels (42).

Detection of luciferase-expressing cells in the mouse

When such luciferase transduced cell pools are injected into the mouse, the cells may be visualized via injection of luciferin intraperitoneally into the mouse. The resulting signal may be used to randomize the mice of a given experiment into treatment groups, as well as to generate tumor growth curves of either treated or untreated mice.

Randomization

Orthotopically implanted cells require a very sensitive detection method to check whether the cells are implanted at the correct location, and measure tumor growth. Although bioluminescence may penetrate 2-3 cm of tissue, the light emitted from the growing tumor depends on the position of the mouse, the depth of the implantation site, on the tissue (highly vascularized tissue, e.g. liver, will quench the signal due to the absorbance of the FLuc signal (at 560 nM) by hemoglobin (400-600 nm)), and on the luciferase expression level of the tumor cells. However, within a given experiment, these parameters may (and should) be kept constant, and the relative apparent size of the tumors may, therefore, be determined. Also, a rough judgment on whether the signal originates from the intended site of implantation is possible.

In the pre-clinical test setting, mice have to be randomized into treatment groups according to their tumor sizes in order to keep the average tumor sizes in the groups constant. The signal strength of the light emitted from the tumor allows for a categorization of the mice according to their apparent tumor sizes. Also, mice with no or aberrant tumors may be excluded.

As in subcutaneously implanted tumor cells, an initial decrease of the signal is often observed. After a cell-type specific incubation period, the signal strength then increases again. With the examples shown, AsPC1 LN, a pancreatic cancer cell line, and PC3 LN, a prostate cancer cell line, cells show comparable lag periods of ca. 2 weeks, whereas RENCA, a syngeneic kidney cell line, grows much faster, with 3-4 days until randomization has to take place. Ideally, randomization is timed at, or shortly after the onset of tumor growth (Figure 2).

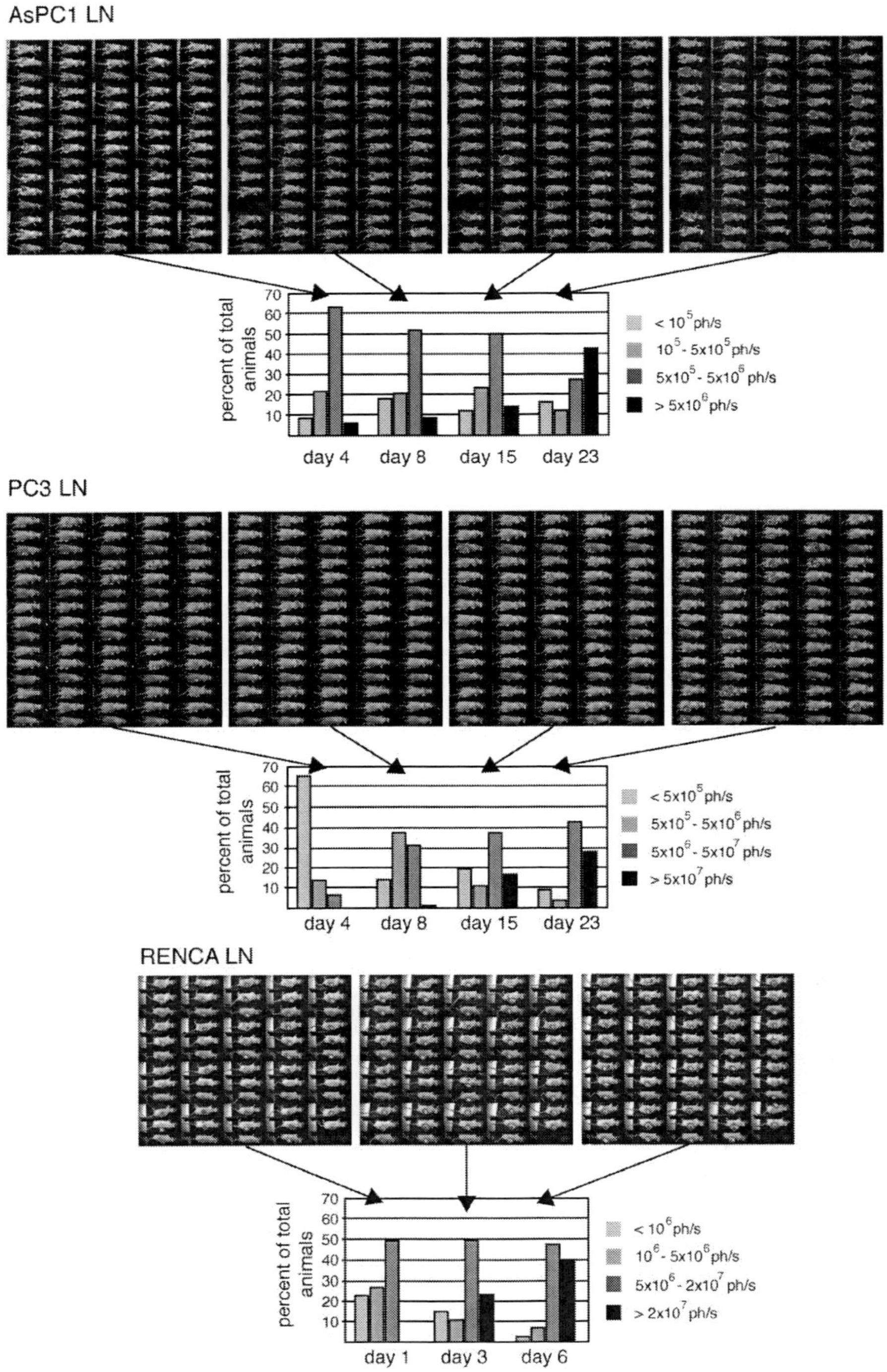

Figure 2. Randomization of mice orthotopically implanted with luciferase-expressing cell lines. AsPC1 LN, PC3 LN, and RENCA LN cells were orthotopically implanted into pancreas, prostate, or spleen, respectively. The upper panels show overlays of mice with bioluminescence signals, the lower panels the quantification, grouped into 4 classes according to signal intensity. Note the time-dependent shift to higher intensity groups.

As in subcutaneously implanted tumor cells, an initial decrease of the signal is often observed. After a cell-type specific incubation period, the signal strength then increases again. With the examples shown, AsPC1 LN, a pancreatic cancer cell line, and PC3 LN, a prostate cancer cell line, cells show comparable lag periods of ca. 2 weeks, whereas RENCA, a syngeneic kidney cell line, grows much faster, with 3-4 days until randomization has to take place. Ideally, randomization is timed at, or shortly after the onset of tumor growth (Figure 2).

Generation of tumor growth curves – solid tumors

After randomization, and the start of treatment, measurement of luciferase signals once weekly is sufficient to generate tumor growth curves. With increasing tumor sizes, the accuracy of the bioluminescence measurements may be affected by some additional factors.

Despite the linearity of the signal over 4 logs (29), the dynamic range is a limiting factor. If a growth curve should be established over the whole period of the experiment, the exposure and camera settings have to be kept constant. In most experiments, tumor signals towards the end will be in the saturation range. A possible way around this limitation is to use two settings, and use the less sensitive setting to establish a growth curve starting at the time of randomization (see Figure 3, RENCA for an example).

The signal appears to be affected by anaesthetics and repetitive positioning. Cui and colleagues found that BLI peak times depended on the anaesthetics and shifted with tumor growth, and also the time course of BLI signals had different shapes, depending on the positioning of the mice (43). Compared to conscious mice kept in a lucid restraining box, the use of mice anesthetized with isofluorene appeared to reduce the bioluminescence signal emitted from luciferase expressing tumors (44). Despite these apparent drawbacks, we have been successfully using isofluorene to anesthetize animals for the imaging of our orthotopically implanted mouse models for many years.

The dosage of luciferin used in *in vivo* bioluminescence studies (ca. 2 mg/mouse) appears to be rate limiting (45). The substrate is usually applied intraperitoneally, which allows rapid uptake and distribution throughout the body. However, if a compartment, or fatty tissue is accidentally hit, the absorption of the substrate may be substantially delayed, resulting in an apparent disappearance of the tumor. Unless this is the final measurement, this ‘spontaneous tumor elimination’ will be identified as an artifact by the next measurement.

Besides luciferin, the luciferase reaction also requires oxygen and ATP. With most tumors developing hypoxic areas once they reach a certain size, these co-factors may become rate-limiting, and affect bioluminescence mediated imaging. However, the K_m’s of luciferase for oxygen (≈1–10 μM) and ATP (≈50 μM) are well below those of the HIF prolyl hydroxylases (≈200 μM), and the normal cellular ATP (≈1 mM), respectively. The measurement of hypoxic tumors, or hypoxic areas may, therefore, work even at relatively low oxygen levels (46). It is, however, not clear whether the resulting signal is still linear to tumor size.

Besides merely hypoxic, many tumors also develop necrotic areas. Since these regions do not contain viable tumor cells, they do not generate light.

Last but not least, tumors with a strong tendency to metastasize locally may generate metastases that produce stronger signals than the primary tumor (47).

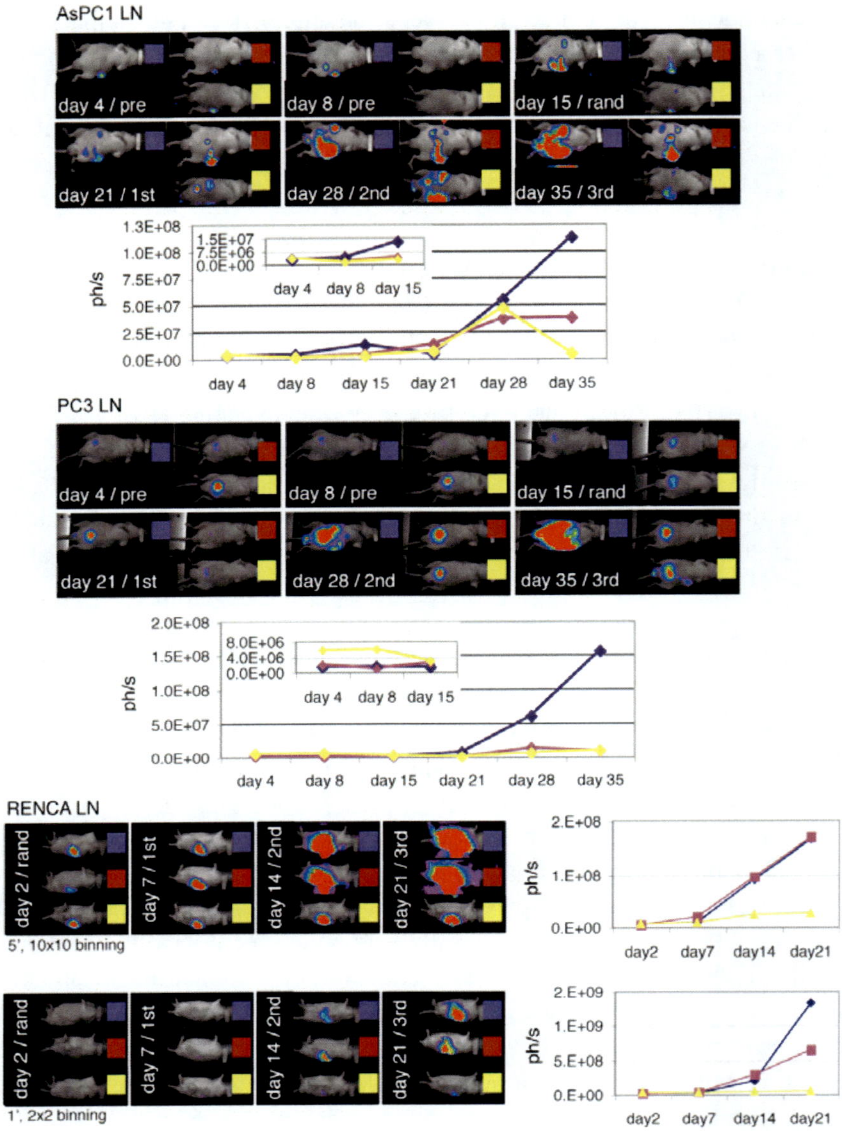

Figure 3. *In vivo* growth curves based upon *in vivo* luciferase measurements. Mice carrying orthotopically implanted pancreatic (AsPC1 LN), prostate (PC3 LN), or kidney (RENCA LN) tumors were randomized and left untreated (blue), or treated with two alternative treatments (yellow, red). The upper (RENCA: left) panels show overlays of mice with bioluminescence signals, the lower (RENCA: right) the growth curves based upon the luciferase signals. Note, predominantly in the untreated controls, the massive spread of the luciferase signal, indicating metastasation. For the RENCA LN tumor growth curve, two sensitivity settings were used. The more sensitive setting allows early detection, but is saturated in the end, whereas the less sensitive setting misses the early signal, but distinguishes between the red treatment and control.

Despite all these complications, luciferase measurements usually provide tumor growth curves that do reflect the development of the tumor sizes, and drug effects may be monitored. Examples for tumor growth curves are shown in Figure 3, including an example using a pancreatic tumor cell line, AsPC1, which shows massive peritoneal metastasation.

Dependent on the grade of local metastasation, the *in vivo* signals usually correlate well with the actual tumor sizes (Figure 4).

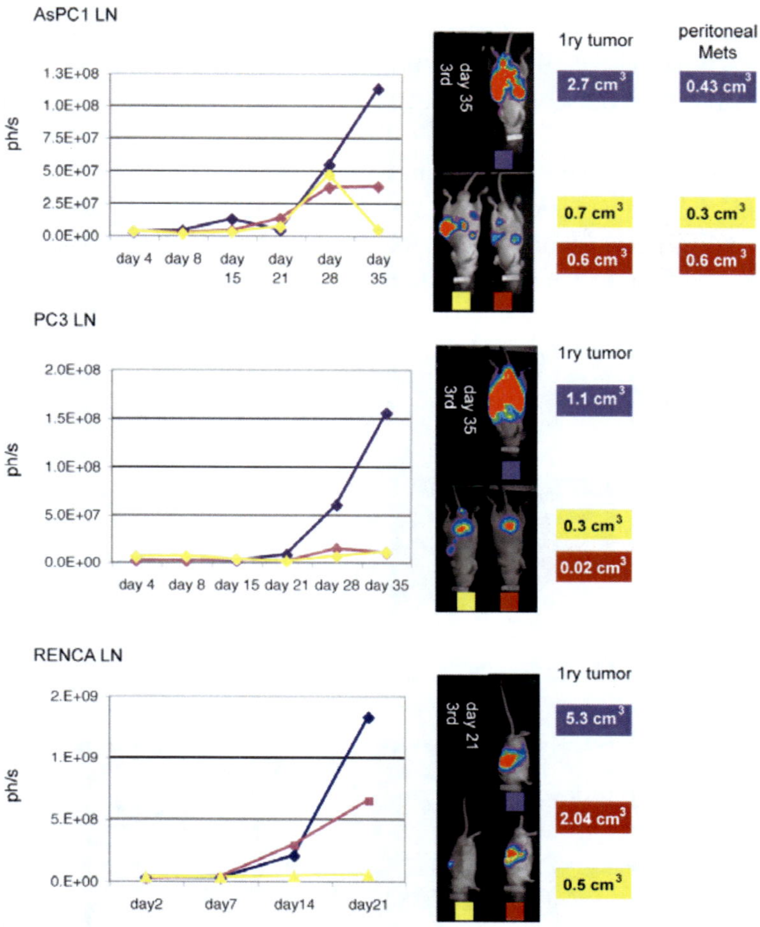

Figure 4. Comparison of *in vivo* bioluminescence signals with necropsy primary tumor sizes. The left hand panel shows the *in vivo* growth curve, the middle panel the final overlay, and the right hand panel the actually measured tumor sizes (and, for AsPC1, peritoneal metastasis).

Detection of metastases *in vivo* – orthotopic models

The pattern of metastasation certainly depends on the site of implantation, but the cell line also appears to be a major determinant. Re-implantation experiments of tumor cells from metastatic sites resulted in tumor cells that metastasized efficiently to specific organs (48, 49); for a review, see (50).

Whether, and how early, metastases may be detected, again depends on the target organ. Peritoneal metastases (as, e.g. often detected in pancreatic tumor models using, e.g. AsPC1 cells), may be detected at a relatively early time-point, since they localize very close to the surface. Liver metastases, however, may be more difficult to visualize due to the localization deeper in the mouse, as well as the strong vascularization of the organ.

The identification of the organ invaded by tumor cells is possible if shape or localization are obvious. Often, however, the identification of the metastatic sites requires sacrificing the animals, and analysis either by eye, by immunohistochemistry, or by assays as shown in the ex vivo metastasis detection section. Metastases from orthotopically implanted tumor cells are shown in Figure 4.

If the primary focus of an experiment is metastasation, removing the primary tumor may help to visualize metastases. An alternative method is to inject tumor cells intravenously or intracardially. A drawback of this approach is that metastases generated that way do not have to escape the primary tumor, so not all aspects of the metastasation process are reflected.

Detection of metastases *in vivo* – dissemination models

Intravenous injection of tumor cells is a well-established method to generate disseminated metastases models. Fidler and others used this method or also intra-cardiac injection - which avoids first passage through the lung -, with B16 cells to demonstrate that the targeting to, as well as the survival and proliferation of tumor cells at metastatic sites is, at least partially, dependent on cellular determinants (51).

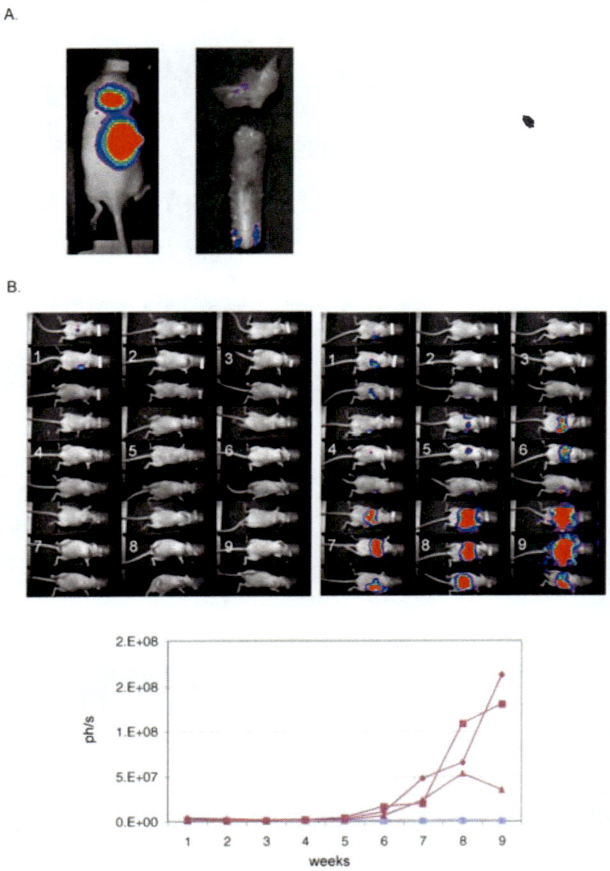

Figure 5. Dissemination models.

A. PC3 LN prostate cells were injected intravenous into nude mice. The left panel shows an *in vivo* bioluminescence picture, indicating spinal cord metastasation, the right hand panel bones from the spinal cord isolated from previously luciferase injected mice.

B. Alexander ELN cells injected into the spleen of NMRI mice (multifocal hepatocarcinoma model). The left hand panel shows three mice injected with 10^6, the right hand panel mice injected with $2x10^6$ tumor cells. Numbers indicate weeks after injection. Below, the quantification of the images.

Prostate tumor cells have a tendency to form bone metastases, and when injected into mice, colonize previously implanted bone fragments, or also the mouse skeleton (52, 53). Our own experiments lead to similar results with very strong signals emanating from the spinal cord. When the spinal cord was isolated from animals injected with luciferase before sacrificing, signals could be detected (Figure 5A).

Smakman and colleagues developed a liver metastasis model using luciferase expressing C26 mouse colon tumor cells. The cells were injected into the spleen, allowing the cells to be transported to the blood vessels and sinusoid system of the liver via the portal vein before resection of the spleen. Tumor cell growth was monitored using BLI and compared, after necropsy, with the percentage of liver replaced by tumor tissue (54). We established a similar model based on the human hepatocarcinoma cell line Alexander/PLC/PRF/5 (Figure 5B). Strikingly, in this model, the number of injected tumor cells appeared absolutely crucial. After injection into the spleen, the cells were readily detected. However, only upon injection of $2x10^6$ cells, tumors developed in the liver. Injection of $3x10^6$ cells lead to the death of the animals, possibly due to embolism.

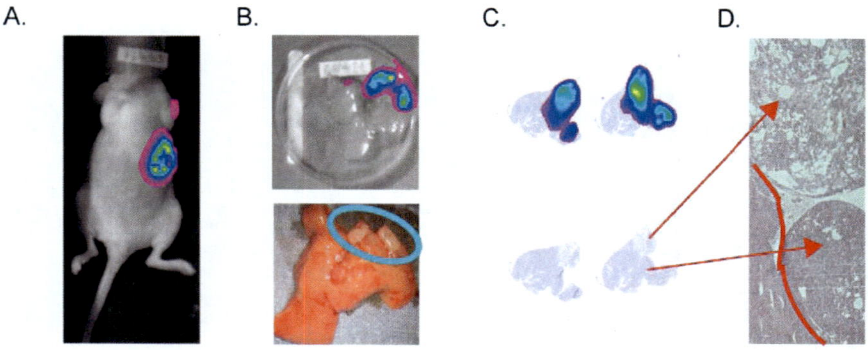

Figure 6. Imaging of Alexander ELN cells in a multifocal hepatocarcinoma model *in vivo* and *in vitro*.
A. *In vivo* bioluminescence signal emanating from the liver.
B. Upper panel, the liver from the animal in A, removed immediately after *in vivo* imaging. Enough luciferin is left to visualize the tumor cells. The blue circle in the lower panel marks some visible metaststatic sites.
C. Bioluminescence imaging of frozen sections. The upper panel shows an overlay of the signal detected from the sections after adding luciferin and ATP with the H&E stain, the lower the H&E stain only.
D. Microscopic magnification of the H&E stained sections with native liver tissue (left of the purple line) and two metaststatic foci.

Detection of luciferase-expressing cells ex vivo and in sections

The use of luciferase expressing cells allows the localization and quantification of tumor cells spread to metastatic sites after sacrificing the animals.

Metastasized organs may be identified via injection of the animals with luciferin just before necropsy followed by exposure of the isolated organs using a CCD camera (e.g. Figure 5A). A more detailed analysis may be performed preparing frozen sections of potential target organs, and overlaying them with luciferin and ATP. The same section may subsequently be stained using, e.g., H&E to reveal the morphology of the organ and metastases (e.g. Figure 6 and (42, 47, 55)).

Homogenizing potential target organs in luciferase assay buffer, and assaying the luciferase activity of potentially invasive tumor cells is a quantitative way to assess the metastatic spread of tumor cells in the mouse. This method yields a quantitative readout of the metastatic spread of tumor cells, and may be used to reveal the distinctive metastatic signature of a tumor cell line (Figure 7). Also, anti-metastatic effects of novel compounds may be assessed (47, 55).

As mentioned above, the metastatic spread of tumor cells derived from orthotopic implantation sites is not always really predictable – which, to a certain degree, also displays the human situation. Specific tumors do have preferences as to which organs they infiltrate, but the process is rarely quantitative.

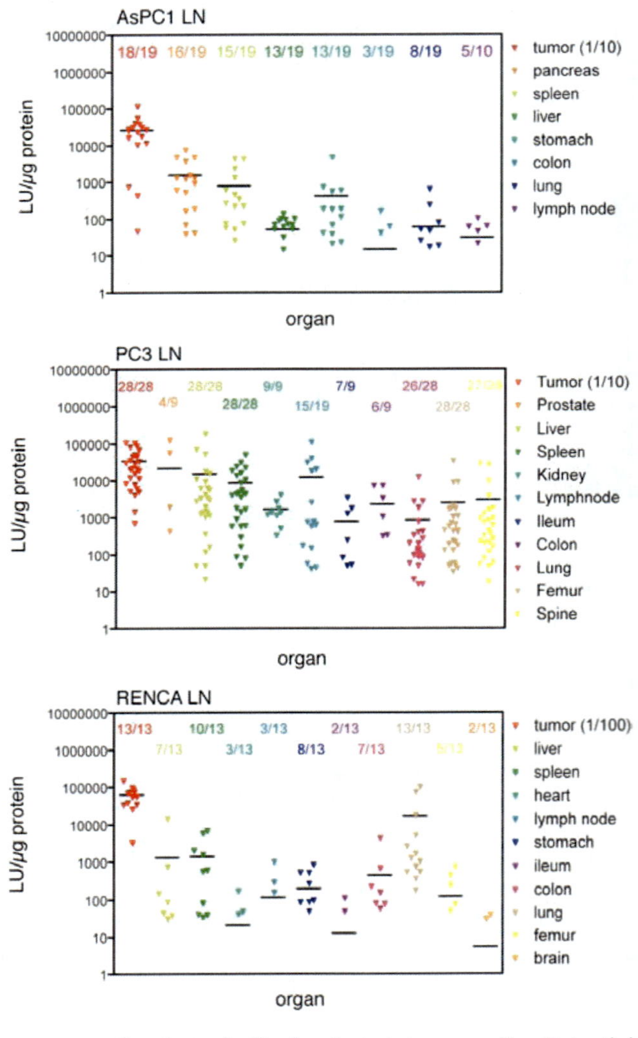

Figure 7. Metastatic pattern of orthotopically implanted tumor cells. Potential target organs were homogenized, and luciferase activity was measured as a proxy for metastatic tumor cells. Note that AsPC1 pancreatic tumor cells invade locally to spleen, liver, and stomach, PC3 prostate tumor cells metastasize liver and spleen, but also femur and spine. RENCA cells mainly target the lung, but also metastasize to the spleen.

Conclusion

Luciferase expressing tumor cells are a powerful tool to generate orthotopic models in which the growth and scattering of tumor cells can be observed *in vivo*, and quantified *in vitro*.

The system does have its drawbacks - due to light scattering, a precise localization of the origin of the signal is difficult. '3D'- bioluminescence imaging systems are being developed that use mirrors to collect the signals from three sides. A combination of luminescence with tomography that would, as in PET/CT systems, provide good spatial resolution, is as yet futuristic. Also, the requirement for substrate injection – at non-saturating concentrations – makes the system susceptible for purely artificial fluctuations. That all said, for the authors, the balance is clearly on the positive side – there is no background, the system is very sensitive, and measurement is fast, which makes it possible to run reasonably large pre-clinical orthotopical mouse studies using bioluminescence to follow tumor growth.

Thus, considering the 3 Rs (reduction, refinement & replacement) for mouse experimental models, the first two are clearly being addressed using the combination of orthotopic implantation with bioluminescence imaging.

Acknowledgment

The authors would like to thank Ulrike Fiedler and Andreas Lingnau for critically reading the manuscript, and the team of the animal facility for excellent work.

References

[1] Suggitt, M. and Bibby, M. C. (2005). *50 years of preclinical anticancer drug screening: empirical to target-driven approaches.* Clin Cancer Res, 11, 971-981,.

[2] Sausville, E. A. and Burger, A. M. (2006). *Contributions of human tumor xenografts to anticancer drug development.* Cancer Res, 66, 3351-3354, discussion 3354.

[3] Kelland, L. R.(2004). Of mice and men: values and liabilities of the athymic nude mouse model in anticancer drug development. *Eur J Cancer, 40,* 827-836.

[4] Fiebig, H. H., Maier, A. and Burger, A. M. (2004). Clonogenic assay with established human tumour xenografts: correlation of *in vitro* to *in vivo* activity as a basis for anticancer drug discovery. *Eur J Cancer, 40,* 802-820,.

[5] Marangoni, E., Vincent-Salomon, A., Auger, N., Degeorges, A., Assayag, F., de Cremoux, P., de Plater, L., Guyader, C., De Pinieux, G., Judde, J. G., Rebucci, M., Tran-Perennou, C., Sastre-Garau, X., Sigal-Zafrani, B., Delattre, O., Dieras, V. and Poupon, M. F. (2007). *A new model of patient tumor-derived breast cancer xenografts for preclinical assays.* Clin Cancer Res, 13, 3989-3998,.

[6] Peterson, J. K. and Houghton, P. J. Integrating pharmacology and *in vivo* cancer models in preclinical and clinical drug development. *Eur J Cancer, 40*, 837-844, 2004.

[7] Hoffman, R. M. (1999*). Orthotopic metastatic mouse models for anticancer drug discovery and evaluation: a bridge to the clinic.* Invest New Drugs, 17, 343-359.

[8] Zechmann, C. M., Woenne, E. C., Brix, G., Radzwill, N., Ilg, M., Bachert, P., Peschke, P., Kirsch, S., Kauczor, H. U., Delorme, S., Semmler, W. and Kiessling, F. (2007).

Impact of stroma on the growth, microcirculation, and metabolism of experimental prostate tumors. Neoplasia, 9, 57-67.

[9] Wilmanns, C., Fan, D., O'Brian, C. A., Bucana, C. D. and Fidler, I. J. (1992). Orthotopic and ectopic organ environments differentially influence the sensitivity of murine colon carcinoma cells to doxorubicin and 5-fluorouracil. *Int J Cancer*, *52*, 98-104, 1992.

[10] Villarroel, M. C., Tan, A., Garrido-Laguna, I., Rubio-Viqueira, B., De Oliveira, E., RajeshKummar, N., Jimeno, A. and Hidalgo, M. (2009). *Orthotopic cancer models are better predictors of clinical response than s.c. models.* Proceedings of the 100th Annual Meeting of the American Association for Cancer Research.

[11] Shimomura, O., Johnson, F. H. and Saiga, Y. (1962). Extraction, purification and properties of aequorin, a bioluminescent protein from the luminous hydromedusan, Aequorea. *J Cell Comp Physiol.*, *59*, 223-239.

[12] Prasher, D. C., Eckenrode, V. K., Ward, W. W., Prendergast, F. G. and Cormier, M. J. (1992). *Primary structure of the Aequorea victoria green-fluorescent protein.* Gene., 111, 229-233.

[13] Chishima, T., Miyagi, Y., Wang, X., Tan, Y., Shimada, H., Moossa, A. and Hoffman, R. (1997). *M. Visualization of the metastatic process by green fluorescent protein expression*. Anticancer Res, 17, 2377-2384.

[14] Chishima, T., Miyagi, Y., Wang, X., Yamaoka, H., Shimada, H., Moossa, A. R. and Hoffman, R. M. (1997). *Cancer invasion and micrometastasis visualized in live tissue by green fluorescent protein expression.* Cancer Res., 57, 2042-2047,.

[15] Yang, M., Jiang, P., An, Z., Baranov, E., Li, L., Hasegawa, S., Al-Tuwaijri, M., Chishima, T., Shimada, H., Moossa, A. R. and Hoffman, R. M. (1999). *Genetically fluorescent melanoma bone and organ metastasis models.* Clin Cancer Res, 5, 3549-3559.

[16] Yang, M., Baranov, E., Jiang, P., Sun, F. X., Li, X. M., Li, L., Hasegawa, S., Bouvet, M., Al-Tuwaijri, M., Chishima, T., Shimada, H., Moossa, A. R., Penman, S. and Hoffman, R. M. (2000*). Whole-body optical imaging of green fluorescent protein-expressing tumors and metastases.* Proc Natl Acad Sci U S A, 97, 1206-1211.

[17] Weissleder, R. (2001). *A clearer vision for in vivo imaging.* Nat Biotechnol., 19, 316-317.

[18] Yang, T. T., Sinai, P., Green, G., Kitts, P. A., Chen, Y. T., Lybarger, L., Chervenak, R., Patterson, G. H., Piston, D. W. and Kain, S. R. (1998). Improved fluorescence and dual color detection with enhanced blue and green variants of the green fluorescent protein. *J Biol Chem*, *273*, 8212-8216.

[19] Matz, M. V., Fradkov, A. F., Labas, Y. A., Savitsky, A. P., Zaraisky, A. G., Markelov, M. L. and Lukyanov, S. A. (1999). *Fluorescent proteins from nonbioluminescent Anthozoa species.* Nat Biotechnol., 17, 969-973.

[20] Yang, M., Li, L., Jiang, P., Moossa, A. R., Penman, S. and Hoffman, R. M. (2003). *Dual-color fluorescence imaging distinguishes tumor cells from induced host angiogenic vessels and stromal cells.* Proc Natl Acad Sci., U S A, 100, 14259-14262.

[21] Egeblad, M., Ewald, A. J., Askautrud, H. A., Truitt, M. L., Welm, B. E., Bainbridge, E., Peeters, G., Krummel, M. F. and Werb, Z. (2008). *Visualizing stromal cell dynamics in different tumor microenvironments by spinning disk confocal microscopy.* Dis Model Mech, 1, 155-167; discussion 165.

[22] Glinskii, A. B., Smith, B. A., Jiang, P., Li, X. M., Yang, M., Hoffman, R. M. and Glinsky, G. V. (2003). *Viable circulating metastatic cells produced in orthotopic but not ectopic prostate cancer models.* Cancer Res., 63, 4239-4243.

[23] Katz, M. H., Takimoto, S., Spivack, D., Moossa, A. R., Hoffman, R. M. and Bouvet, M. (2004). *An imageable highly metastatic orthotopic red fluorescent protein model of pancreatic cancer.* Clin Exp Metastasis., 21, 7-12.

[24] Yang, M., Baranov, E., Wang, J. W., Jiang, P., Wang, X., Sun, F. X., Bouvet, M., Moossa, A. R., Penman, S. and Hoffman, R. M. (2002). *Direct external imaging of nascent cancer, tumor progression, angiogenesis, and metastasis on internal organs in the fluorescent orthotopic model.* Proc Natl Acad Sci., U S A, 99, 3824-3829.

[25] Yang, M., Jiang, P. and Hoffman, R. M. (2007). *Whole-body subcellular multicolor imaging of tumor-host interaction and drug response in real time.* Cancer Res., 67, 5195-5200.

[26] Bouvet, M., Spernyak, J., Katz, M. H., Mazurchuk, R. V., Takimoto, S., Bernacki, R., Rustum, Y. M., Moossa, A. R. and Hoffman, R. M. (2005). *High correlation of whole-body red fluorescent protein imaging and magnetic resonance imaging on an orthotopic model of pancreatic cancer.* Cancer Res., 65, 9829-9833.

[27] de Wet, J. R., Wood, K. V., Helinski, D. R. and DeLuca, M. (1985). *Cloning of firefly luciferase cDNA and the expression of active luciferase in Escherichia coli.* Proc Natl Acad Sci U S A, *82*, 7870-7873.

[28] Edinger, M., Sweeney, T. J., Tucker, A. A., Olomu, A. B., Negrin, R. S. and Contag, C. H. (1999). *Noninvasive assessment of tumor cell proliferation in animal models.* Neoplasia, *1*, 303-310.

[29] Sweeney, T. J., Mailander, V., Tucker, A. A., Olomu, A. B., Zhang, W., Cao, Y., Negrin, R. S. and Contag, C. H. (1999). *Visualizing the kinetics of tumor-cell clearance in living animals.* Proc Natl Acad Sci., U S A, 96, 12044-12049.

[30] Rehemtulla, A., Stegman, L. D., Cardozo, S. J., Gupta, S., Hall, D. E., Contag, C. H. and Ross, B. D. (2000). *Rapid and quantitative assessment of cancer treatment response using in vivo bioluminescence imaging.* Neoplasia., 2, 491-495.

[31] Paroo, Z., Bollinger, R. A., Braasch, D. A., Richer, E., Corey, D. R., Antich, P. P. and Mason, R. P. (2004). *Validating bioluminescence imaging as a high-throughput, quantitative modality for assessing tumor burden. Mol Imaging.*, *3*, 117-124.

[32] Lorenz, W. W., McCann, R. O., Longiaru, M. and Cormier, M. J. (1991). *Isolation and expression of a cDNA encoding Renilla reniformis luciferase.* Proc Natl Acad Sci., U S A, 88, 4438-4442.

[33] Bhaumik, S. and Gambhir, S. S. (2002). *Optical imaging of Renilla luciferase reporter gene expression in living mice.* Proc Natl Acad Sci., U S A, 99, 377-382.

[34] Wetterwald, A., van der Pluijm, G., Que, I., Sijmons, B., Buijs, J., Karperien, M., Lowik, C. W., Gautschi, E., Thalmann, G. N. and Cecchini, M. G. (2002). Optical imaging of cancer metastasis to bone marrow: a mouse model of minimal residual disease. *Am J Pathol.*, 160, 1143-1153.

[35] Mouchess, M. L., Sohara, Y., Nelson, M. D., Jr., De, C. Y. A. and Moats, R. A. (2006). Multimodal imaging analysis of tumor progression and bone resorption in a murine cancer model. *J Comput Assist Tomogr.*, 30, 525-534.

[36] Szentirmai, O., Baker, C. H., Lin, N., Szucs, S., Takahashi, M., Kiryu, S., Kung, A. L., Mulligan, R. C. and Carter, B. S. (2006). *Noninvasive bioluminescence imaging of*

luciferase expressing intracranial U87 xenografts: correlation with magnetic resonance imaging determined tumor volume and longitudinal use in assessing tumor growth and antiangiogenic treatment effect. Neurosurgery., 58, 365-372; discussion 365-372.

[37] Ray, P., De, A., Min, J. J., Tsien, R. Y. and Gambhir, S. S. (2004). *Imaging tri-fusion multimodality reporter gene expression in living subjects.* Cancer Res., 64, 1323-1330.

[38] Ray, P., Tsien, R. and Gambhir, S. S. (2007). *Construction and validation of improved triple fusion reporter gene vectors for molecular imaging of living subjects.* Cancer Res., 67, 3085-3093.

[39] Teicher, B. A. (2006). *Tumor models for efficacy determination.* Mol Cancer Ther., 5, 2435-2443.

[40] Goto, H., Yang, B., Petersen, D., Pepper, K. A., Alfaro, P. A., Kohn, D. B. and Reynolds, C. P. (2003). *Transduction of green fluorescent protein increased oxidative stress and enhanced sensitivity to cytotoxic drugs in neuroblastoma cell lines.* Mol Cancer Ther, 2, 911-917.

[41] Brutkiewicz, S., Mendonca, M., Stantz, K., Comerford, K., Bigsby, R., Hutchins, G., Goebl, M. and Harrington, M. (2007). *The expression level of luciferase within tumour cells can alter tumour growth upon in vivo bioluminescence imaging.* Luminescence, 22, 221-228.

[42] Bornmann, C., Graeser, R., Esser, N., Ziroli, V., Jantscheff, P., Keck, T., Unger, C., Hopt, U. T., Adam, U., Schaechtele, C., Massing, U. and von Dobschuetz, E. (2008). *A new liposomal formulation of Gemcitabine is active in an orthotopic mouse model of pancreatic cancer accessible to bioluminescence imaging.* Cancer Chemother Pharmacol, 61, 395-405.

[43] Cui, K., Xu, X., Zhao, H. and Wong, S. T. (2008). *A quantitative study of factors affecting in vivo bioluminescence imaging.* Luminescence, 23, 292-295.

[44] Schnell, C., Samuel, A., Axelle, W., Michael, J., Carlos, G. and Robert, C. (2009). *Effects of anesthesia on host and tumor physiology: impact on bioluminescence measurements when compared to conscious mice.* Proceedings of the 100th Annual Meeting of the American Association for Cancer Research.

[45] Rettig, G. R., McAnuff, M., Liu, D., Kim, J. S. and Rice, K. G. (2006). *Quantitative bioluminescence imaging of transgene expression in vivo.* Anal Biochem, 355, 90-94.

[46] Lembert, N. and Idahl, L. A. (1995). Regulatory effects of ATP and luciferin on firefly luciferase activity. *Biochem J.*, 305 (Pt 3), 929-933.

[47] Graeser, R., Bornmann, C., Esser, N., Ziroli, V., Jantscheff, P., Unger, C., Hopt, U. T., Schaechtele, C., von Dobschuetz, E. and Massing, U. (2009). *Antimetastatic Effects of Liposomal Gemcitabine and Empty Liposomes in an Orthotopic Mouse Model of Pancreatic Cancer.* Pancreas.

[48] Bresalier, R. S., Raper, S. E., Hujanen, E. S. and Kim, Y. S. (1987). A new animal model for human colon cancer metastasis. *Int J Cancer.*, 39, 625-630.

[49] Morikawa, K., Walker, S. M., Nakajima, M., Pathak, S., Jessup, J. M. and Fidler, I. J. (1988). *Influence of organ environment on the growth, selection, and metastasis of human colon carcinoma cells in nude mice.* Cancer Res., 48, 6863-6871.

[50] Fidler, I. J. (1990). *Critical factors in the biology of human cancer metastasis: twenty-eighth G.H.A.* Clowes memorial award lecture. Cancer Res., 50, 6130-6138.

[51] Fidler, I. J. and Nicolson, G. L. (1976). Organ selectivity for implantation survival and growth of B16 melanoma variant tumor lines. *J Natl Cancer Inst*., 57, 1199-1202.

[52] Nemeth, J. A., Harb, J. F., Barroso, U., Jr., He, Z., Grignon, D. J. and Cher, M. L. (1999). *Severe combined immunodeficient-hu model of human prostate cancer metastasis to human bone.* Cancer Res., 59, 1987-1993.

[53] Chu, K., Cheng, C. J., Ye, X., Lee, Y. C., Zurita, A. J., Chen, D. T., Yu-Lee, L. Y., Zhang, S., Yeh, E. T., Hu, M. C., Logothetis, C. J. and Lin, S. H. (2008). *Cadherin-11 promotes the metastasis of prostate cancer cells to bone.* Mol Cancer Res., 6, 1259-1267.

[54] Smakman, N., Martens, A., Kranenburg, O. and Borel Rinkes, I. H. (2004). Validation of bioluminescence imaging of colorectal liver metastases in the mouse. *J Surg Res*., 122, 225-230.

[55] Graeser, R., Chung, D. E., Esser, N., Moor, S., Schachtele, C., Unger, C. and Kratz, F. (2008). Synthesis and biological evaluation of an albumin-binding prodrug of doxorubicin that is cleaved by prostate-specific antigen (PSA) in a PSA-positive orthotopic prostate carcinoma model (LNCaP). *Int J Cancer*., 122, 1145-1154.

In: 3D Imaging: Theory, Technology ... ISBN: 978-1-60876-885-1
Editors: E. H. Duke and S. R. Aguirre, pp.159-174

Chapter 6

3D MEDICAL IMAGING APPLICATIONS - RECONSTRUCTION AND AUTOMATIC ANALYSIS

***Rajasvaran Logeswaran**[*]*
Faculty of Engineering, Multimedia University, 63100 Cyberjaya, Malaysia

ABSTRACT

3D imaging has become commonplace in the medical field, with its routine use in the better established institutions for pre-natal observations, diagnosis of ailments, work-up prior to surgery, recovery monitoring and many other medical procedures. In an example such as ultrasound, the difference between 2D and 3D is dramatic as the 3D visualisation of the foetus is apparent even to the uninitiated, whereas the 2D visualisation is only discernable by experts. This chapter starts by introducing some of the common 3D equipment and the type of diagnosis for which they cater. The following section takes a retro look into examples of research work that have been undertaken in the past to produce 3D reconstructions from 2D. This is an important issue as most imaging devices still reproduce images of 3D volume as a series of 2D slice images. Description of a 3D setup for 2D ultrasound probe is provided as an example of a cost-effective means of using existing 2D equipment. The next level is to then undertake 3D processing for automatic diagnosis. This chapter discusses the research methodology required in the reconstruction of 3D volume and employing computer-aided diagnosis to identify various diseases. Details of the different stages of processing, along with the promising results achieved are presented. The chapter concludes with some considerations for future trends of 3D imaging in the medical field.

1. INTRODUCTION

3D is the preferred visualisation technique for volume data. Such visualisation in the medical field allows the medical practitioner to better study the anatomy of the affected region or organ, leading to more accurate diagnosis. For surgery, such visualisation is paramount in the pre-surgical workup, intra-operative imaging and in post-operative evaluation of the disease and healing. It overcomes the shortcomings of 2D visualisation in terms of correlation between series of slices, loss due to partial volume, obstructions due to the limited field of view (FOV) and is more definitive in artifact elimination.

[*] E-mail: loges@ieee.org

Of late, there have been many advances in the development of equipment that not only scans the volume, but also has the ability to visualise it in 3D. Examples include 3D ultrasound, functional MRI, 3D CT etc. There has also been a lot of work in the reconstruction of 3D volume visualisation from equipment that originally acquired data in the native 2D format. Such an example for ultrasound is described later on in this chapter, where the system serves as a cost-effective means of 3D visualisation using the less expensive 2D probes that are available in most medical institutions. There have also been efforts towards 3D surface reconstruction in the medical field, targeted at telemedicine applications.

The next section describes some of the medical equipment that facilitate direct 3D visualisation. This is followed by examples of 3D reconstruction applications, and a cost-effective setup to enable 3D reconstruction using a 2D ultrasound probe and a digital camera. Then, some of the important aspects in automated 3D image analysis are described in terms of the major phases required, supported by an example of a computer-aided diagnosis (CAD) system. Discussions on the expected future trends precede the conclusion of the chapter.

2. 3D Medical Equipment

The main theme of this chapter is to present some of the work undertaken in the reconstruction and automated analysis of 3D volumes in the medical context. Due to its obvious advantages in intuitive visualisation and diagnosis, recent modern medical diagnostic imaging equipment come factory-built for the scanning and presentation of the data in 3D, rather than just producing the traditional series of 2D slice images. Some of the well known diagnostic equipment are discussed below.

2.1 Ultrasound

Ultrasound is one modality that has gained immensely from 3D imaging. The 3D ultrasound [Nelson et al., 1990; Downey & Fenster, 1998], produces high-resolution images that allow the objects of interest to be clearly distinguished from the background even to the layman, as opposed to the grainy greyscale conventional 2D images in the past that require a trained eye. Its lower cost as compared to the other 3D modalities makes the 3D ultrasound a popular diagnostic imaging tool in many medical institutions.

Nowadays, 3D ultrasound is routinely used in foetal [Goncalves et al., 2003; Merz et al., 1995], cardiac [Nelson et al., 1996] and gynaecological [Jurkovic et al., 1995] diagnosis. It has also been successfully used in other clinical areas such as imaging of the vascular anatomy, prostate and bladder volume measurement [Riccabona et al., 1996], in the assessment of seed placement, guidance of interventional needles and catheters [Rose et al., 1999], neonatal head evaluation, and evaluation of breast mass vascularity [3D USIG, 2009]. 3D ultrasound can be enhanced with additional parameters to represent further dimensions that aid to improve diagnosis. Figure 1(a) [Maadiagnostic, 2009] shows a 4D ultrasound scanner displaying a snapshot of the 3D foetal image.

2.2 Computed Tomography (CT)

Computed Tomography (CT) has long been the preferred modality for clear high-resolution images. The modern spiral helical 3D CT scanners have not only improved the quality of the image acquisition, but advances in technology have enabled such scanners to operate faster, reducing the ionizing exposure to the patient. In addition, modern 3D CT scanners have a more open structure, as shown in Figure 1(b) [GSMI, 2009], which eases the sense of claustrophobia in patients.

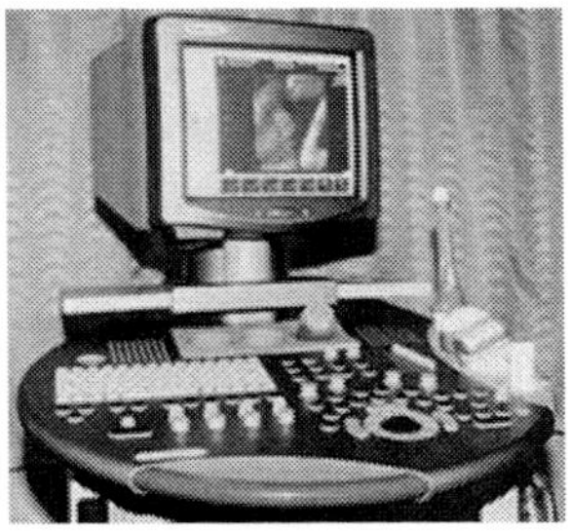

(a) Ultrasound scanner

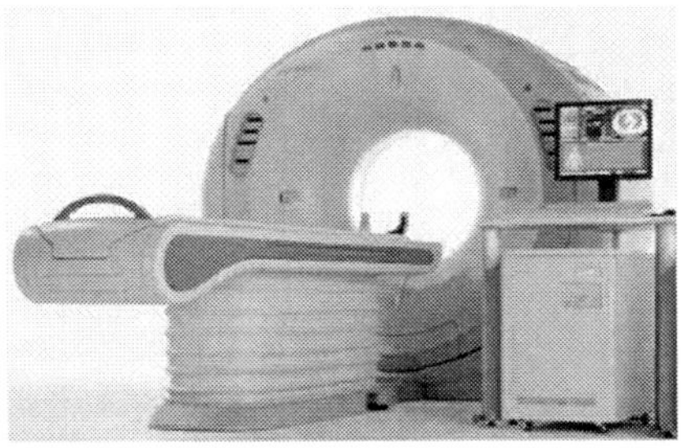

(b) typical CT scanner

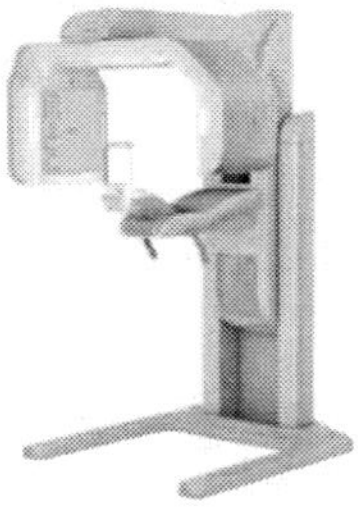

(c) CT dental scanner

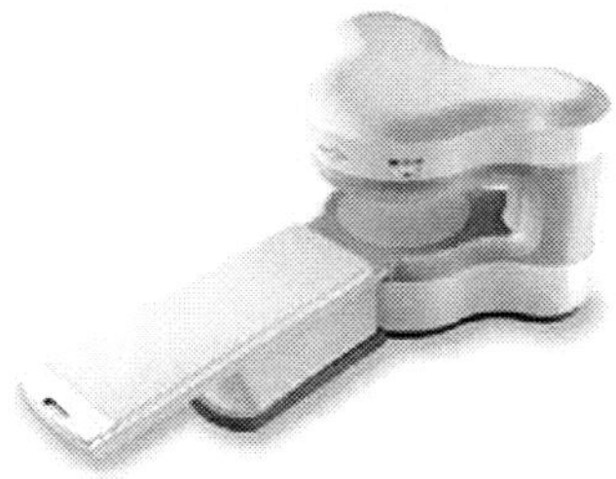

(d) open MRI scanner

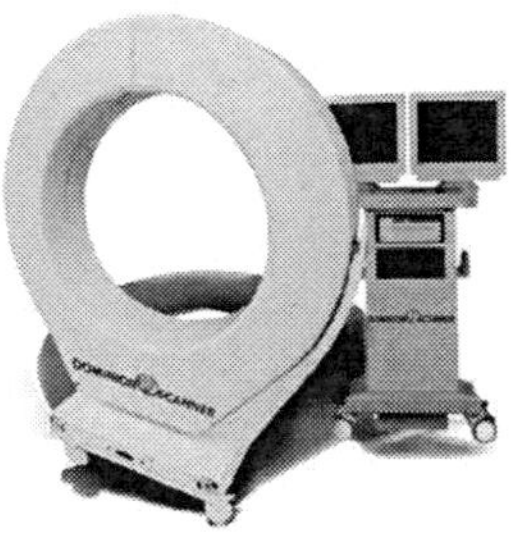

(e) photo-fluoroscopy scanner

Figure 1. Popular 3D medical diagnostic imaging scanners.

Popular uses of the 3D CT include angiogram, colonography, orthodontics [Valiathan et al., 2008], scanning of the ankle, head, neck, knee, varicose veins, cleft lip, tendons, lung, colon/renal [Gössl et al., 2006] and many other parts of the anatomy. Customised open 3D CT scanners have been built for different parts of the anatomy, such as the E-Woo Master 3DS dental scanner shown in Figure 1(c) [Ascend Media, 2009] that is able to complete a 3D CT scan in just 15 seconds.

2.3 Magnetic Resonance Imaging (MRI)

3D Magnetic Resonance Imaging (MRI) provides clear images without ionizing side effects as it uses electromagnets instead of radiation. However, this type of equipment is not suitable for those with magnetisable metallic implants. 3D MRI has become a popular alternative for angiogram (known as MRA or magnetic resonance angiogram), liver and bile duct imaging, diagnosing the deadly pancreatic cancer [ARRS, 2005], scanning of the lumbar spine [Hoad et al., 2001], cranial nerves [Rabinov et al., 2004], brain and foetal heart, and recently, even in detecting bleeding in the carotid arteries [HealthImaging, 2008]. The use of MRI in breast imaging has also gained popularity as a painless alternative to the conventional mammogram. Figure 1(d) [GSMI, 2009] shows an example of a 2D/3D open MRI scanner that reduces the incidence of claustrophobia.

2.4 Photo-Fluoroscopy

A newly introduced real-time 3D imaging equipment in the market is the Dominion, shown in Figure 1(e) [Imaging3, 2008]. This type of scanner produces high resolution photo-fluoroscopy 3D images instead of using x-ray or magnets. It is reported to be able to emulate 3D CT scans, thus providing a less ionizing version of the 3D CT.

3. Reconstruction of 3D Volume Using 2D Equipment

Actual 3D scanners are fast becoming popular, but they are still a costly investment, especially for less affluent medical institutions that already have older 2D scanners. Conventional scanners such as the earlier CT and MRI equipment were capable of scanning the 3D volume data but were not factory-equipped to represent them in 3D. Instead, most systems only succeeded in producing series of 2D images. Although computer graphics techniques for simple 3D reconstruction were available, image acquisition kinks such as partial volume, artefacts and noise made it a challenge for the equipment manufacturers to provide sufficiently advanced 3D tools in the past.

3.1 3D Volume Reconstruction Applications

Consequently, there has been much research carried out by various academic and research institutions, and the industry, in developing suitable tools and applications for the segmentation and 3D reconstruction of such images. One such well-known commercial software that has gained FDA (Food and Drug Administration authority, USA) approval for 3D medical visualisation applications is 3D-Doctor [2009]. Examples of successful 3D reconstruction include its use in the modelling of various body parts such as bone (from CT), soft tissues (from MRI), foetus (from ultrasound), brain, liver, breast (from mammogram), tumours, lung and many more including microscopy imaging of blood cells and vessels, alveoli and nerves. The 3D models generated are also useful in the calculation of size and volume of body parts. Other examples of segmentation-based 3D reconstruction products include TeleMed-VS, SeeThrough and 3D-Generator [Meinel, 2009].

3.2 Cost-effective 3D Setup using 2D Ultrasound

In the case of CT and MRI, it is relatively easy to obtain the location information of each 2D slice image as its relative location could be obtained from the equipment and is often stored in the electronic header of the images. In paperless institutions, or those equipped with hospital information systems (HIS), patient information inclusive of the diagnostic images, are stored electronically. The accepted file format used adheres to the DICOM (Digital Imaging and Communications for Medicine) 3 (Part-10) standard, that allows for storage of the acquisition information. With the location-based information derived from these headers, the 3D reconstruction applications are able to approximate the rendered volume of the organ or part of anatomy under examination. However, in the case of typical ultrasound, the probe is handled manually and in various orientations, without the location information recorded. This poses a problem in 3D reconstruction.

Efforts have been undertaken to create a cost-effective solution to overcome this limitation. One method is to use a simple conventional digital camera or webcam to photograph the acquisition. In the case of a digital camera, a photo of the probe would be taken at each location during the examination. As the probe is relatively static at each position, the physician could easily handle this without assistance by using the camera's remote control or delay timer. In the case of a video camera or webcam, the entire examination could be recorded and the relevant frames selected. If the ultrasound equipment supports a timing mechanism, a simple synchronization method would then be to have a clock in the field of view (FOV) of the webcam, or use the computer's internal clock, and the relevant frames would be selected based on the time.

In order to use the above setup, the individual equipment would need to be calibrated. In most cases, the calibration steps would only need to be performed once, and repeated only if any of the equipment is replaced or settings changed. A brief description of an example setup, calibration and reconstruction steps is given below.

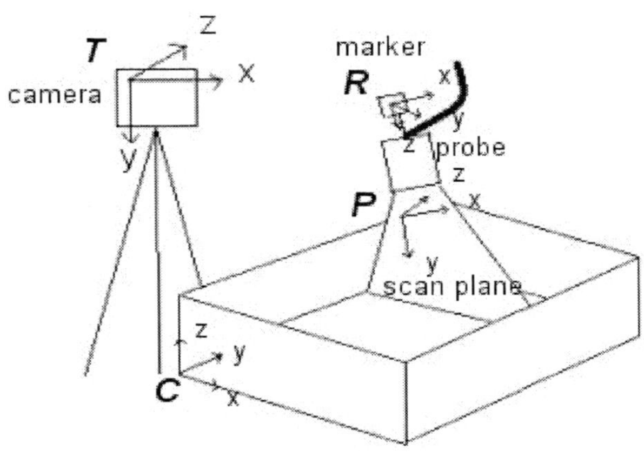

Figure 2. 3D ultrasound setup using a 2D probe and camera, along with the different coordinate systems identified.

3.2.1 Setup

The main parts of this setup are: the ultrasound probe (P), the camera (C), the volume (V) scanned and to be reconstructed, and a marker (M) affixed to the probe. The purpose of the marker is to allow for the orientation of the probe to be determined accurately. Experimentally, it was found that a small black and white chessboard-design cube made a suitable marker. Figure 2 shows a diagram of the setup, along with the reference coordinate system of each of the items in the setup. The volume in the figure represents a basin of warm water used for the calibration testing. This would be replaced at implementation with the actual object, i.e. body part, to be scanned.

3.2.2 Calibration

The purpose of the calibration is to unify the various reference coordinates in order to produce the reconstruction. The calibration of this system consists of calibration of the coordinate systems of the various parts of the setup with respect to each other, and then standardising them to correspond to the final reference coordinates of V. Several tested and readily available tools are used. Firstly, the camera calibration is undertaken to identify the real-world coordinates of the probe with respect to the camera. Then, probe calibration is tasked with identifying its position with respect to the 2D ultrasound scans. Using these, the actual position of the area being scanned is identified and can be fed into a 3D reconstruction application for 3D visualisation of a series of 2D ultrasound scans.

The whole calibration process entails that each pixel (u,v) on the ultrasound scan, represented by the probe in the P plane as x_p through scaling, be first transformed to the marker's coordinates (M plane), which in turn is transformed to the camera coordinates (C plane), and finally transformed to the volume to be reconstructed (V plane) to produce the x_v coordinates. This process can be summarised and represented by the following, as given in [Ali & Logeswaran, 2007a]:

$$x_v = T_v\, T_c\, T_m\, x_p \qquad (1)$$

where

$$x_p = \begin{pmatrix} s_x u \\ s_y v \\ 0 \\ 1 \end{pmatrix} \qquad (2)$$

xv = coordinates in the V (volume) plane,

xp = coordinates in the P (probe) plane,

T_v = transformation matrix for the V plane,

T_c = transformation matrix for the C (camera) plane,

T_m = transformation matrix for the V plane,

(u,v) = image pixel coordinates on the ultrasound scan,

sx and sy = scaling factors of the coordinates.

As the orientation is in 3D, i.e. in the three axes x, y and z, there are 6 degrees of freedom. These are the translations along each axis and the rotations (R) about those axes (i.e. α, β, γ, respectively). Thus, the general transformations can be represented by:

$$T(x,y,z,\alpha,\beta,\gamma) = \begin{bmatrix} R_{11} & R_{12} & R_{13} & x \\ R_{21} & R_{22} & R_{23} & y \\ R_{31} & R_{32} & R_{33} & z \\ 0 & 0 & 0 & 1 \end{bmatrix} \quad (3)$$

where

$$R_{11} = \cos\alpha \cos\beta \quad (4)$$

$$R_{12} = \sin\gamma \sin\alpha \cos\beta - \cos\gamma \sin\beta \quad (5)$$

$$R_{13} = \cos\gamma \sin\alpha \cos\beta + \sin\gamma \sin\beta \quad (6)$$

$$R_{21} = \cos\alpha \sin\beta \quad (7)$$

$$R_{22} = \sin\gamma \sin\alpha \cos\beta + \cos\gamma \cos\beta \quad (8)$$

$$R_{23} = \cos\gamma \sin\alpha \cos\beta - \sin\gamma \cos\beta \quad (9)$$

$$R_{31} = -\sin\alpha \quad (10)$$

$$R_{32} = \sin\gamma \cos\alpha \quad (11)$$

$$R_{33} = \cos\gamma\cos\alpha \tag{12}$$

It is not the intention of this chapter to provide a complete analysis of the mathematics involved in the calibration steps, as these utilise standard matrix transformations (**T**), consisting of rotations (R) and scaling (s), and can be solved using readily-available tools that exist. For solving $\mathbf{T_c}$, a good camera calibration toolbox in MATLAB [Bouguet, 2008] was used in this work. For readers interested in a more extensive description of the formulae and various experiments for determining the optimal camera calibration parameters, please refer to [Ali & Logeswaran, 2007b]. $\mathbf{T_v}$ is included for convenience to eliminate the need to construct a large (mostly empty) voxel (volume pixel in 3D) array when the reconstructed volume is aligned with the camera coordinate system.

For probe calibration, only $\mathbf{T_m}$ and the estimates of s_x and s_y need to be solved. A physical setup adapted from the well-known Cambridge phantom [Prager et al., 1998] was used as described in [Ali & Logeswaran, 2007a] and shown in Figure 3(a). A simpler setup by just attaching the marker to the probe and taking the scans at corresponding snapshots with the camera would do in practice, but the phantom allows more accurate measurements that are less prone to human error due to movement. Scans were taken using the phantom immersed in warm water (appropriate simulation of human tissue) in various orientations. By identifying the steel ruler in the resulting ultrasound scans (see Figure 3(b)), the values of the variables for the six degrees of freedom are determined through solving of the simultaneous equations. Substituting them back into equations (4)-(12) and then into equation (3) gives the transformation matrix $\mathbf{T_m}$.

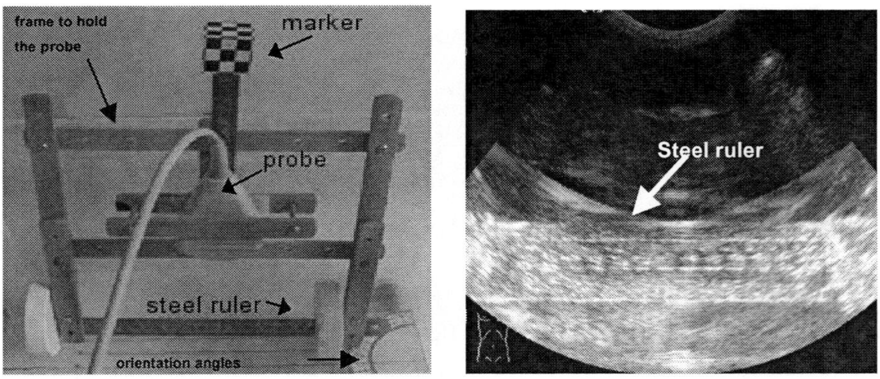

(a) simple probe calibration phantom (b) steel ruler in ultrasound scan

Figure 3. Probe calibration setup based on the Cambridge phantom.

3.2.3 Results

The calibrated setup can then be used to acquire actual ultrasound scans, retrieving the location information from each scan and reconstructing a 3D representation from the series of scans. For the purposes of this work, a simple surface fitting is undertaken to observe the results.

Figure 4 shows the 3D reconstruction results obtained. The first two are for ultrasound scans on the human body, i.e. (a) gallbladder, and (b) part of the aorta. These were verified by medical experts as acceptable representations. Higher quality reproductions are possible with more scans and better interpolation algorithms, but simple surface fitting was deemed sufficient for this work. An example of a test case conducted using a PVC (polyvinyl chloride) cylindrical pipe immersed in jelly produced the result in Figure 4(c), which was used to verify the accuracy of the setup, in terms of diameter and shape. The use of jelly in this case follows the accepted convention used to simulate tissue, and allows for the cylinder to be suspended in the jelly.

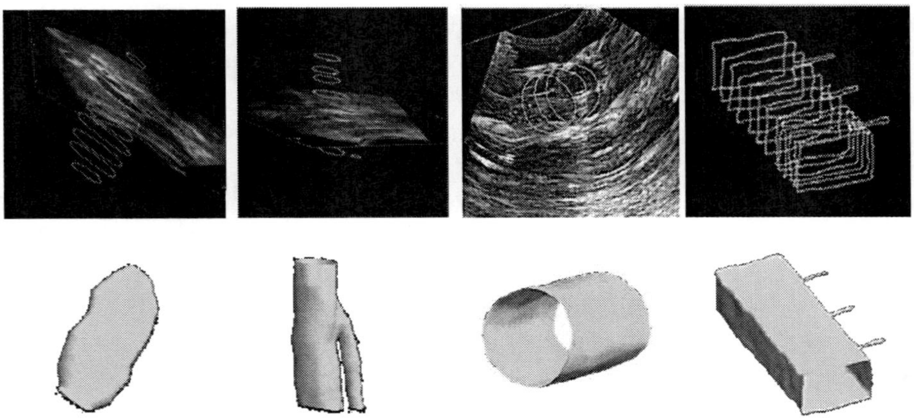

(a) gallbladder (b) aorta (c) cylindrical pipe (d) block with nails

Figure 4. Segments from ultrasound images (above) and the corresponding preliminary reconstructions using simple 3D surface fitting (below).

Other more extensive experiments using a block of wood affixed with nails at various intervals, see Figure 4(d), were also undertaken. Details of these are available in [Ali & Logeswaran, 2007b]. From all the experiments, it was determined that the proposed system with simple surface fitting was able to accurately reconstruct the 3D volume within 1 mm of the actual dimensions of the object being scanned. More precision, if desired, could be achieved by more sophisticated 3D applications such as those discussed earlier in this section.

4. Automatic Analysis

In medical applications, the purpose of 3D reconstruction is to aid in the diagnosis. With the advent of more powerful computer methods and artificial intelligence, CAD systems are more widespread and can assist the medical practitioner in preliminary detection of diseases and abnormalities. This is particularly useful when taking into consideration the large volume of images acquired at medical institutions. A typical MRI examination of a patient routinely produces 100-200 images, ranging from location images to series of slice images for acquisitions in various orientations.

This section provides a brief discussion of the typical automatic image processing and analysis steps undertaken in the preliminary diagnosis of diseases by CAD systems for 3D capable imaging devices. Most 3D reconstruction applications do incorporate at least some of the steps below, and allow controlled manipulation of some of the parameters. The purpose of this section is to briefly introduce the main stages in the analysis of the 3D volume imaging.

4.1 Image Enhancement

Acquisition equipment usually allow, and may even cause, the influence of some noise on the images. The common ambient noise due to environmental radiation is one such influence. The movement of parts of the equipment, fluctuations in the electromagnetic field or beam strength, the inaccuracies in calculations and parameter selection, usage wear and tear, and partial volume due to the representation of a 3D slab of certain thickness into a flat 2D image, are some possible influences that reduce the quality of the image. Additionally, artifacts may be caused by the subject (patient) due to breathing, movement, irregular heart beat, body fat composition, abnormalities and injuries. All these contribute to lower quality images, and thus lead to lower quality 3D volume, which may impair the diagnosis.

Image enhancement is carried out as the first stage of the process to reduce image noise and normalize the images. The algorithms used would depend on the characteristics of the noise and the image, but some popular noise removal techniques include filtering using the Gaussian or median distribution functions. Gaussian filtering generally blurs the image, removing high frequency noise. Median filtering is effective for removal of salt and pepper type noise. In cases where the edges are to be preserved (these are otherwise destroyed by isotropic functions such as Gaussian), anisotropic filters such as the Perona-Malik or Euclidean Shortening Flow (ESF) may be used. It has been shown in [Choong et al., 2006] that blurring or filtering, by itself, can help improve the diagnosis stage, in addition to reducing the image size and saving on storage space.

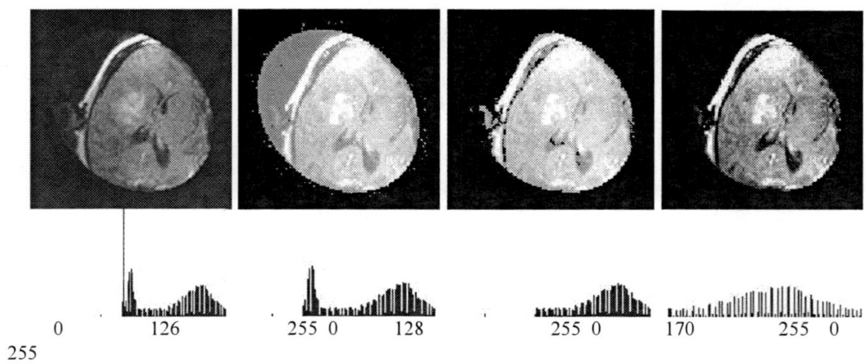

(a) original (b) peak 1 eliminated (c) peak 2 eliminated (d) normalized

Figure 5. Enhancement of a low-field MRI brain image through histogram truncation.

The size and intensity of the various parts of the images may vary depending on the depth and field of view (FoV) of the acquisition. It is usually sensible to normalize the images with respect to these at this stage, in order to ensure more consistent treatment in later stages. One effective method of normalization is through histogram analysis, where parts of the histogram may be truncated to reduce the influence of unwanted parts (e.g. noise, artifacts, bright spots etc.). An example of such treatment on a low-field MRI image of the brain is shown in Figure 5 [Ishak et al., 2008]. Truncating parts of the histogram not only reduces the influence of unwanted parts of the image, it can also be very useful in detecting other adverse parts, such as the artifact that has become more visible in Figure 5(b) due to the improved contrast once the high frequency lower intensity background was truncated.

The intensity range may then be stretched (see Figure 5(d)) to enhance the visibility of the region of interest (ROI). This is noticeable in Figure 5(d), where the bleeding in the brain is more prominent, and the tissue structure is more clearly discernable. This step also normalizes the image intensity with respect to the other images in a test set. Cropping of the background and any padding that may exist on the images also leads to standardization of the size of the ROI, enabling more consistent treatment of the images in the remaining stages.

4.2 Structure Detection

Before any disease or abnormality can be detected automatically, it is necessary to detect and label the structures within the image. The choice of conducting this processing before or after 3D reconstruction depends on the complexity of the volume to be studied. 3D reconstruction allows for the 3D object (c.f. 2D image) to be studied, but at the cost of much higher processing power and time. Generally, if sufficient structure detection is possible using the individual 2D slice images, it would be recommended to conduct this analysis in 2D. Once the structures of interest have been detected in 2D, 3D reconstruction could be limited to these structures rather than rendering the volume to include the background and other parts of the image.

For detection, the images are first segmented into homogenous parts. A popular segmentation algorithm in medical applications is watershed, which is applied on the image gradients. Alternative edge detection algorithms may also be used. For labeling, some additional (often statistical) knowledge is incorporated to determine the segments that correspond to different structures. Features, in terms of colour (or intensity), size, location, neighbouring segments etc., may be used for this purpose.

More advanced algorithms such as wavelets, scale-space [Logeswaran, 2005] and other multiresolution techniques may also be used to map various levels of information in a portion of the image to determine its energy and thus, its significance. Structure identification in terms of hierarchy or growing from significant portions of the identified structure to locate other connected and/or less significant parts may be undertaken, in 2D [Logeswaran, 2008c] or 3D [Logeswaran & Eswaran, 2005], using such an approach. An example of the 3D structure detection for a thick slab magnetic resonance cholangiopancreatography (MRCP) image is shown in Figure 6(b). The erroneous parts (i.e. not bile ducts) of the detection are eliminated through known statistics such as size, location and connectedness, reproducing the 3D result in Figure 6(c).

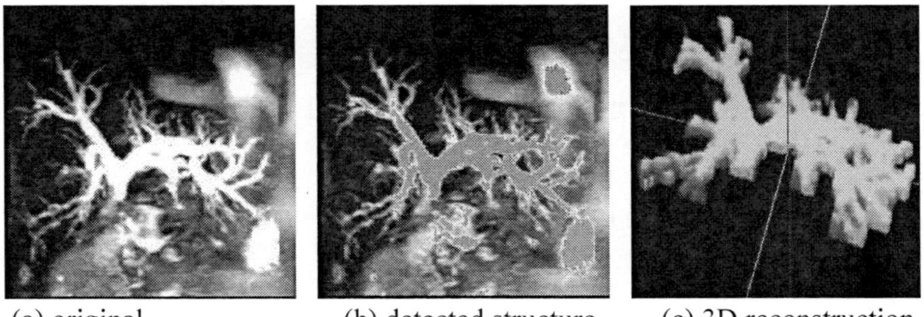

(a) original (b) detected structure (c) 3D reconstruction

Figure 6. Results of multiresolution biliary structure detection and 3D reconstruction.

4.3 Automated Diagnosis

From the previous operations, the structures of interest that represent the organs or other parts of the anatomy would have been accurately detected, or at least approximated. Diseases and abnormalities may be physically represented in a large number of ways, depending on the specific disease or abnormality. Some diseases are fairly obvious, such as detecting the presence of a large cyst in the brain. Some diseases may be observed in relation to their influence on other parts of the image, such as a blockage causing the vessel to swell up. A tumour mass in a T2-weighted MRCP image is dark and may not be seen against the dark background, but can be inferred by the position and lack of visibility of the surrounding structures. Some diseases may be observed through the change of tissue texture or colour, and abnormalities may be detected through comparison with "normal" cases. In biology, "normal" can be rather broad as biological objects inherently vary at least slightly from each other - an example being that even identical twins are not exactly identical. As such, there has to be a certain amount of variation allowable in the range of normality.

Straightforward algorithms may be developed for the automated detection. This includes the selection and shortlisting of features and parameters to identify a certain disease. Often, statistics and empirical methods are used to decide on the optimum parameter values. As an example, a bile duct, vessel or organ, may be considered distended (swollen) if it is larger than a certain percentage of its expected size. The expected size may be a known threshold or a scaled value based on clues from other aspects of the patient, such as age, physical size, known disorders etc. An example of a successful multi-disease detection system using such an approach is given in [Logeswaran, 2008a].

Artificial neural networks (ANN) have been used in many medical applications to successfully identify various medical conditions (e.g. stones detection in [Logeswaran, 2006c]), as well as in many other non-medical applications [Chung & Logeswaran, 2006]. In most cases, it has been found that more advanced artificial intelligence techniques such as these, as well as strong statistical methods such as Support Vector Machines (SVM), improve the accuracy of the diagnosis. An example of employing a trained ANN to improve detection accuracy can be found by comparing the work in [Logeswaran, 2006a] with that in [Logeswaran, 2006b]. In the latter, ANN was used to enhance the detection of choledocol cysts and managed to improve the overall performance accuracy from 89.55% (without ANN in the former) to 94.77% (with ANN in the latter) for the same test set.

5. Discussion and Future Trends

There is much more that is being done and can be done in terms of 3D imaging and 3D visualisation in the medical field. Some of the efforts being taken include development of telemedicine applications including webcam-based tools such as 3D imaging of external injuries, patient locator [Logeswaran, 2008b], holographic projection on a transparent surface and many more. In terms of equipment, we will see smaller, quieter and more open (reduced incidence of claustrophobia) instruments capable of producing clearer images and representations of objects even with minimal or no use of contrast agents. As the trend is for non-invasive diagnosis methods, and technology in this respect has matured to be up to par with the gold standard invasive procedures in diagnosis, more practitioners (and patients) would opt for the use of these 3D imaging devices.

One should not forget the vast developments that are being made in CAD applications, whether embedded into the equipment, packaged by the manufacturer, or developed by third-party researchers. These applications have been fine-tuned so much that in many aspects, it allows for visualisation and diagnostic assistance (medical knowledgebase, image manipulation tools, artificial intelligence) that many medical specialist rely on them. Most equipment now are equipped with at least some amount of CAD tools, more so for 3D imaging devices. These have become extremely user-friendly, that with little training, the medical practitioner is able to produce very in-depth representations of the ROI under study.

Of course, as with any assisted technology, care must be exercised with regards to its use. A pitfall in many institutions, especially when cash strapped, is the lack of proper regular calibration and maintenance of the equipment. These can have severe consequences if there are defects, miscalibration, degradation of the quality of shielding etc., and should be monitored.

CONCLUSION

This chapter has provided a brief overview of some of the developments involving 3D imaging in the medical field. Beginning with an introduction to the currently available 3D medical equipments, the chapter progressed into reconstruction of 3D volume objects from the acquired and stored as 2D slice data. Sample 3D reconstruction applications were surveyed and an experimental setup using the conventional 2D ultrasound probe to reconstruct 3D visualisation was described. The discussion then moved on to the various stages of activities required for the automatic treatment of images in order to conduct automated computer-aided diagnosis for preliminary detection of diseases and abnormalities. An example of using neural networks to improve the diagnosis performance was also mentioned, with relevant references provided. Finally, discussions on the expected future trends were given in the previous section.

Overall, 3D imaging has seen much innovation in the medical field, in addition to many other fields, the most prominent being entertainment. With the exposure to 3D, patients expect such visualisation when they undergo an examination. It is also more convenient for the discussion of patient cases and history when 3D data is available. Its use will continue to grow, and augmented with other "dimensions" such as time, signals from other equipment (e.g. heartbeat data used during MRI or CT to compensate for motion artifacts and correlate the reconstruction). It is hoped that some of the 3D and hologram technology portrayed in the entertainment industry would soon become a reality in the medical world, as it would certainly add value and accuracy in conducting diagnosis.

REFERENCES

[1] 3D USIG – Ultrasound Interest Group (2009). 3D/4D *ultrasound imaging* [online]. 1 Feb 2009 [7 July 2009]. Available from: http://3dviz.ucsd.edu/ ~3DUS/Home.html.

[2] 3D-Doctor (2009). *FDA-approved, vector-based 3D imaging, modeling and measurement software [online].* [7 July 2009]. Available from: http://www.ablesw.com/3d-doctor/.

[3] Ali, A. and Logeswaran, R. (2007a). *A Visual Probe Localization and Calibration System for Cost-Effective Computer-Aided 3D Ultrasound.* Computers in Biology and Medicine, 37(8), 1141-1147 (DOI: 10.1016/j.compbiomed.2006.10.003).

[4] Ali, A. and Logeswaran, R. (2007b). Implementing Cost-effective 3D Ultrasound Using Visual Probe Localization. *Journal of Digital Imaging, 20*(4), 352-366 (DOI: 10.1007/s10278-006-0624-6).

[5] ARRS - American Roentgen Ray Society (2005). *3D MRI useful in detecting most lethal of all major cancers [online].* ScienceDaily 8 September 2005 [9 May 2009]. Available from: http://www.sciencedaily.com /releases/2005/09/050907103046.htm.

[6] Ascend Media (2009). *E-WOO Master 3DS [online].* [10 July 2009]. Available from: http://www.orthodonticproductsonline. com/newsbites/2009-03-02_06.asp.

[7] Bouguet, J. Y. (2008*). Camera Calibration Toolbox for Matlab [online].* 2 June 2008 [12 July 2009]. Available from: http://www.vision.caltech.edu/bouguetj/calib_doc/index.html.

[8] Choong, M. K., Logeswaran, R. and Bister, M. (2006). Improving Diagnostic Quality of MR Images Through Controlled Lossy Compression using SPIHT. *Journal of Medical Systems, 30(3)*, 139-143.

[9] Chung, S. H. and Logeswaran, R. (2006). Neural Networks in Image Processing: A Review of Current Applications. *INTI Journal, 2*(1), 582-592.

[10] Downey, D. B. and Fenster, A. (1998). Three-dimensional ultrasound: A maturing technology. *Ultrasound Quarterly,* 14, 25-40.

[11] Goncalves, L. F., Lee, W., Chaiworapongsa, T., Espinoza, J., Schoen, M. L., Falkensammer, P., Treadwell, M. and Romero, R. (2003). Four-dimensional ultrasonography of the fetal heart with spatiotemporal image correlation. *American Journal of Obstetrics and Gynecology,* 189(6), 1792-802.

[12] Gössl, M., Bentley, M. D. and Lerman, L. O. (2006). *Review - 3D micro CT imaging of renal micro-structural changes.* Nephron Clinical Practice, 103, c66-c70 (DOI: 10.1159/000090611).

[13] GSMI (2009). *Garden State Medical Imaging [online].* [10 July 2009]. Available from: http://thegsmi.com/.

[14] HealthImaging (2008). *3D MRI technique helps detect high-risk carotid disease [online].* HealthImaging.com 15 September 2008 [9 May 2009]. Available from: http://www.healthimaging.com/index.php?
option=com_articlesandview=articleandid=12121:3d-mri-technique-helps-detect-high-risk-carotid-disease.

[15] Hoad, C. L., Martel, A. L., Kerslake, R. and Grevitt, M. (2001). A 3D MRI sequence for computer assisted surgery of the lumbar spine. *Physics in Medicine and Biology,* 46, N213-N220 (DOI: 10.1088/0031-9155/46/8/403).

[16] Imaging3 (2008). *3D real-time medical imaging - Dominion Vi 3D medical imaging scanner - medical imaging technology [online].* [7 July 2009]. Available from: http://www.imaging3.com/.

[17] Ishak, N. F., Logeswaran, R. and Tan, W. H. (2008). Artifact and Noise Stripping on Low-Field Brain MRI. *International Journal of Biology and Biomedical Engineering,* 2(2), 59-68.

[18] Jurkovic, D., Geipel, A., Gruboeck, K., Jauniaux, E., Natucci, M. and Campbell, S. (1995). Three-dimensional ultrasound for the assessment of uterine anatomy and detection of congenital anomalies: A comparison with hysterosalpingography and two-dimensional sonography. *Ultrasound Obstetrics and Gynecology*, 5, 233-237.

[19] Logeswaran, R. (2005). Scale-space Segment Growing For Hierarchical Detection of Biliary Tree Structure. *International Journal of Wavelets, Multiresolution and Information Processing, 3*(1), 125-140.

[20] Logeswaran, R. (2006a). Choledochol Cyst – An Automated Preliminary Detection System using MRCP Images. 6th WSEAS International Conference on Signal, *Speech and Image Processing*, 162-167.

[21] Logeswaran, R. (2006b). Choledochol Cyst Preliminary Detection System for MRCP Images using Neural Networks. *WSEAS Transactions on Signal Processing,* 2(9), 1299-1305.

[22] Logeswaran, R. (2006c). *Neural Networks Aided Stone Detection in Thick Slab MRCP Images.* Medical and Biological Engineering and Computing, 44(8), 711-719.

[23] Logeswaran, R. (2008a). A Computer-Aided Multi-Disease Diagnostic System using MRCP. *Journal of Digital Imaging, 21(2)*, 235-242.

[24] Logeswaran, R. (2008b). Cost Effective Patient Location Monitoring System using Webcams. *Journal of Medical Systems.* DOI: 10.1007/s10916-008-9202-4.

[25] Logeswaran, R. (2008c). Reconstruction of Biliary Structure in 2D MRCP Images using Multi-Scale Analysis. *Computers in Biology and Medicine,* 38(3), 391-400.

[26] Logeswaran, R. and Eswaran, C. (2005). Application of 3D Multiresolution Analysis for Structure Detection in 2D. *Multimedia Cyberscape Journal,* 3(4), 30-34.

[27] Maadiagnostic (2009). 4D Ultrasound [online]. [10 July 2009]. *Available from: http://www.maadiagnostic.com/4dus.htm.*

[28] Meinel, C. (2009*). 3D medical image processing [online].* [7 July 2009]. Available from: http://www.hpi.uni-potsdam.de/meinel/projects/ telemedicine_and_security/ 3d_ medical_image_processing.html.

[29] Merz, E., Bahlmann, F. and Weber, G. (1995). Volume scanning in the evaluation of fetal malformations: A new dimension in prenatal diagnosis. *Ultrasound Obstetrics and Gynecology*, 5, 222-227.

[30] Nelson, T. R., Downey, D. B., Pretorius, D. H. and Fenster, A. (1990). *Three-dimensional Ultrasound.* New York: Lippincott.

[31] Nelson, T. R., Pretorius, D. H., Sklansky, M. and Hagen-Ansert, S. (1996). Three-dimensional echocardiographic evaluation of fetal heart anatomy and function: acquisition, analysis, and display. *Journal of Ultrasound Medicine,* 15(1), 1-9.

[32] Prager, R. W., Rohling, R. N., Gee, A. H. and Berman, L. (1998). Rapid Calibration for 3-D Free-hand ultrasound. *Ultrasound in Medicine and Biology,* 24(6), 885-869.

[33] Rabinov, J. D., Barker, F. G., McKenna, M. J. and Curtin, H. D. (2004). Virtual cisternoscopy: 3D MRI models of the cerebellopontine angle for lesions related to the cranial nerves. *Skull Base*, 14(2), 93–99 (DOI: 10.1055/s-2004-828701).

[34] Riccabona, M., Nelson, T. R., Pretorius, D. H. and Davidson, T. E. (1996). Three-dimensional sonographic measurement of bladder volume. *Journal of Ultrasound Medicine,* 15, 627-632.

[35] Rose, S. C., Pretorius, D. H., Kinney, T. B., Nelson, T. R., Valji, K., D'Agostino, H. R., Forsythe, N. M., Roberts, A. C. and Manco-Johnson, M. L. (1999). 3D sonographic guidance of transvenous intrahepatic invasive procedures: Feasibility of a new technique. *Journal of Vascular Intervention Radiology,* 10, 189-198.

[36] Valiathan, A., Dhar, S. and Verma, N. (2008). 3D CT imaging in orthodontics: Adding a new dimension to diagnosis and treatment planning. Trends in Biomaterial Artificial Organs, 21(2), 116-120.

In: 3D Imaging: Theory, Technology … ISBN: 978-1-60876-885-1
Editors: E. H. Duke and S. R. Aguirre, pp.175-188

Chapter 7

BONE MACROARCHITECTURE BY 3D IMAGING AND OSTEOPOROSIS

Sami Kolta**, *Jacques Fechtenbaum and Christian Roux
Paris-Descartes University, Cochin Hospital, Rheumatology Department, Paris, France.

ABSTRACT

Exploration of bone using two-dimensional (2D) techniques is widely used by plain x-rays, dual x-ray absorptiometry (DXA), CT scan and magnetic resonance imaging (MRI). Evaluation of fracture risk does not depend only on the bone mineral density (BMD, g/cm²) but also on its structure as its micro and macroarchitecture. Bone is a three-dimensional (3D) structure. Using 2D imaging systems will cause loss of information. For example BMD measured by DXA depends on bone size. Patients' height reflects bone size and therefore affects BMD results and this information should be available for a proper interpretation of the BMD results. Bone geometry (macroarchitecture) is a very important parameter in the evaluation of bone strength. It has been evaluated from DXA scans or plain X-rays. Much progress has been made in 3D imaging and 3D reconstruction from several 2D images. We can nowadays evaluate geometric parameters of bone in 3D using CT scans or a new low-radiating device (EOS®). We have also recently described a method of 3D reconstruction using 2 perpendicular DXA scans: the 3D-XA (3 Dimensional X-ray Absorptiometry). Cross-sectional area, cortical thickness, cross-sectional moment of inertia, section modulus, buckling ratio, bone size and bone diameter can be measured in vivo using 3D imaging techniques. Finite element models have also been calculated from 3D images and allows the prediction of a personalized fracture risk. The recent progress in 3D imaging has greatly improved the evaluation of bone structure. BMD, microarchitecture parameters as well as geometric parameters predict failure load and improve the calculation of an individualized risk of fracture. In vivo 3D imaging will allow longitudinal studies in animals and in humans. The effect of antiosteoporotic drugs on BMD is very heterogeneous and can't explain their antifracture effect. This can be better understood by the effect of therapeutic agents on bone micro and macroarchitecture. Three dimensional imaging of bone may contribute in the field of osteoporosis to a better prediction of a personalized risk of fracture as well as a better understanding of the mechanism of action of antiosteoporotic agents.

* Corresponding author : CEMO – Hôpital Cochin, 27, rue du faubourg Saint Jacques, 75014 Paris, France, e.mail : sami.kolta@cch.aphp.fr

Osteoporosis is a worldwide disease with a great epidemiological and economic burden (1), that will increase due to the aging of the world population. Osteoporotic fractures increase morbidity (2), mortality (3,4) and affects the quality of life of patients (5). All the bones are concerned. The main osteoporotic fractures are those affecting the hip, wrist and vertebrae. About two-thirds of vertebral fractures are asymptomatic. Even asymptomatic, vertebral fractures are an important risk factor for new vertebral and non-vertebral fractures. About one woman out of four aged 50 years or more will sustain a vertebral fracture (6). The incidence of vertebral fractures increases with age (7). Risk factors for osteoporotic fractures include the risk of fall, the parental history of hip fracture, the personal history of peripheral fracture or the number (8) and severity (9,10) of prevalent vertebral fractures. The occurrence of osteoporotic fractures depends on bone strength which results from bone quantity and quality parameters. Bone mineral density (BMD, g/cm^2) measured by Dual X-ray Absorptiometry (DXA) assesses the bone quantity. One standard deviation decrease in BMD doubles the risk of fracture (11). However, there is an overlap between BMD of fractured and non-fractured individuals (12). Moreover, if treatment decision is based on BMD alone, about half of the postmenopausal women who will sustain a fracture will not be selected for treatment. The majority of patients with fracture are indeed osteopenic. Effective anti-osteoporotic drugs are available and should be given to patients at risk. It is therefore important to recognize these patients and treat them.

Measurement of BMD by DXA is in two dimensions (2D) and cannot differentiate between cortical and trabecular bone density. Using a three-dimensional (3D) technique as CT scanner, allows this differentiation (13).

The strength of bone tissue is not only determined by its mass, but also by other properties usually referred to as bone quality, such as microarchitecture, macroarchitechture, distribution of bone tissue in space, ... (14). Other parameters should therefore be evaluated in order to determine bone strength. This chapter will deal with 3D measurement of bone macroarchitecture (geometry) in the field of osteoporosis. Bone geometry has been evaluated in 2D by plain X-rays (15) and DXA scans (16,17). Anterior-posterior (AP) with or without lateral DXA scans were used to calculate 3D results as vertebral body volume (cm^3), but these calculations necessitate some assumptions as to the form of bone. For example, vertebral body was assumed to be either cylindrical, ellipsoid or cubic. Calculation of volumetric bone density (g/cm^3), based on paired AP and lateral DXA scans was found to have a better discriminatory capability for the presence or absence of vertebral fracture than 2D BMD (18). Recent DXA devices are equipped with a software allowing automatic measurement of geometric parameters of the hip with a standard hip BMD scan. Hologic devices (Hologic Inc, Bedford, MA, USA) are equipped with the HSA (Hip Structural Analysis) software and GE-Lunar (Madison, WI, USA) are equipped with the AHA (Advanced Hip Analysis) software. However, bone being a 3D structure, in order to use a 2D method such as DXA to measure these geometrical parameters, several assumptions are made. These assumptions include the shape of the bone (cylindrical, ellipse, ...), its composition (cortical to trabecular bone ratio), homogeneity of the cortical wall thickness, etc ... Moreover, the influence of patient positioning and individual anatomic variation on the accuracy of these 2D measurements have been pointed out (19,20). Three-dimensional assessment of these geometric parameters is a way to bypass the dependence on patient positioning (21).

The aims of adding 3D macroarchitecture of bone to the standard BMD results are:

A To improve the fracture risk prediction and therefore allow a more precise selection of patients at high risk of fracture as candidates for anti-osteoporotic treatment.
B To get a better understanding of the mechanism of action of anti-osteoporotic drugs.

Several devices allow measurement of 3D macroarchitecture of bone:

1. CT (Computerized Tomography) Scanners

Quantitative CT (QCT) can be done by most of CT scanners at the spine. Some of them can perform these measurements on peripheral bones. This technique has the advantage of separating the cortical and the trabecular bones and being widely available around the world. Its disadvantage is the relatively high radiation dose to the patients (effective dose of about 100-1000 μSv for spine and hip) compared to other techniques as DXA (< 5 μSv) or MRI (no radiation) (22). In vivo 3D QCT precision errors of bone density measurement are about 1-1.5% for trabecular and 2.5-3% for cortical bone in postmenopausal women (23).

Differentiating cortical and trabecular bone is important in the evaluation of the contribution of each type of bone in bone strength as cortical bone is known to play a central role in bone strength of the proximal femur (13,24). The measurement of 3D geometric variables allows also the evaluation of their contribution to bone strength. Alone, they explained 43% of femoral failure load variance compared with 72% for densitometric variables. Combining densitometric and geometric variables measured by QCT explained 76% of the failure load compared to 69% with DXA alone (13). QCT can measure cortical thickness to a level of approximately 1.5–2 mm. Even below these values, a 10-20% change of thickness can still be measured accurately (25). CT scanners have also been used to calculate individualized geometric parameters from the 3D bone reconstruction as 3D femoral neck length.

At the spine, the cross-sectional area of the vertebral bodies is a macrostructural parameter of interest, since it is likely that larger vertebrae can sustain load better than smaller ones. Perisoteal apposition, which may occur at the spine and the femur, has the potential to offset the increase in fragility caused by loss of bone mass by increasing cross-sectional area (26). In a cross-sectional study using volumetric QCT (vQCT), it has been shown that women had smaller vertebrae, they lose bone mass faster and they also increase cross-sectional area slower than men (27). As in the spine, this study showed that periosteal apposition causes the cross-sectional areas of the femoral neck and shaft to expand with age (27). The magnitude of the changes reported by vQCT were inconsistent with DXA findings (28). They explain femoral strength partially independently from BMD (29). Geometric parameters with higher femoral neck and lumbar spine volumetric BMD but lower cross-sectional areas in African-Americans, have also been shown which might explain some of the ethnic difference in the epidemiology of hip and spine fracture (30). The 3D reconstruction of bone can also be used to calculate individualized Finite Element Model (FEM) that give a computer-based simulation of strains and stresses induced by mechanical loading and therefore can help the estimation of individualized fracture risk (31).

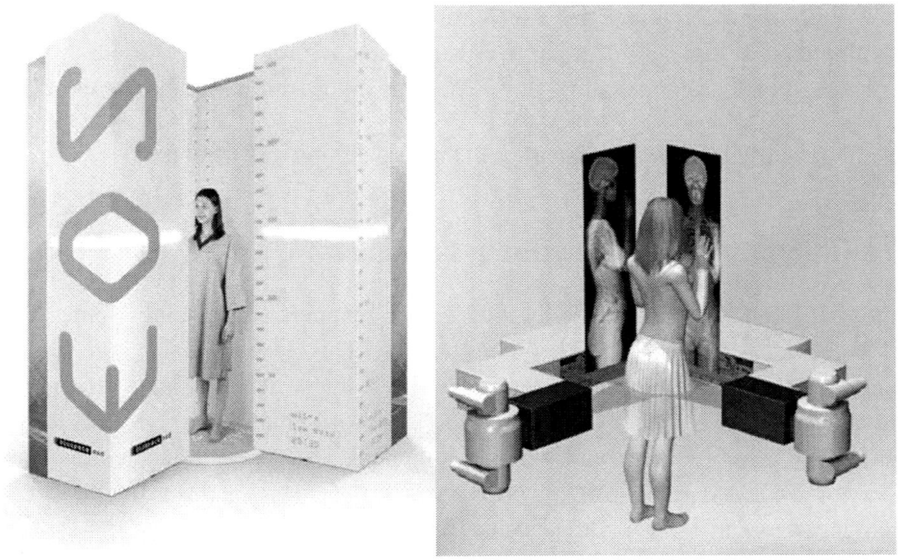

Figure 1. EOS device (Biospace Med, Paris, France) allowing simultaneous acquisition of anterior-posterior and lateral views of whole body x-rays in the standing position.

2. EOS™

This is a new device based on the technique described by the 1992 Nobel price of physics Georges Charpak. This ultra low dose 2D/3D digital X-ray system, is a new imaging system developed by Biospace Med (Paris, France). This technique has the advantage of being very low radiating to the patient. The radiation dose necessary to obtain a 2D image has been reduced 8 to 10 times, while that required to obtain a 3D reconstruction from CT slices has fallen by a factor of 800 to 1000 with a comparable accuracy (32). Follow-up of certain patients as children, or certain pathologies needing repeated x-rays as in scoliosis, osteoporotic vertebral fracture, ankylosing spondylitis, ... can therefore be done without any ethical concern.

EOS allows for the simultaneous acquisition of two orthogonal planar images in a vertical, weight-bearing standing or sitting position (Figures 1, 2). The gantry is composed of two sets of detectors and two X-ray tubes positioned orthogonally and supported by a mobile C-arm which moves vertically. The patient is positioned at the intersection of the two X-ray fan-beams which scan the patient vertically. A single scan will simultaneously produce both posterior-anterior and lateral views of the patient, without any distortion to the image. Full spine images are easily created in about 8 seconds for an adult and 5 seconds for a child.

Reconstruction of the 3D bone envelope of the spine and lower limbs (Figures 3, 4) is performed with a good accuracy using EOS low dose biplane images, and a priori statistical information about the 3D bones. The user initiates the reconstruction process by positioning a few anatomical landmarks on the posterior-anterior and lateral views with the help of epipolar constraint. These landmarks, with the help of edge detection algorithms and statistical inference, allow the software to produce a 3D envelope of the bone. The user then adjusts the model to minimize the distance between the corresponding observed model and anatomical features. The intra and inter observer reproducibility of 3D reconstruction are good (33).

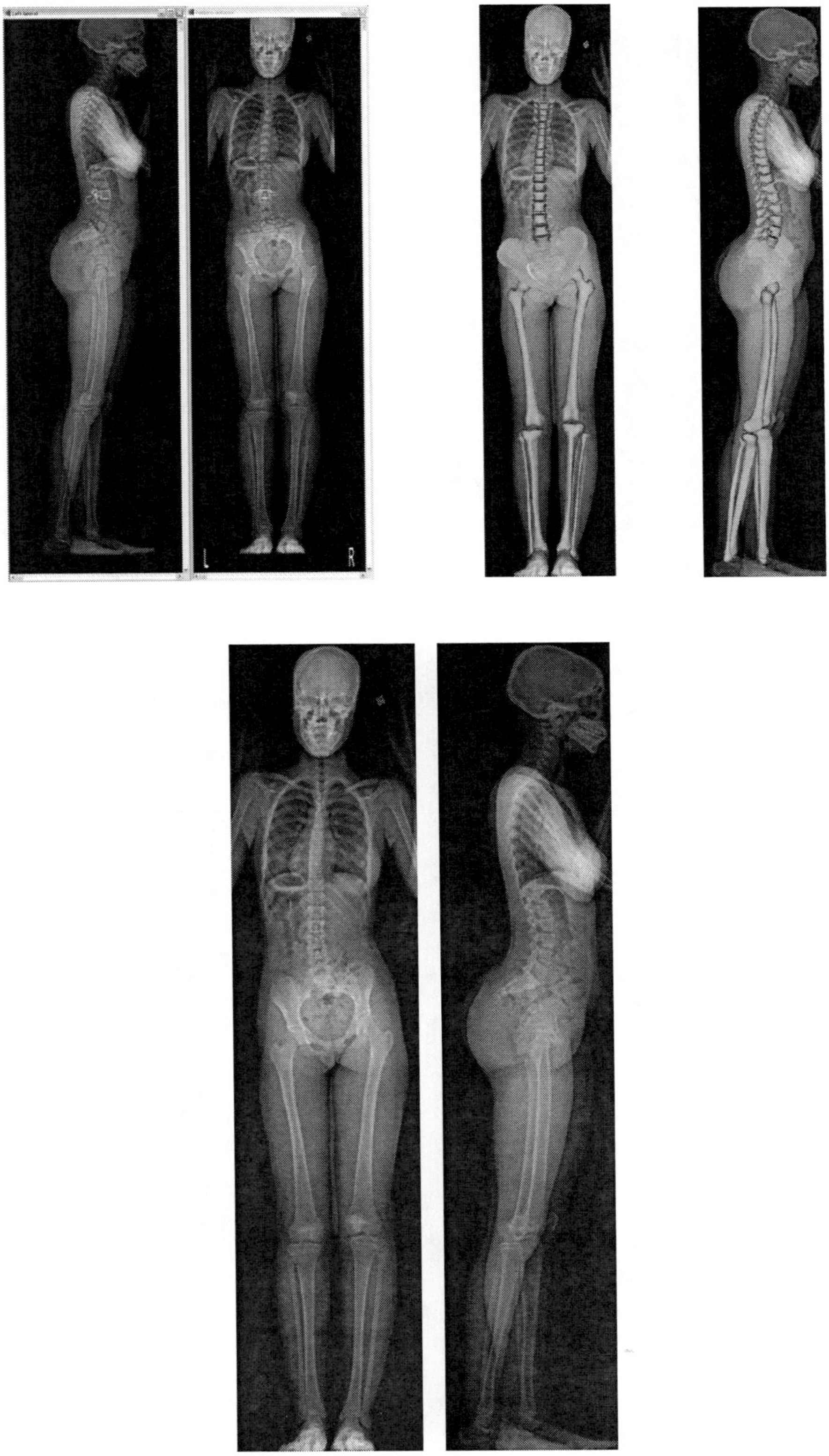

Figure 2. Anterior-posterior and lateral views of the skeleton on an EOS device; Biospace Med, Paris, France (Courtesy of Dr Ana Presedo – Robert Debré hospital, Paris, France).

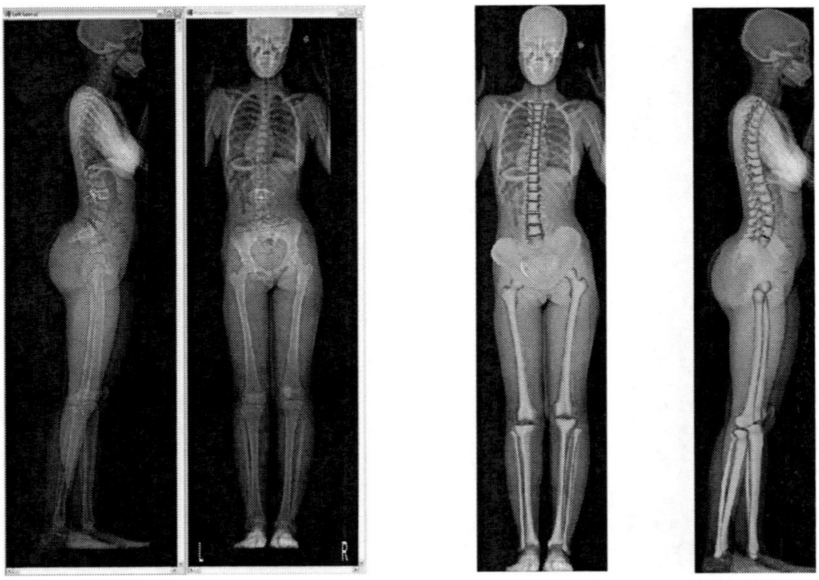

Figure 3. Lateral and anterior-posterior views leading to 3D reconstruction of the skeleton on an EOS device; Biospace Med, Paris, France (Courtesy of Dr Ana Presedo – Robert Debré hospital, Paris, France).

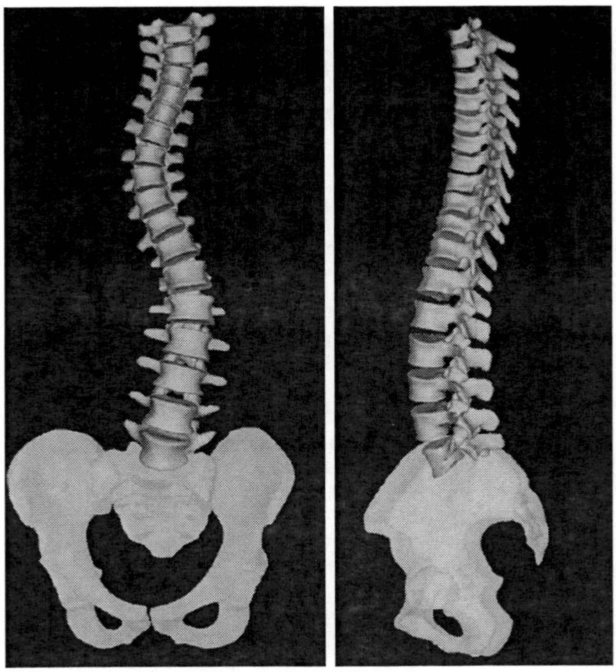

Figure 4. Anterior-posterior and lateral views of 3D reconstruction of the spine by an EOS device; Biospace Med, Paris, France (Courtesy of Pr Vital – Bordeaux, France).

The advantage of the acquisition of the x-ray views with the patient in the standing position is to allow the measurement of spinal curvatures as in scoliosis, kyphosis, … Once the 3D model is complete, the software can automatically generate over 100 angle and length calculations, which have been pre-programmed into the system, such as kyphosis and lordosis, pelvic parameters, vertebral and intervertebral rotations and Cobb angle, leg length, femoral and tibial torsion, etc ... Unlike calculations made from 2D X-ray images which are distorted by the conical projection inherent to 2D detector usage, these calculations are accurate because they have been computed from within 3D space and should enable more accurate and effective diagnosis, treatment and surgical planning. The 3D reconstruction makes also possible the calculation of Finite Element Models (FEM) leading to the evaluation of individualized fracture risk prediction. In addition to the 3D geometric parameters, the possibility of measuring BMD ex vivo with the EOS system with a good accuracy has been shown (34).

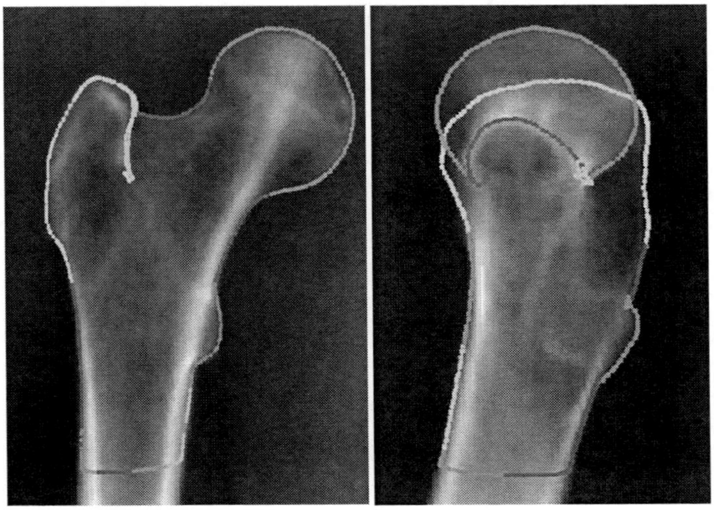

Figure 5. Anterior-posterior and lateral views of ex-vivo human femur by DXA (authors' collection).

3. Three-Dimensional X-ray Absorptiometry (3D-XA)

Recent advances in stereoradiographic techniques of reconstruction have allowed to obtain 3D geometry of bones using 2D contours identified on biplanar radiographs (35,36). We published in 2005 a new technique: the three-dimensional x-ray absorptiometry (3D-XA), which allows the 3D reconstruction of human bones using 2 perpendicular DXA scans obtained from a standard DXA device. It has been applied on excised human femurs (Figure 5) using a dedicated non-stereo-corresponding contours (NSCC) algorithm applied to the proximal femur (37,38). The validation of this technique has been done by comparison with 3D reconstruction with CT scanners. Quantitative comparison on the whole specimen between the 3D-XA reconstructions and the CT reconstructions (processed on approximately 10 000 points per specimen) yielded a mean difference of 0.06 ± 1.02 mm. Mean absolute error was 0.8 mm and 95% of errors were less than 2.1 mm. This 3D reconstruction (Figure 6) allows the measurement of real geometric parameters as femoral neck length, femoral head diameter, neck-shaft angle, cross-sectional area (CSA, cm^2) and cross-sectional moment of inertia (CSMI, cm^4). These parameters can be measured at the hip in 2D on DXA devices using special softwares, but, bone being a 3D structure, several assumptions are made in order to use a 2D method such as DXA to measure these geometrical parameters,. These assumptions reduce the precision and accuracy of the 2D method. Using a 3D technique as 3D-XA would reflect the real bone geometry. We suggested that to use 3D-XA of the femur in vivo, the lateral view will not be optimal (as there will be a superposition of the contralateral femur and the pelvis). The C-arm should therefore be stopped at various positions as +/- 30° or 45° in addition to the AP view. We also suggested that the use of more than 2 views would improve the accuracy and the precision of the reconstruction (37).

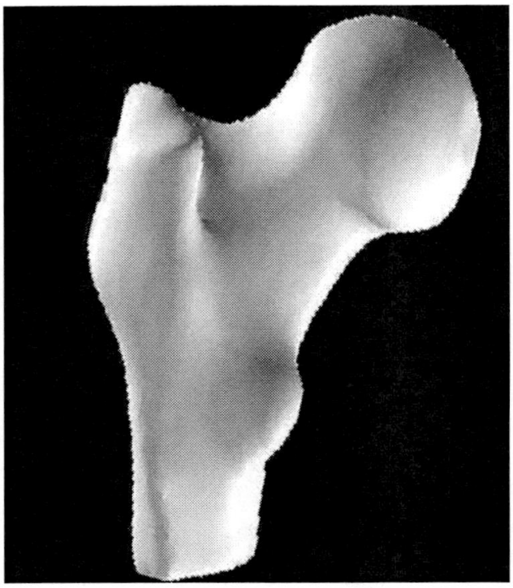

Figure 6. 3D reconstruction of ex-vivo human femur by 3D-XA (authors' collection).

These geometric parameters reflect bone strength. They provide additional information to areal BMD. We evaluated the geometric parameters obtained by 3D-XA by mechanical testing. These tests done using stance phase configuration revealed that failure load tests were correlated to age, femoral head diameter, neck-shaft angle, and BMD measurements. Multiple regression analysis showed that adding femoral head diameter and mid-femoral neck CSA to femoral neck BMD, improved the failure load prediction to $r^2 = 0.84$ ($p<0.0001$) compared to $r^2 = 0.50$ for femoral neck BMD alone (39).

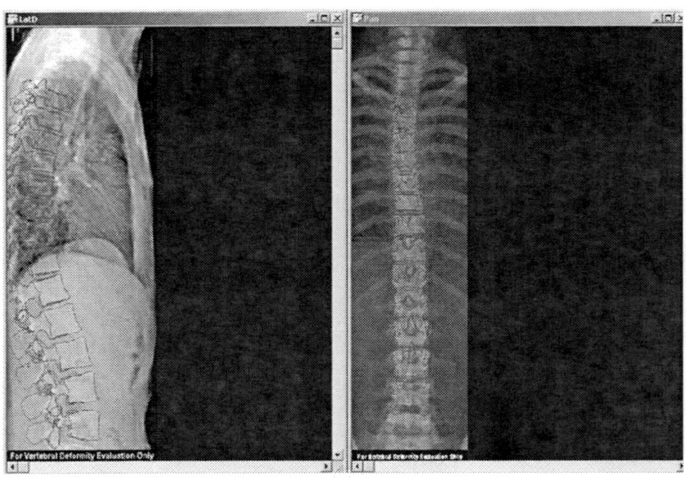

Figure 7. In vivo anterior-posterior and lateral views of the thoracic and lumbar spine by DXA (Vertebral Fracture Assessment software) (authors' collection).

Vertebral body size and shape are important predictors of their strength (40). Women have smaller vertebrae than men (41). CSA of non-fractured vertebrae measured by a CT scanner is 4.9% to 11.5% smaller in postmenopausal women with fractures than in age, weight, height and BMD adjusted women without fractures (42). Vertebral dimensions such as vertebral height, width, CSA and volume are smaller in patients with vertebral fractures compared to controls even after adjustment on the different confounding factors (43). We have applied the 3D-XA technique to human vertebrae in vivo using a standard DXA device (Hologic QDR 4500 A) equipped with a rotating arm (C-arm) (44). The Vertebral Fracture Assessment software allows the acquisition of anterior-posterior and lateral images of the thoracic and lumbar spines from the 4th thoracic to the 4th lumbar vertebrae with the patient lying on his back without any movement in between (Figure 7). The 3D-XA reconstruction method of the vertebrae can briefly be summarized as follows:

(a) it is based on vertebral body volume reconstruction,
(b) definition of a local referential associated to this volume,
(c) reliable a priori knowledge of the vertebral shape using 8 morphologic descriptors of the vertebral body to estimate, from a multiple linear regression, 21 3D-landmarks coordinates per vertebra, and
(d) kriging (non-linear shape deformation using a specific interpolation technique) of 2000-point model with regard to the 21 landmarks.

This method allows in vivo 3D reconstruction of the vertebrae (Figure 8) based on routine DXA exams and the real measurement of the geometric parameters of the vertebral bodies: heights, depths, widths, minimal CSA and volume with an acceptable variability. In vivo precision was calculated by reconstructing 20 human spines by 2 different observers. The mean absolute difference between 2 observers for the whole vertebral bodies is 0.6 mm, with 2 RMS of 1.7 mm. The mean relative difference was –0.1 ± 1.5 mm. For the geometric parameters, the mean relative difference between the 2 observers ranged from –0.3 to + 0.5 mm for the heights, depths and widths. It was –11.0 mm^2 for minCSA and –0.7 mm^3 for the vertebral body volume. The accuracy of the measurement has been evaluated by reconstructing 16 dry human vertebrae by 3D-XA and CT scanner. The mean difference was –0.2 ± 1.3 mm (44). The 3D-XA method is therefore a good way – readily applicable in vivo - for the real measurement of the vertebral body geometry with a good accuracy and precision. It yields complementary information on bone geometry. Further studies are needed to evaluate if, coupled with BMD, it improves vertebral fracture risk prediction.

Anti-osteoporotic drugs increase BMD to various degrees. The contribution of BMD increase in vertebral fracture risk reduction varies greatly between different anti-osteoporotic drugs (45). Therefore, the reduction of fracture risk cannot only be explained by the increase in BMD. Three dimensional bone imaging allows a better understanding of the mechanism of action of anti-osteoporotic drugs by showing their effect on bone micro and macroarchitecture. Such studies show that different anti-osteoporotic drugs reduce fracture risk by different mechanisms of action.

Few studies used vQCT technique to evaluate the effect of anti-osteoporotic drugs as parathyroid hormone and alendronate alone or in combination on bone macroarchitecture in postmenopausal osteoporosis. Femoral cortical volume was found to increase with a 1-year treatment with parathyroid hormone followed by 1-year treatment with alendronate (46,47).

CT examination showed also an increase in volumetric trabecular BMD at total hip and femoral neck in parathyroid hormone treated postmenopausal women with osteoporosis (48).

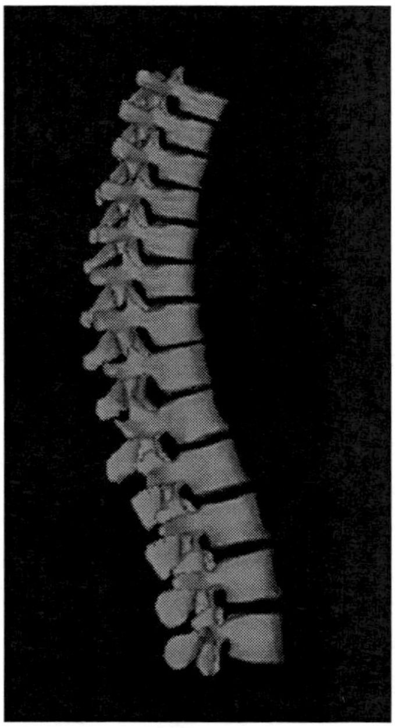

Figure 8. In vivo 3D reconstruction of thoracic and lumbar spine by 3D-XA method (authors' collection).

In another study, 3D reconstruction of femurs of mice allowed the evaluation of the effect of alendronate on femoral macroarchitecture in a model of osteogenesis imperfecta and controls. Alendronate appears to increase cortical volumetric BMD and diaphyseal cortical thickness but not femoral length and growth. Predicted material strength and elastic modulus were negatively impacted by 12 weeks of treatment by alendronate. Femoral brittleness was unimproved (49).

The 3D evaluation of the effect of different anti-osteoporotic treatments on the cortical bone, trabecular bone, macro architecture and microarchitecture may help to understand in a better way the mechanism of action by which they decrease the fracture risk. This may also improve the management of osteoporotic patients by a better selection of the most adapted anti-osteoporotic drug according to its mechanism of action.

Conclusion

Three-dimensional imaging methods have the potential to improve osteoporosis diagnosis and our understanding in the way anti-osteoporotic drugs decrease fracture risk. They are more accurate as they do not use model assumptions necessary for 2D techniques and therefore are unbiased. They are non-invasive, provide a direct measurement of the real 3D structure and allow biomechanical testing in a longitudinal way. Continuous improvement in these technologies should allow a better selection of patients to treat by a more precise evaluation of individualized fracture risk as well as a the selection of the most adapted anti-osteoporotic drug according to its mechanism of action.

REFERENCES

[1] Melton, L. J. 3rd. Adverse outcomes of osteoporotic fractures in the general population. *J Bone Miner Res.*, 2003, 18, 1139-1141.

[2] Nevitt, MC; Thompson, DE; Black, DM; Rubin, SR; Ensrud, K; Yates, AJ; Cummings, SR. Effect of alendronate on limited-activity days and bed-disability days caused by back pain in postmenopausal women with existing vertebral fractures. Fracture Intervention Trial Research Group. *Arch Intern Med.*, 2000, 160, 77-85.

[3] Bliuc, D; Nguyen, ND; Milch, VE; Nguyen, TV; Eisman, JA; Center, JR. Mortality risk associated with low-trauma osteoporotic fracture and subsequent fracture in men and women. *JAMA*, 2009, 301, 513-521.

[4] Ensrud, KE; Thompson, DE; Cauley, JA; Nevitt, MC; Kado, DM; Hochberg, MC; et al. Prevalent vertebral deformities predict mortality and hospitalization in older women with low bone mass. Fracture Intervention Trial Research Group. *Am Geriatr Soc.*, 2000, 48, 241-2419.

[5] Lips, P; Cooper, C; Agnusdei, D; Caulin, F; Egger, P; Johnell, O; et al; and for the Working Party for Quality of Life of the European Foundation for Osteoporosis. Quality of Life in Patients with Vertebral Fractures: Validation of the Quality of Life Questionnaire of the European Foundation for Osteoporosis (QUALEFFO). *Osteoporos Int,* 1999, 10, 150-160.

[6] O'Neill, TW; Felsenberg, D; Varlow, J; Cooper, C; Kanis, J; Silman, AJ. The prevalence of vertebral deformity in european men and women: the European Vertebral Osteoporosis Study. *J Bone Miner Res.*, 1996, 11, 1010-1018.

[7] Melton, LJ; 3rd; Lane, AW; Cooper, C; Eastell, R; O'Fallon, WM; Riggs, BL. Prevalence and incidence of vertebral deformities.. *Osteoporos Int.*, 1993, 3, 113-119.

[8] Lindsay, R; Silverman, SL; Cooper, C; Hanley, DA; Barton, I; Broy, SB; et al. Risk of new vertebral fracture in the year following a fracture. *JAMA.*, 2001, 17, 320-323.

[9] Delmas, PD; Genant, HK; Crans, GG; Stock, JL; Wong, M; Siris, E; Adachi, JD. Severity of prevalent vertebral fractures and the risk of subsequent vertebral and nonvertebral fractures: results from the MORE trial. *Bone.*, 2003, 33, 522-532.

[10] Roux, C; Fechtenbaum, J; Kolta, S; Briot, K; Girard, M. Mild prevalent and incident vertebral fractures are risk factors for new fractures. *Osteoporos Int.*, 2007, 18, 1617-1624.

[11] Marshall, D; Johnell, O; Wedel, H. Meta-analysis of how well measures of bone mineral density predict occurrence of osteoporotic fractures. *Br Med J.*, 1996, 312, 1254-1259.

[12] Cummings, S. Are patients with hip fractures more osteoporotic? *Am J Med.*, 1985, 78, 487-94.

[13] Bousson, V; Le Bras, A; Roqueplan, F; Kang, Y; Mitton, D; Kolta, S; et al. Volumetric quantitative computed tomography of the proximal femur: relationships linking geometric and densitometric variables to bone strength. Role for compact bone. *Osteoporos Int.*, 2006, 17, 855-864.

[14] Lotz, JC; Chael, EJ; Hayes, WC. Stress distributions within the proximal femur during gait and falls: implications for osteoporotic fractures. *Osteoporos Int.*, 1995, 5, 252-261.

[15] Glüer, CC; Cummings, SR; Pressman, A; Li, J; Glüer, K; Faulkner, KG; Grampp, S; Genant, HK. Prediction of hip fractures from pelvic radiographs: the study of

osteoporotic fractures. The Study of Osteoporotic Fractures Research Group. *J Bone Miner Res*., 1994, 9, 671-677.

[16] Faulkner, KG; Cummings, SR; Black, D; Palermo, L; Glüer, CC; Genant, HK. Simple measurement of femoral geometry predicts hip fracture: the study of osteoporotic fractures. *J Bone Miner Res*., 1993, 8, 1211-1217.

[17] Faulkner, KG; McClung, M; Cummings, SR. Automated evaluation of hip axis length for predicting hip fracture. *J Bone Miner Res*., 1994, 9, 1065-1070.

[18] Jergas, M; Breitenseher, M; Glüer, CC; Yu, W; Genant, HK. Estimates of volumetric bone density from projectional measurements improve the discriminatory capability of dual X-ray absorptiometry. *J Bone Miner Res*., 1995, 10, 1101-1110.).

[19] Cheng, XG; Nicholson, PH; Boonen , S; Brys, P; Lowet, G; Nijs, J; Dequeker, J. Effects of anteversion on femoral bone mineral density and geometry measured by dual energy x-ray absorptiometry: a cadaver study. *Bone*., 1997, 21, 113-17.

[20] Michelotti, J; Clark, J. Femoral neck length and hip fracture risk. *J Bone Miner Res*, 1999, 14, 1714-1720.

[21] Kim, JS; Choi, KW; Kim, SI. Femoral anteversion: estimation by 3D modelling. *Medinfo*., 1998, 2, 1025-1029.

[22] Genant, HK; Engelke, K; Pervrhal, S. *Advanced CT bone imaging in osteoporosis*. Rheumatology, 2008, 47, iv9-iv16.

[23] Engelke, K; Mastmeyer, A; Bousson, V; Fuerst, T; Laredo, JD; Kalender, WA. Reanalysis precision of 3D quantitative computed tomography (QCT) of the spine. *Bone*, 2009, 44, 566-572.

[24] Mazess, RB. *Fracture risk: a role for compact bone*. Calcif Tissue Int., 1990, 47, 191-193.

[25] Prevrhal, S; Engelke, K; Kalender, WA. Accuracy limits for the determination of cortical width and density: the influence of object size and CT imaging parameters. *Phys Med Bio*., 1999, 44, 751-764.

[26] Genant, HK; Engelke, K; Pervrhal, S. Advanced CT bone imaging in osteoporosis. *Rheumatology,* 2008, 47, iv9-iv16.

[27] Riggs, BL; Melton, LJ; 3rd; Robb, RA; Camp, JJ; Atkinson, EG; Peterson, JM; et al. Population-based study of age and sex differences in bone volumetric density, size, geometry, and structure at different skeletal sites. *J Bone Miner Res*., 2004, 19, 1945-1954.

[28] Duan, Y; Beck, TJ; Wang, XF; Seeman, E. Structural and biomechanical basis of sexual dysmorphism in femoral neck fragility has its origins in growth and aging. *J Bone Miner Res*., 2003, 18, 1766-1774.

[29] Lang, TF; Keyak, JH; Heitz, MW; Augat, P; Lu, Y; Mathur, A; Genant, HK. Volumetric quantitative computed tomography of the proximal femur: precision and relation to bone strength. *Bone*., 1997, 21, 101-108.

[30] Marshall, LM; Lang, TF; Lambert, LC; Zmuda, JM; Ensrud, KE; Orwoll, ES. Dimensions and volumetric BMD of the proximal femur and their relation to age among older U.S. men. *J Bone Miner Res*., 2006, 21, 1197-1206.

[31] Van Rietbergen, B; Majumdar, S; Pistoia, W; Newitt, DC; Kothari, M; Laib, A; Rüegsegger, P. *A*ssessment of cancellous bone mechanical properties from micro-FE models based on micro-CT, pQCT and MR images. *Technol Health Care*., 1998, 6, 413-420.

[32] Dubousset, J; Charpak, G; Dorion, I; Skalli, W; Lavaste, F; Deguise, J; et al. A new 3D and 3D imaging approach to musculoskeletal physiology and pathology with low-dose radiation and the standing position: the EOS system. *Bull Acad Natl Med.*, 2005, 189, 287-297.

[33] Rousseau, MA; Laporte, S; Chavary-Bernier, E; Lazennec, JY; Skalli, W. Reproducibility of measuring the shape and three-dimensional position of cervical vertebrae in upright position using the EOS stereoradiography system. *Spine.*, 2007, 32, 2569-2572.

[34] Sapin, E; Briot, K; Kolta, S; Gravel, P; Skalli, W; Roux, C; Mitton, D. Bone mineral density assessment using the EOS low-dose X-ray device: a feasibility study. *Proc Inst Mech Eng.*, 2008, 222, 1263-1271.

[35] Laporte, S; Skalli, W; De Guise, JA; Lavaste, F; Mitton, D. A biplanar reconstruction method based on 2D and 3D contours: Application to distal femur. *Comput Methods Biomech Biomed.*, 2003, 6, 1-6.

[36] Le Bras, A; Laporte, S; Bousson, V; et al. *Personnalised 3D reconstruction of proximal femur from low-dose digital biplanar radiographs. CARS. Computer Assisted radiology and surgery.* Proceedings of the 17th international congress and exhibition., 2003, 1256, 214-219.

[37] Kolta, S; Le Bras, A; Mitton, D; Bousson, V; De Guise, JA; Fechtenbam, J; et al. Three-dimensional x-ray absorptiometry (3D-XA): a method for reconstruction of human bones using a dual x-ray absorptiometry device. *Osteoporos Int.*, 2005, 16, 969976.

[38] Le Bras, A; Laporte, S; Bousson, V; Mitton, D; De Guise, JA; Laredo, JD; Skalli, W. 3D reconstruction of the proximal femur with low-dose digital stereoradiography. *Comput Aided Surg.*, 2004, 9, 51-57.

[39] Le Bras, A; Kolta, S; Soubrane, P; Skalli, W; Roux, C; Mitton, D. Assessment of femoral neck strength by 3-Dimensional X-ray Absorptiometry. *J Clin Densitom.*, 2006, 9, 425-430.

[40] Ruyssen-Witrand, A; Gossec, L; Kolta, S; Dougados, M; Roux, C. Vertebral dimensions as risk factors of vertebral fracture in osteoporotic patients: a systematic literature review. *Osteoporos Int.*, 2007, 18, 1271-1278.

[41] Riggs, BL; Melton, LJ; III; Robb, RA; Camp, JJ; Atkinson, EJ; Peterson, JM; et al. Population-based study of age and sex differences in bone volumetric density, size, geometry, and structure at different skeletal sites. *J Bone Miner Res.*, 2004, 19, 1945-1954.

[42] Gilsanz, V; Loro, M; Roe, TF; Sayre, J; Gilsanz, R; Schulz, EE. Vertebral size in elderly women with osteoporosis. *J Clin Invest.*, 1995, 95, 2332-2337.

[43] Gilsanz, V; Boechat, M; Roe, T; Loro, M; Sayre, J; Goodman, W. Gender differences in vertebral body sizes in adults: biomechanical implications. *Radiology.*, 1994, 190, 678-3682.

[44] Kolta, S; Quiligotti, S; Ruyssen-Witrand, A; Amido, A; Mitton, D; Le Bras, A; et al In vivo 3D reconstruction of human vertebrae with the three-dimensional x-ray absorptiometry (3D-XA) method). *Osteoporos Int.*, 2008, 19, 185-192.

[45] Sarkar, S; Mitlak, BH; Wong, M; Stock, JL; Black, DM; Harper, KD. Relationships between bone mineral density and incident vertebral fracture risk with raloxifene therapy. *J Bone Miner Res.*, 2002, 17, 1-10.

[46] Black, DM; Greenspan, SL; Ensrud, KE; Palermo, L; McGowan, JA; Lang, TF; et al. The effects of parathyroid hormone and alendronate alone or in combination in postmenopausal osteoporosis. *N Engl J Med.*, 2003, 349, 1207-1215.

[47] Black, DM; Bilezikian, JP; Ensrud, KE; Greenspan, SL; Palermo, L; Hue, T; et al. One year of alendronate after one year of parathyroid hormone (1-84) for osteoporosis. *N Engl J Med.*, 2005, 353, 555-565.

[48] Greenspan, SL; Bone, HG; Ettinger, MP; Hanley, DA; Lindsay, R; Zanchetta, JR; et al. Effect of recombinant human parathyroid hormone (1-84) on vertebral fracture and bone mineral density in postmenopausal women with osteoporosis: a randomized trial. *Ann Inter Med.*, 2007, 146, 326-339.

[49] Uveges, TE; Kozloff, KM; Ty, JM; Ledgard, F; Raggio, CL; Gronowicz, G; et al Alendronate treatment of the Brtl osteogenesis imperfecta mouse improves femoral geometry and load response before fracture but decreases predicted material properties and has detrimental effects on osteoblasts and bone formation. *J Bone Miner Res.*, 2009, 24, 849-859.

In: 3D Imaging: Theory, Technology … ISBN: 978-1-60876-885-1
Editors: E. H. Duke and S. R. Aguirre, pp.189-198

Chapter 8

Clinical Relevance of CT- Based Computer Aided 3D- Planning in Hepatobiliary, Pancreatic Surgery and Living Donor Liver Transplantation

Jens Harms[1*], Holger Bourquain[2] and Heinz-Otto Peitgen[2]
[1]Klinik für Visceral-, Transplantations-, Thorax- und Gefäßchirurgie, Universitätsklinikum Leipzig AöR, 04103 Leipzig, Liebigstrasse 20, Germany
[2]MeVis- Center for Medical Diagnostics and Visualization, 28359 Bremen, Universitätsallee 29, Germany

Abstract

Multiple imaging approaches are currently used for diagnosis and surgery planning of hepatobiliary tumors and living donor liver transplantations. Conventional imaging studies remain insufficient to demonstrate the individual anatomy. Refinements in CT technology with the introduction of "multidetector-row" CT scanners and implementation of mathematical methods on computerized digital data enabled CT based 3D-visualizations. This renders preoperative surgery planning more reliable and reproducible. Since the application in oncological liver surgery has been studied previously, our interest focussed on pancreatic- and biliary tract tumors including preoperative work-up in living donor liver transplantation. CT based 3D- display provided accurate preoperative visualization and computerized risk analyses for safety margins of pancreatic- and biliary- tract tumors. In living related liver transplantation the 3D- procedure may help to recognize vascular variants and to define the splitting line. The results may have major impact on patient selection and in our opinion allow better planning of the appropriate surgical approach.

Introduction

Hepatobiliary and pancreatic surgery as well as liver transplantation have shown considerable developments, mainly due to improvements of surgical techniques, diagnostic imaging modalities and postoperative care. Technical advances with the use of surgical devices such

---

* Corresponding author: 04416 Markkleeberg , Colkwitzer Weg 10, Germany , e-mail dr.jens.harms@gmx.de

as ultrasonic dissectors, argon beam coagulators improved accuracy of surgical procedures. Recent developments of imaging techniques with the implementation of computer technologies have enabled a new quality of visualization consisting in 3D- representation to realize image guided and computer assisted surgery. These developments allow enhanced precision in preoperative planning and image guided surgery using intraoperative navigation tools. This is already practiced in neuro-, maxillo-facial and orthopaedic surgery.

3D- visualizations of visceral organs failed in the past because of technological limitations to create image data with minimal motion artifacts and lack of stable computerized image processing technologies. The introduction of «multidetector- row» helical CT, however, has offered the opportunity to create digital data with minimal motion artifacts [1]. The application of a variety of dedicated and robust computerized image processing steps succeeded in visualizations, which enable precise localization and exact in- depth representation of tumors especially in surgery of liver cancers [2,3]. So far there is no consensus among surgeons about the indicative value for treatment planning. Points of criticisms are the time lag needed for computed visualizations, non-availability of real-time display required in the operating room, the lack of specialized medical computer scientists and costs.

Applications of laparoscopic techniques in hepatobiliary surgery are limited so far. Improvements in the field of 3D- visualization and navigation techniques may allow major liver resections via a laparoscopic approach. This development is already underway in upper gastrointestinal tract surgery.

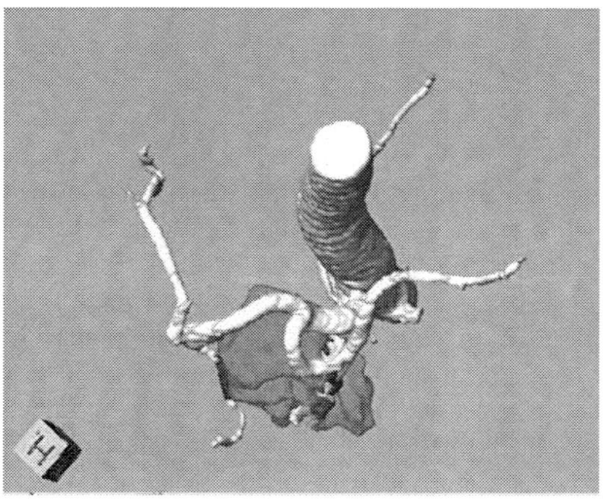

Figure 1. 3D- CT based visualization of pancreatic head tumor and its relation to the arteries originating from the celiac trunk.

Because of limited availability of postmortal liver donors, the challenging technique of living related liver donor transplantation (LDLT) has gained increasing application worldwide. Especially this field reinforced the interest in computerized preoperative 3D- visualizations. Adult-to-adult LDLT is technically demanding. The liver has to be splitted into in a well preserved right lobe representing the graft and a remnant left liver lobe without any damage to the donor. To achieve these aims accurate anatomical and functional work- up for surgical planning is mandatory. The same holds true for planning of oncological resections in biliary- and pancreatic tumors. In this field experiences with 3D- visualization are limited. To analyze the clinical impact of computerized 3D- visualizations in hepatobiliary – pancreatic surgery and LDLT we performed a collaborative study with the IT- research institute MeVis, Bremen, Germany.

A total of 27 patients were assessed by CT based 3 D- visualization techniques. 12 patients were analysed for pancreatic- (head n= 9, corpus n= 2, tail n = 1), 4 patients for biliary tract tumors and 10 patients for LDLT. In addition 3 liver transplant recipients were analysed. CT scans were performed with a 4 slice «multirow-detector» helical scanner machine (Siemens Volume Zoom®, Siemens Erlangen ,Germany). For computer assisted 3D- viszualisation data were transferred to the IT- Research Institute MeVis, Bremen, Germany. 3D- image processing of original CT- data included segmentation of specific anatomic and pathologic structures. For relevant vascular structures centre lines were calculated. A hierarchical mathematical model representing the vascular tree was created. This allowed calculation of individual vascular territories. Computerized "surgery planning" included virtual insertion of splitting lines in LDLT and safety margins in oncologic patients. Results were displayed either one by one or in arbitrary combinations in both, 3D- and overlayed to the original CT data [2,3].

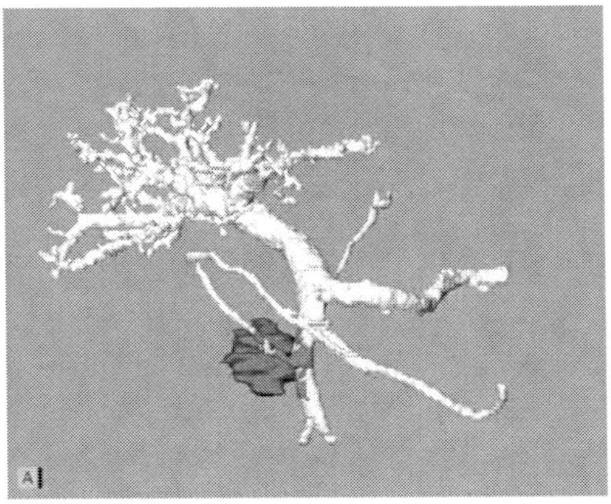

Figure 2.Visualization of the venous mesenterico-portal trunk. The pancreatic head tumor is closely attached the vicinity of the superior mesenteric vein.

Pancreatic Tumors

3D- visualization of pancreatic tumors succeeded in 11 of 12 cases. In a single case of cancer of the papilla of Vater with the tumor mass localized within the duodenum visualization was unsatisfactory. In 2 patients arterial variants of the common hepatic artery originating from the superior mesenteric artery could be displayed. Visualization of vascular structures in the vicinity of the tumor succeeded in all cases. Involvement of regional arteries by the tumor (A. gastroduodenalis n= 3, Superior Mesenteric Artery n= 1, Celiac trunk n= 1, A. lienalis n=1) and/ or of the venous mesenterico- portal trunk (portal vein n= 1, confluens n= 2, Superior Mesenteric Vein n= 1, V. lienalis n= 1) could be shown in 5 patients. On the basis of computerized surgery planning, resection of the tumor seemed likely in 9 cases. Operative procedures included duodenopancreatectomy in 7 and extended left sided pancreatic resection in 2 patients. Palliative surgery was carried out in 2 patients because of multivisceral tumor infiltration. In all patients the specific findings (tumor size, localization, vascular involvement) obtained by 3D– CT visualization could be reconfirmed intraoperatively. Because of non-resectability one patient was treated with palliative chemotherapy.

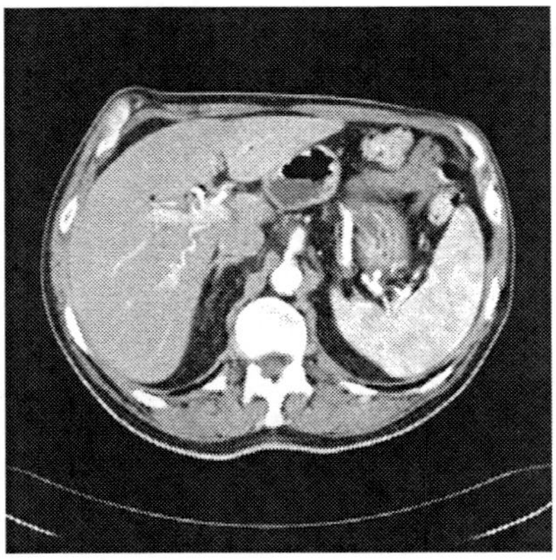

Figure 3. Preoperative CT –scan .Tortous course of the right hepatic branch artery.Tumor mass within the liver hilum.

Biliary-Tract Tumors

3D- CT based visualizations demonstrated localization, extraluminal extend and involvement of adjactend vascular structures within the liver hilum and the hepatoduodenal ligament. Longitudinal ductal tumor extension could be demonstrated as well. ERC- and MRC-examination revealed biliary- tract tumors classified as Bismuth type IV in 1, Bismuth type I in 2 and tumor of the distal common hepatic duct in one case. 3D- CT based visualizations were discrepant in 2 cases. ERC- and MRC classified Bismuth type I tumors appeared as Bismuth type II/IIIa in 1 and as a tumor originating from the gall bladder in 1 case. Compared to conventional radiological methods, 3D- CT based visualizations seem to be more precise to determine the extend of tumor spread, vascular involvement and the possibility of dissociation of the liver remnant bile ducts. Thus 3D- CT based visualizations representing the advantage of a single non- invasive examination of biliary tumors may complement conventional diagnostic tools and may improve treatment planning.

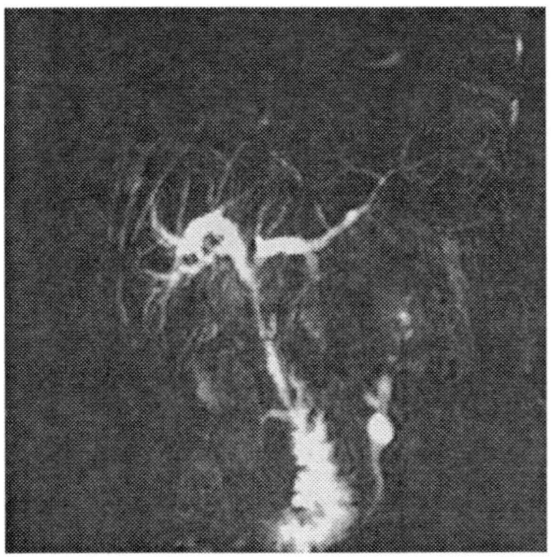

Figure 4. MRCP illustrates hilar stenoses mimicking Bismuth type IV- Klatskin tumor. MRCP reveals no information of the extra-, intraluminal tumor extend, dissociation of the peripheral bile ducts of the left remnant liver after extended right hemihepatectomy and of vascular tumor involvement.

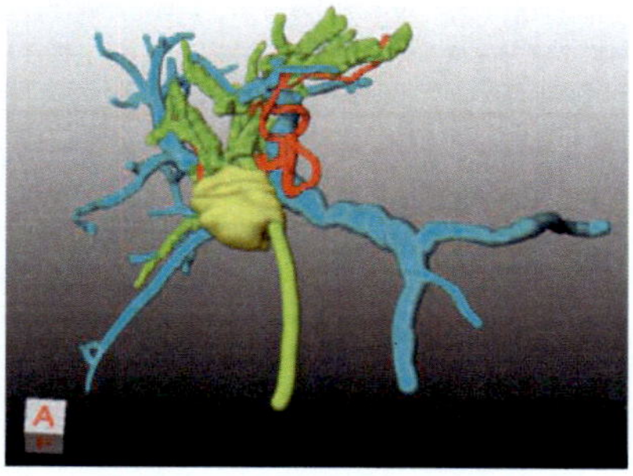

Figure 5. Summarized representation of the arterial (red), the portal venous (blue), the biliary tract (green) and the biliary tract tumor originating from the main the right hepatic bile duct system by 3D CT- based reconstruction.

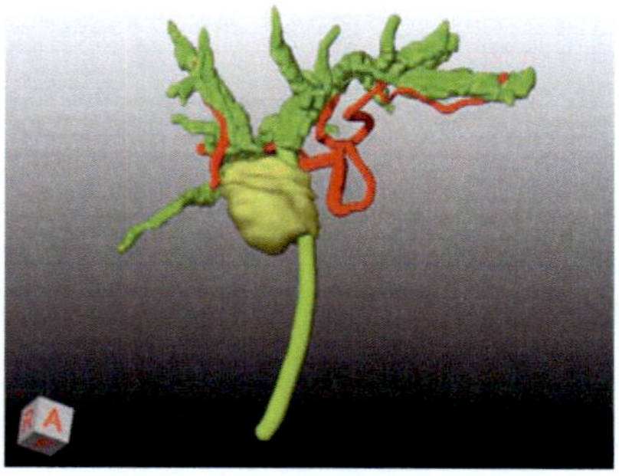

Figure 6. Selective visualization of the intrahepatic course of the right and left proper hepatic artery (red), its interface to the bile duct system and the tumor (green).

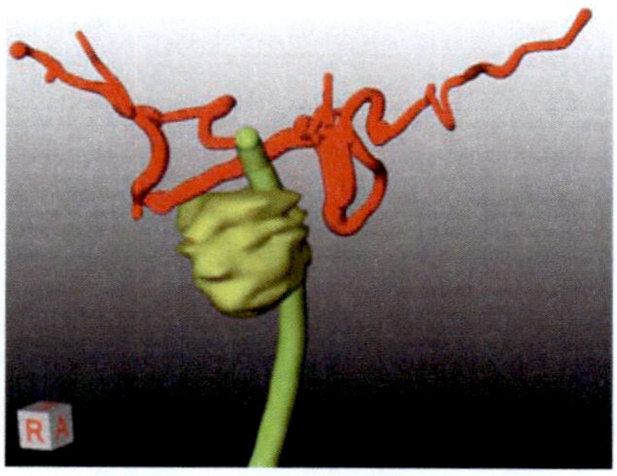

Figure 7. Angulated 3D CT-based visualizations illustrates lack of dissociation of the non- tumor compromised left hepatic bile duct system.

Living Donor Liver Transplantation: 3D- imaging studies were performed in 10 consecutive candidates evaluated for adult-to-adult living donor liver transplantation. Appropriate 3D-visualizations of the arterial anatomy succeeded in 8, of the portal vein anatomy in all, of the hepatic vein anatomy in 9, of the hepatic vein confluens in 9 and of the bile duct anatomy in all 5 patients in which biliary tract visualizations were performed. Hepatic arteries, veins and liver segments could be displayed in a multidirectional 3D- view. Course and branching points of hepatic arteries, veins and their relation to the intended splitting line (full right split and left lobe remnant liver) could be visualized in arbitrary combinations. Anatomic variants detected were: (1.) accessory left hepatic arteries in 2, hepatomesenteric trunk in 1; (2.)

trifurcation of the portal vein in 2; (3.) variant hepatic veins (HV) in 6 (intraparenchymal entry of LHV in MHV n= 3, RHV in MHV n=1, accessory RHV n= 1, two RHV n=1); (4.) normal anatomy and branching patterns of bile ducts in 5 patients examined. On the basis of the individual anatomic findings 9 candidates were assumed appropriate for LDLT. 3 patients were excluded from the procedure because of steatosis hepatis in 2 donors and tumor progression in one potential recipient. In summary, data indicate that 3D-CT based visualization facilitates diagnostic work-up with high accuracy. Multiple examinations especially with regard to invasive diagnostics may be avoided in future.

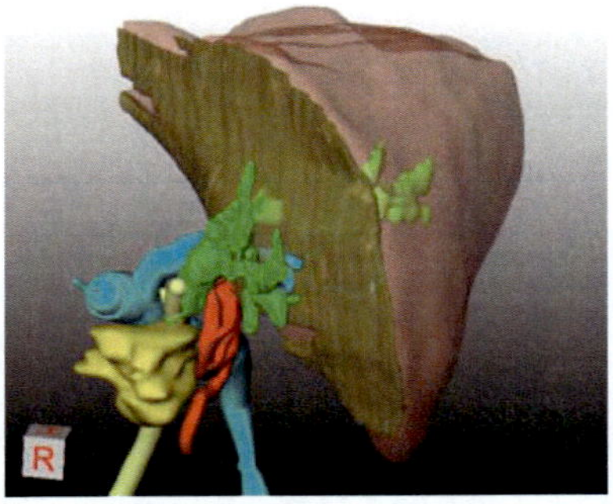

Figure 8. Virtual 3D CT - based surgery planning. Resection plane of extended right sided hemi-hepatectomy as the only oncologic treatment of choice is simulated on the same CT data set.

Liver Transplant Recipients: 3D- CT imaging studies were also conducted in 3 liver transplant recipients. Examinations were requested for assessment of tumor progress in 1, confirmations of portal vein thrombosis and deleneation of consequtive venous collaterals in another and in a 6- months old infant suffering from progressive hepatic failure due to Alagille syndrome. The patient with a substantial tumor progress was excluded from transplantation. The suspected portal vein thrombosis was confirmed. Impressive results were obtained in the 6- months old infant. Alagille syndrome is associated with multiple anatomic anomalies. Beside other diagnostics 3D- CT based visualization revealed abnormal course of the inferior caval vein, lack of hepatic venous confluens and an arterial hepatomesenteric trunk. In this case results obtained were more conclusive than other imaging studies. Intraoperative display allowed image guided surgery with the consequence that the operative risk during surgical dissection could be kept low.

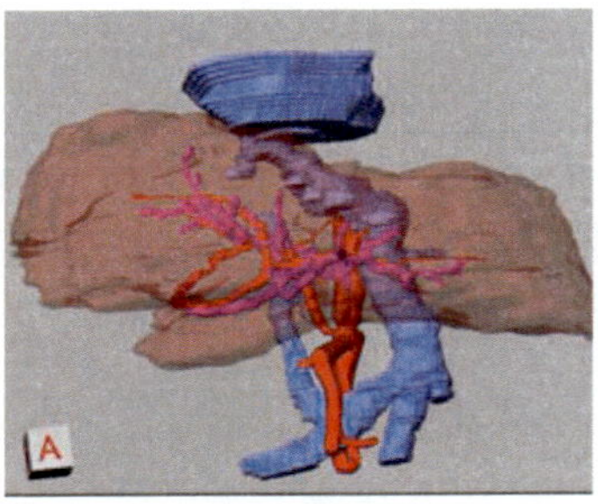

Figure 9. Preoperative 3D- CT based visualization of the complex intraabdominal vascular variants in a child suffering from end-stage liver disease by Allagile syndrome. Arterial variants with a common celiaco- mesenteric trunk (red) and abnormal course of the inferior caval vein (blue).

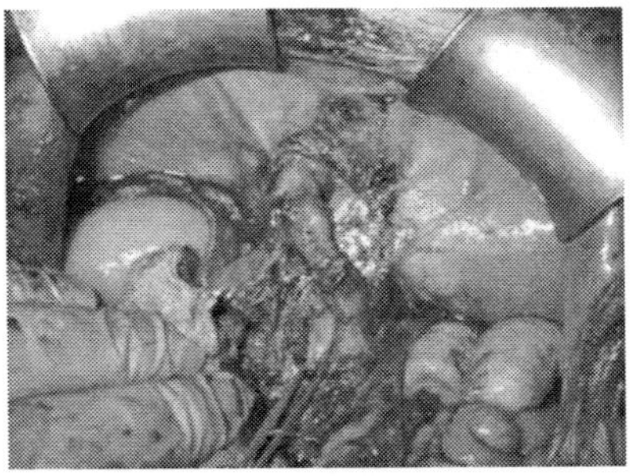

Figure 10. Intraoperative view after hepatectomy for living donor liver transplantation confirmed vascular courses as obtained by computerized 3D- display.

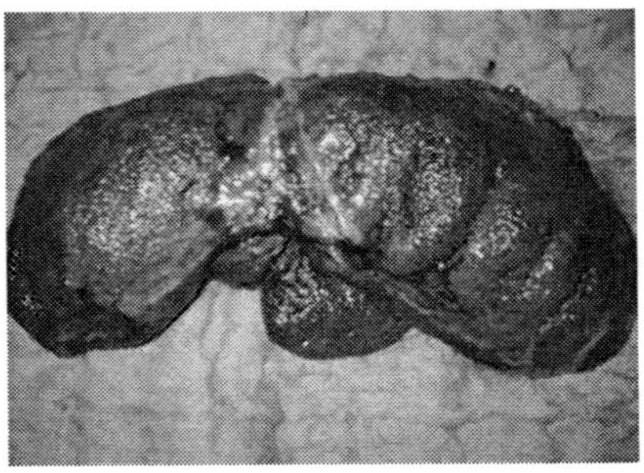

Figure 11. Removed cirrhotic liver.

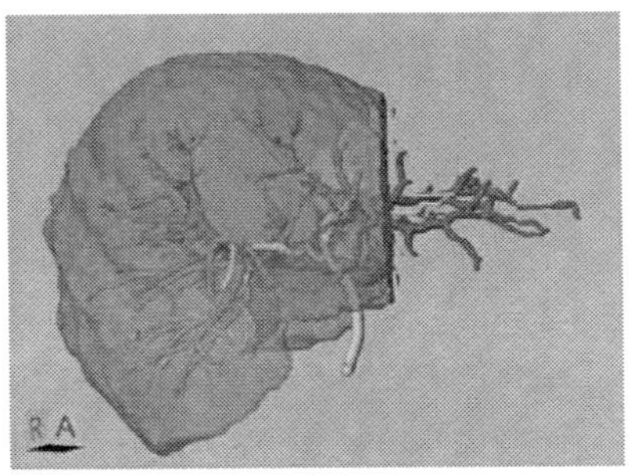

Figure 12. Preoperative CT based computer aided 3D- planning of the LDLT. The splitting line follows the falciform ligament for removal of a graft consisting of left lateral liver segments. Areas of arterial malperfusion of the remnant liver are visualized.

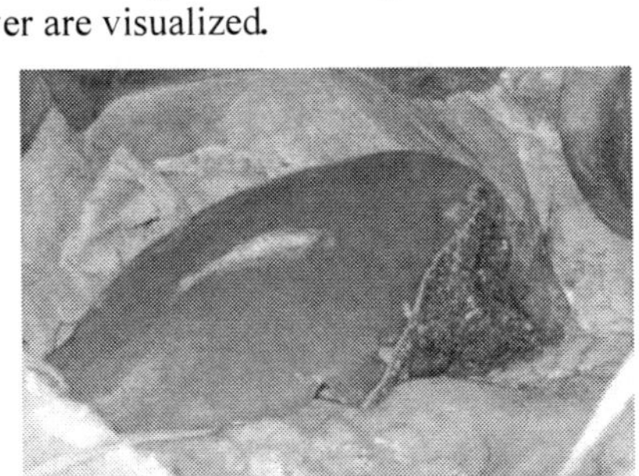

Figure 13. Intraoperative view after removal of a left lateral graft (liver segments II + III).

Conclusion

Research on computer assisted surgery has expanded rapidly allowing application for clinical procedures on routine basis. Two fields of engineering technologies are required to realize computer assisted surgery in visceral organs: (1) a surgical simulation system to realize planning according to the condition and anatomical feature of the patient, (2) an image fusion system which is applicable for visceral organ surgery and acts as an apparatus for image guided surgery.

Application of computerized segmentation techniques on digital data derived from computer tomography facilitate 3D- geometrical and structural organ analyses. Computer simulations permit multiple viewing perspectives. Interactive insertion of resection lines ensures preoperative identification of "saftey margins" and "areas of risk" in oncological patients and in living related liver donors. Results achieved are accurate and robust. Data may be used as a "virtual road map" during surgery.

Because of the inability of precise intraoperative registration image fusion during visceral surgery render computer assisted surgery presently impossible. Physiologic organ shifting and soft organ composition with deformation during surgical manipulation are obstacles. The actual manual operating process is guided by fusion of visual and tactile information. For image assistance and representation during surgery developments in the design of modern operating rooms with the operational availability of computer technologies offer an interim solution. Consequently computerized 3D- visualizations can be transferred and displayed on flat screen monitors near to the surgical field.

Pancreatic Tumors

Imaging of pancreatic tumors shows considerable progress. About 35% of pancreatic tumors are demonstrated to be resectable with curative intent [4]. Assessment of resectability, in most cases remains unclear until surgical exploration. Conventional diagnostics often fail to provide accurate assessment of regional tumor infiltration. Further limitation is the inability to depict small hepatic and peritoneal metastases. Neither conventional CT techniques, nor MRI and angiography can rule out these problems. From the surgical point of view 3 issues have to be addressed clearly by the preoperative staging of pancreatic tumors: (1.) local resectability; (2.) lymph node metastases and (3.) distant metastases. Accuracy for these determinants can be established by CT- and MRI in 71% and 70% ,respectively [5]. Computerized CT based 3D- visualization techniques may allow improved precision of staging pancreatic tumors that includes: (1.) interactive visualization of the pancreatic tumor (2.) tumor size (3.) display of the vascular anatomy; i.e. variants which are essential for surgical dissection and lymphadenectomy; (4.) tumor involvement of vessels; (5.) preoperative computerized resection planning in order to ensure adequate "safety margins". The potential of CT based 3D- visualizations to detect metastatic lymph nodes remains to be shown. In summary, our preliminary experience suggests that 3D- modeling of CT data should be included in staging of pancreatic tumors in selected cases. Small peritoneal and hepatic metastases can not be visualized sufficiently. In such suspected cases laparoscopy is useful and favourable compared to diagnostic laparotomy.

Biliary- Tract Tumors

Evaluation of biliary- tract tumors is an assessment of resectability, since resection is the only effective therapy. Resectability ranges between 10- 50% with 5-year survival rates of 20%. Preoperative staging must assess 4 critical issues: (1.) extend of tumor within the biliary tree, (2.) vascular invasion, (3.) hepatic lobar atrophy, (4.) metastatic disease, (5.) hepatic lobar increase in the case of preoperative portal vein embolization for hypertrophy induction[6]. Cholangiography (ERC) demonstrates the location of the tumor and the ductal extent of the disease. The procedure however carries a considerable risk. In addition MRC provides information regarding patency of hiliar vascular structures, presence of nodal and distant metastases and of lobar atrophy. There are a few limtations including cost, availability, operator dependence, patient tolerance and representation. In biliary- tract tumors experience with 3D- CT based visualizations is rare. CT based 3D- visualization meet above mentioned requirements. Quality and accuracy in the accomplished investigations in our opinion was superior to MRC. CT based 3D- visualizations provide improved tumor localization and a virtual view of vascular structures within the liver hilum and the hepatoduodenal ligament. 3D- mapping probably allows meticulous tumor dissection and effective protection of crucial vascular structures. In hilar bile duct tumors preoperative visualization of the course, the caliber and the branching of bile ducts will facilitate intraoperative identification for bilidigestive reconstruction. Application of the procedure is limited due to possible side effects of the contrast medium [7]. The procedure however may be indicated in cases of non-obstructed bile ducts (living donor liver candidates) or in patients with contraindications to PTC and MRC.

Living Donor Liver Transplantation

3D- CT based visualizations achieved increasing acceptance in the work-up of in living donor liver transplantation. The complex anatomy of the liver with high incidence of vascular variants reinforces the necessity for accurate preoperative vascular imaging. Up to one-third of potential donors may not be eligible for the procedure because of unsuitable vascular anatomy [8]. CT based 3D- visualization is non- invasive. Our data presented suggest that the method has achieved a robust standard. The procedure gives essential and detailed information about: variants of the hepatic artery, origin of the artery to segment IV, anatomy of portal and hepatic veins, variants of the biliary- tract. In addition the liver volume can be calculated. In our opinion the results of 3D- visualization of CT- based cholangiograms were as good as those by ERC and seem to be superior than MRC- scans. According to our experience preoperative interactive simulation of the splitting line in the donor liver is of major value because it identifies "areas at risk". These are margins along the splitting line of potential arterial devascularization or venous congestion. In conclusion, 3D- CT based visualization seems to be a valuable tool in order to perform this surgical procedure with high accuracy and to minimize potential risks to the donor and the graft.

REFERENCES

[1] Kamel, IR; Kruksal, JB; Pomfret, EA; Keogan, MT; Warmbrand, G; Raptopoulos, V. Impact of multidetector CT on donor selection and surgical planning before living adult right lobe liver transplantation. *AJR*, 2003, 176, 193-200.

[2] Bourquain, H; Schenk, A; Link, F; Preim, B; Prause, G; Peitgen, HO. HepaVision2-a software assistant for preoperative planning in living-related liver transplantation and oncologic liver surgery. In: Lembke HW, editor; CARS 2002; Computer-Assisted Radiology and Surgery. Proc of the 16th International Congress and Exhibition, Paris June 26-29; 2002, *Leiden University Medical Center*, 2002, Vol 1, 341-346.

[3] Preim, B; Bourquain, H; Selle, D; Peitgen, HO; Oldhafer, KJ. Resection proposals for oncologic liver surgery based on vascular territories. In: Lembke HW, editor; CARS 2002; *Computer-Assisted Radiology and Surgery.* Proc of the 16th International Congress and Exhibition, Paris June, 26-29. 2002, Leiden University Medical Center, 2002, Vol 1, 353-358.

[4] Baulieux, J; Delpero, JR; Surgical treatment of pancreatic cancer: curative resections. *Ann Chir.*, 2000, 125, 609- 614.

[5] Schwarz, M; Pauls, S; Sokiranski, R; Brambs, HJ; Glasbrenner, B; Adler, G; Dierichs, C.G; Reske, SN; Moller, P; Beger, HG. Is preoperative multidiagnostic approach to predict surgical respectability of periampullary tumors still effective? *Am J Surg.*, 2001, 182, 243-249.

[6] Blumgart, LH; Fong, Y. Biliary tumors; In: Blumgart, LH; Fong, Y. *Surgery of the liver and biliary tract*, WB. Saunders Co Ltd, GB, Vol. 1, 1021-1028.

[7] Ott, DJ; Geland, DW. Complications of gastrointestinal radiologic procedures II. Complications related to biliary tract studies. *Gastrointest Radiol* 1981, 6,47-52.

[8] Winter, TC; Freeny, PC; Nghiem, HV. Hepatic arterial anatomy in transplantation candidates: evaluation with three-dimensional CT arteriography. *Radiology* 1995, 195, 363-370.

In: 3D Imaging: Theory, Technology … ISBN: 978-1-60876-885-1
Editors: E. H. Duke and S. R. Aguirre, pp.199-230

Chapter 9

ELECTRICAL RESISTIVITY IMAGING: OVERVIEW AND A CASE STUDY IN STONE CULTURAL HERITAGE

***Edite Martinho*[*1], *Francisco Alegria*[‡1], *Carlos Grangeia*[*†2], *Amélia Dionisio*[≠1] and *Fernando Almeida*[£2]**

[1] Technical University of Lisbon (TULisbon), Lisboa, Portugal

[2] Universidade de Aveiro, Campus Universitário de Santiago, Aveiro, Portugal

ABSTRACT

Electrical resistivity imaging (ERI) is a geophysical technique used to obtain images of geological structures from electrical measurements made at the surface or in boreholes. This technique has been widely used for environmental and engineering studies.

A 3-D electrical subsurface image can be obtained with 2-D or 3-D surveys. Since all geological structures are 3-D in nature, a fully 3-D resistivity survey using a 3-D interpretation model gives most accurate results. Here we describe the basic resistivity theory, compare the 3-D interpretation made from 2-D versus 3-D data sets, discuss the possible arrangements of the electrodes for a 3-D surveys, present equipment used for signal injection and automatic data acquisition and review signal processing algorithms used to process the acquired data.

We present the results of applying ERI in stone Cultural Heritage conservation. Two Portuguese renascence panels made of porous limestone showing severe decay phenomenon, located in the cloister of Santa Cruz Church in Coimbra, were studied in order to locate the origin of one of the most dangerous causes of stone decay – moisture.

We show the data acquisition system developed, which uses multichannel data acquisition boards, relays for electrode switching, DC and AC sources for current injection and LabVIEW software for data processing. The survey was carried out using a pole-pole array with electrodes arranged in a 5-by-7 rectangular grid, with the same electrode spacing in both directions (0.36 m). The electrodes were numbered consecutively from left to right and top to bottom; odd-numbered electrodes were used for potential measurement and even-numbered electrodes were used for current injection.

* E-mail address: emar@mail.ist.utl.pt
‡ E-mail address: falegria@lx.it.pt
*† E-mail address: cgrangeia@ua.pt
≠ E-mail address: fernandoalmeida@ua.pt
£ E-mail address: amelia.dionisio@ist.utl.pt

This system, with 35 electrodes (18 potential and 17 current) provided 306 measurements in each panel and in a side masonry wall (for comparison). The data was processed using a 3-D inversion program (RES3DINV) and the resulting resistivity distributions were then displayed as volumetric 3-D tomograms.

As a non-destructive and inexpensive tool, the 3-D resistivity imaging technique allowed 1) creation of a resistivity model of the two panels and the wall, where the high levels of the moisture are clearly visible and 2) the estimation of the thickness of the panels. The resistivity is lower in the bottom half of the panels and of the wall (higher levels of moisture) showing that in this case the moisture comes from the ground, rises along the wall and reaches the stone panels.

1. INTRODUCTION

The electrical resistivity imaging (ERI) technique is considered a relatively new geophysical method and of considerable current interest owing to its application to a wide range of geophysical problems [1]. As a non-invasive and inexpensive tool, this technique has been widely used for geological [2, 3, 4, 5], environmental [6, 7, 8], engineering [9] or archaeological [10, 11, 12] studies in recent years. The method aims to determine the distribution of electrical properties in the subsurface by conducting measurements at the ground surface or inside shallow boreholes. Electric imaging combines sounding and profiling, so it can give information about the resistivity distribution as a function of both depth and horizontal distance [13]. Resistivity images are created by inverting hundreds to thousands of individual resistivity measurements [e.g. 14, 15] to produce a graphical representation of the subsurface resistivity.

The development of the technology associated with automatically multiplexed electrode arrangements and automatic measuring systems, that facilitate the acquisition of a large number of measurements in a limited time, with the use of automated resistivity inversion schemes, make the application of the electric imaging method successful, even in complex geological environments. Data in two-dimensional and three-dimensional forms can be collected though full three-dimensional measurements providing the best subsurface information even in complex geological cases. Nowadays the most common practice to obtain the three-dimensional resistivity variation of the subsurface is from parallel two-dimensional lines whose data are interpreted with two-dimensional inversion algorithms and the results combined to generate a quasi-three-dimensional (x, y, z) image. Due to the cost and time involved, three-dimensional surveying is not yet routinely employed for near-surface applications. Moreover, it is still at the stage of active research. In this chapter we present a overview of the method including basic resistivity theory, electrodes array, 2-D versus 3-D data sets, equipment used and automatic data acquisition and also review signal processing algorithms used to process the acquired data.

Generally, geological studies of existing monuments are not easy and whatever the type of investigation used, it should be non-invasive [16]. Many indoors geophysical surveys of existing monuments have been reported using mostly a ground-penetrating radar (GPR). Linford, for instance, investigated the subsurface beneath a mosaic at a Roman villa at Bignor in England [17]. A similar survey was conducted by Piro et al., who tried to detect structures beneath the Emperor Trajan's villa floors near Rome [18]. A GPR survey at the Taj Mahal in India as also been reported [19]. There are also quite a few reports of surveys conducted inside churches like the ones described in [11, 20, 21, 22 and 23]. Investigations in the castle of Lefkas, in Greece [24] and on the wall of the Acropolis in Athens [25] were also reported.

All the above surveys were carried out with GPR because the technique is fully non-invasive and the floors are usually flat, which ensures smooth movement of the antennae which is not the case with uneven terrains where corrections for slope are needed [16].

In the works mentioned above, performed in churches, a severe "back-scatter" and a very limited penetration depth was observed. Furthermore, very subtle diffractions were seen for which it was very hard to indicate a cause [16].

Alternatively to GPR, the other feasible technology that could be applied around and inside churches is the ERI. Carrara et al. investigated the mosaic floor of a Roman villa [26] while Cosentino et al. investigated the damages to walls [27]. Tsokas et al. explored the area inside and around the church of Kapnikarea in Athens (Greece) with the aim of investigating the possible presence of concealed ancient wells and voids or spaces filled with debris and clay, located beneath the floor, which could threaten the stability of the monument due to the construction of the underground [16].

Measurements of the moisture contents of porous material involved in cultural heritage are important because moisture is one of the most dangerous agents to stone decay. Quantitative measurements are scarce, which is partly due to the lack of reliable measurement techniques [28]. Some available techniques are invasive or include various moisture probes based on conductance, resistance or capacitance [29, 30]. Such methods can give good temporal resolution of data, but effectively only provide point samples over space, and installing the sensors may affect the moisture movements [31]. Sass used different techniques for obtaining rock moisture data, including 2-D geoelectric measurements [28] and concluded that the method is reliable in determination of the spatial moisture distribution. Sass et al. also used successfully the 2-D electrical resistivity method to investigate moisture contents of walls at two ruined abbeys [31]. Viles et al. used the resistivity survey to provide 2-D information of moisture contents within historical masonry walls (Wren Wall, Sheldonian Theatre, Oxford) [32]. The works mentioned above show that the ERI method, as a non-invasive technique, has been successfully used to investigate existing monuments. Here we present the results of applying the 3-D resistivity imaging technique in two Portuguese renascence panels (*Descent from the Cross* and *Ecce Homo* Retable) located in Santa Cruz Monastery (Coimbra, Portugal), made of a porous limestone. The ERI survey was done in order to locate the origin of the moisture that is causing severe deterioration of the panels. Measurements in a side masonry wall were also carried out in order to compare moisture distribution on the panels with that of neighbouring walls.

2. Overview

2.1 Basic Resistivity Theory

Electrical resisitivity surveys are used to map the resistivity of geological structures. Rock resistivity is related to various geological parameters such as the mineral and fluid content, porosity and degree of water saturation in the rock. The method is used in hydrogeological investigations to search for suitable groundwater sources and to monitor types of groundwater pollution, in engineering to locate sub-surface cavities, faults and fissures, mineshafts, etc., in archaeology for mapping out the areal extent of remnants of buried foundations of ancient buildings, and in environmental studies for defining contamination plumes amongst other applications.

Resistivity is determined by injecting electric currents into the ground and measuring the resulting potential differences at the surface. Two pairs of electrodes are required: electrodes C_1 and C_2 are used for current injections, while electrodes P_1 and P_2 are for potential differences measurements.

For a continuous medium, the current density **J** is related to the electric field **E** and the resistivity ρ through Ohm's law

$$\mathbf{J}=\sigma\mathbf{E} \tag{1}$$

where σ is the conductivity of the medium defined as 1/ρ, the reciprocal of its resistivity. In geophysical surveys the medium resistivity is more commonly used. The electric field is the gradient of the scalar electric potential,

$$\mathbf{E}=-\nabla V \tag{2}$$

Combining equations (1) and (2), we have

$$\mathbf{J}=-\sigma\nabla V \tag{3}$$

For an elemental volume ΔV surrounding the current source I, located at (x_s, y_s, z_s) the relationship between the current density and the current [33] is given by

$$\nabla \bullet \mathbf{J} = \left(\frac{I}{\Delta V}\right)\delta(x-x_s)\delta(y-y_s)\delta(z-z_s) \tag{4}$$

where δ is the Dirac delta function. Thus, the equation that gives the potential distribution in the ground due to a point current source is

$$-\nabla \bullet [\sigma(x,y,z)\nabla V(x,y,z)] = \left(\frac{I}{\Delta V}\right)\delta(x-x_s)\delta(y-y_s)\delta(z-z_s) \tag{5}$$

A large number of techniques have been developed to solve this equation [33].

For a single point source of the current at the surface of the homogeneous isotropic medium, the current flows radially away from the source and at any instant its distribution will be uniform over a hemispherical shell of an underground region of resistivity ρ.

At a distance, r, away from the current source, the potential is given by [e. g. 34]

$$V = \frac{\rho I}{2\pi r} \tag{6}$$

In practice, all resistivity surveys use at least two current electrodes, a positive current +I (entry point C1) and a negative current –I (exit point C2) source, and two potential electrodes (P1 and P2). From Eq. (6), we have that difference in potential between points P1 and P2 caused by current +I is

$$\Delta V = \frac{\rho I}{2\pi}\left(\frac{1}{C1P1} - \frac{1}{C1P2}\right) \tag{7}$$

and by current –I is

$$\Delta V = -\frac{\rho I}{2\pi}\left(\frac{1}{C2P1} - \frac{1}{C2P2}\right) \tag{8}$$

where CxPx is the distance between the current and potential electrodes. The total potential difference is given by the sum of the right-hand sides of Eqs (7) and (8) and is

$$\Delta V = \frac{I\rho}{2\pi}\left(\frac{1}{C1P1} - \frac{1}{C1P2} - \frac{1}{C2P1} + \frac{1}{C2P2}\right) \tag{9}$$

Such an arrangement corresponds to the four-electrode spreads normally used in resistivity field work.

The field surveys are invariably conducted over an inhomogeneous medium where the subsurface resistivity has a 3-D distribution. The resistivity measurements are made by injecting current into the ground through the two current electrodes (C1 and C2) and measuring the resulting voltage difference at two potential electrodes (P1 and P2). From the current (I) and potential (ΔV) values, a resistivity (ρ) value is calculated

$$\rho = 2\pi \frac{\Delta V}{I}\frac{1}{(G)} \tag{10}$$

where (G) is an abbreviation for the expression in parentheses in Eq. (9). The 2π/(G) denotes the geometric factor of an electrode configuration.

Over homogeneous isotropic ground this resistivity will be constant for any current and electrode configuration (true resistivity). For inhomogeneous earth the resistivity ρ, as computed from Eq. (10), will vary with different geometrical arrangements of the electrodes or on moving them on the ground surface without altering their geometry. The resistivity obtained from Eq. (10) for an inhomogeneous underground is, therefore, designated as the apparent resistivity, ρa. The relationship between the "apparent" resistivity and the "true" resistivity is a complex one. The determination of the true subsurface resistivity from the apparent resistivity values is called the "inversion problem".

2.2. Electrode Arrays

An enormous number of electrode dispositions can be used in electrical resistivity imaging. In principle it is not necessary to use a collinear array. However, the electrodes are almost always in line; otherwise interpretation of results becomes difficult and the field work complicated. Several commonly used linear array types are Wenner, Schlumberger, gradient, pole-dipole and dipole-dipole [e. g. 35, 36]. For each arrangement the apparent resistivity equation can be obtained by using the appropriate geometrical factor in Eq. 10. The choice of the best array for a field survey depends on the type of structure to be mapped, the sensitivity of the resistivity meter and the background noise level. Among the characteristics of an array that should be considered are [33]: 1) the depth of investigation, 2) the sensitivity of the array to vertical and horizontal changes in the subsurface resistivity, 3) the horizontal data coverage and 4) the signal strength.

In 3-D surveys, the pole-pole, pole-dipole and dipole-dipole arrays are frequently used because other arrays have poorer data coverage near the edges of the survey grid [33]. The pole-pole array is used for small survey grids (less than 12 by 12 electrodes) with relatively small spacing (less than 10 metres) between the electrodes, while pole-dipole array is used for surveys with medium size grid (12 by 12 electrodes). The dipole-dipole array is the least used of the three arrays mentioned above. This array can be recommended only for grids that are larger than 12 by 12 because of the poorer horizontal data coverage at the sides.

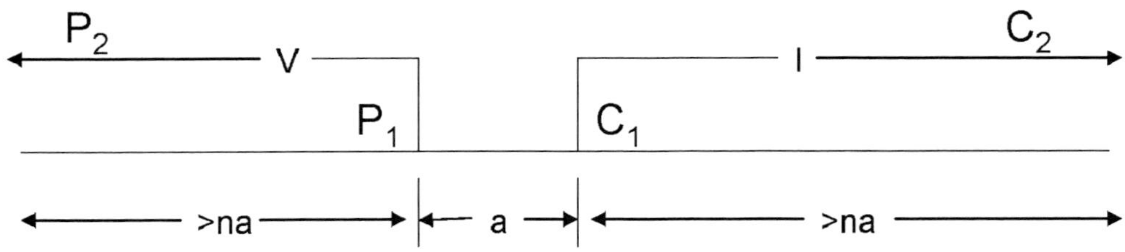

Figure 1. – Pole-pole array. C_1, C_2 and P_1, P_2 denote the positions of the current and potential electrodes, respectively.

Pole-pole array – one of the current electrodes and one of the potential electrodes are placed at a great distance from the other two (Figure 1). The apparent resistivity value is given by

$$\rho_a = 2\pi a R \qquad (11)$$

where R is the measured resistance and a is the spacing between C1 and P1 electrodes. For 3-D surveys, the electrodes are usually arranged in a square grid, as shown in Figure 2 [33], with the same electrode spacing in the x and y directions. To map slightly elongated bodies, a rectangular grid with different numbers of electrodes and spacings in both directions could be used. The maximum number of independent measurements that can be made with P electrodes is [37]

$$n_{max} = P(P-1)/2 \tag{12}$$

In the measurement sequence, each electrode is in turn used as a current electrode and the potential at all the other electrodes are measured. One problem with this type of survey is the time taken (at least several hours) to make such a large number of measurements. For the example, in the case of Figure 2, there are 1176 possible measurements. An alternative measurement sequence, without seriously degrading the quality of the model obtained, is the cross-diagonal survey method [33], where the potential measurements are only made at the electrodes along the x-direction, the y-direction and the 45 degrees diagonal lines passing through the current electrode (Figure 3). The number of data points with this arrangement for 7 by 7 grid is reduced to 476 which is about one-third of that required by a complete data set survey [14].

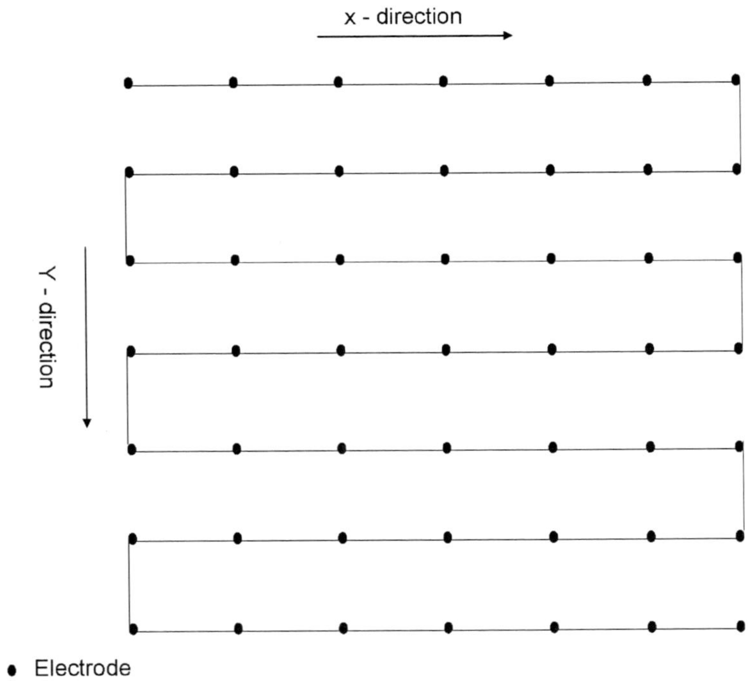

Figure 2. – Possible arrangement of the electrodes with a pole-pole array for a 3-D survey using a multi-electrode system with 49 nodes (Modified from [33]).

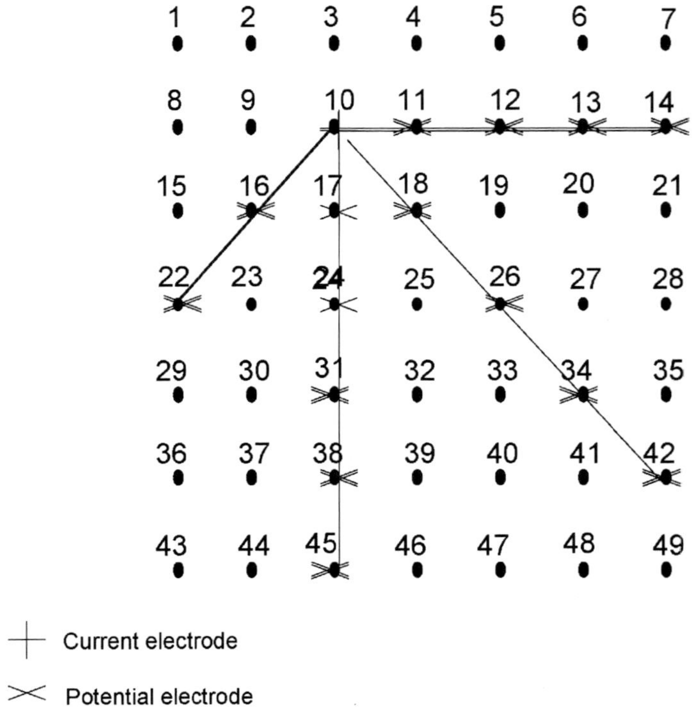

Figure 3. – Cross-diagonal survey method (Modified from [33]).

In the pole-pole array, the loss of data points near the sides of the grid is kept to a minimum, and provides better horizontal data coverage compared to any other array. However, it has two main disadvantages [33]: 1) it has much poorer resolution compared to other arrays; 2) requires that two electrodes (second current and potential electrode) must be placed at a sufficiently large distance (at least 10 times the maximum electrode spacing used) from the survey grid. Due to the large distance between the two potential electrodes, this array is more sensitive to telluric noise.

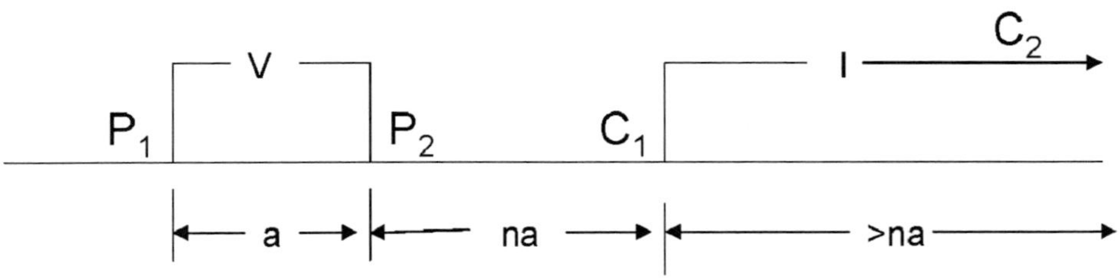

Figure 4. – Pole-dipole array. C_1, C_2 and P_1, P_2 denote the positions of the current and potential electrodes, respectively.

Pole-dipole array – one of the current electrodes is fixed at a great distance from the other three (infinite electrode), all of which can have various spacings (Figure 4).

The apparent resistivity value is given by

$$\rho_a = 2\pi n(n+1)aR \tag{13}$$

where R is the measured resistance, a is the spacing between the potential electrodes (P_1 and P_2) and n is the ratio of the distances between the C_1 and P_1 electrodes to the P_1 - P_2 spacing.

As the pole-dipole array is an asymmetrical array, the measurements should be made with the forward and reverse arrangements of the electrodes. This allows, in some situations, the elimination of the effect of the asymmetry in the measured apparent resistivity values and which may influence the model obtained after inversion. For large values of the n factor (exceeding 8) the signal strength is low. To increase the signal strength, the a spacing between P_1 – P_2 dipole should be increased to get a deeper depth of investigation with a smaller n factor. This increases the data density and, in some cases, as in noisy areas, improves the resolution of the resulting inversion model.

The pole-dipole array has a higher resolution than the pole-pole array; it requires only one remote electrode and is much less sensitive to telluric noise. Compared to the dipole-dipole array, it has much stronger signal strength.

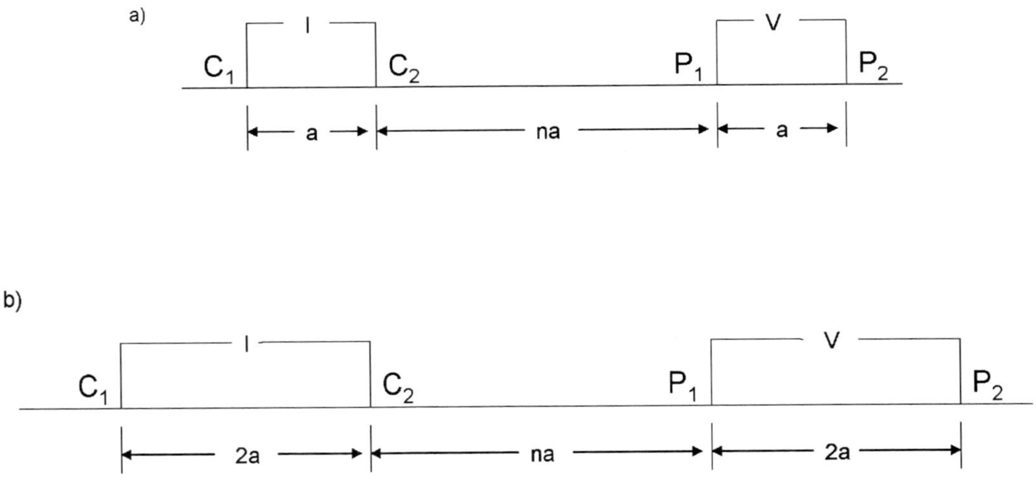

Figure 5. – a) Dipole-dipole array. b) Increasing the spacing between the dipoles (C_1-C_2 and P_1-P_2) to increase the signal strength. C_1, C_2 and P_1, P_2 denote the positions of the current and potential electrodes, respectively.

Dipole-dipole array – the potential electrodes, P_1 and P_2, are outside the current electrodes, C_1 and C_2, each pair having a constant mutual separation, a (Figure 5). In this case, the apparent resistivity is given by

$$\rho_a = \pi a n(n+1)(n+2)R \tag{14}$$

where R is the measured resistance, a is the spacing between the electrodes of each dipole and n is the ratio of the distances between the C_1 and P_1 electrodes to the a spacing. This array has the advantage of very good horizontal resolution; the main problem is its relatively low signal strength. Like the pole-dipole array, to get a deeper depth of investigation, the spacing between current and potential electrodes pairs is increased. To reduce the effect of noise, different combinations of the n and a spacing can be used. The dipole-dipole array is more sensitive to 3-D effects compared to the other common arrays [33].

Other arrays which can also be used, as the dipole-dipole array, are the Wenner and Schlumberger.

2.3. Two versus Three-Dimensional Resistivity Imaging Surveys

The two-dimensional electrical resistivity image (ERI) can be obtained from the collection of the data along a profile, with continuously increasing inner-electrode spacing (pseudo-section) or as a series of successive vertical electrical soundings along a line. In practice, a number of electrodes with a given spacing between them are inserted into the ground along a line and various measurements are obtained for different electrode spacing. The result is a model of the subsurface based on the resistivity changes in the vertical and horizontal direction along the survey line (2-D model).

At sites of complex geology, the 2-D assumption may introduce significant error because artefacts may be generated in the two-dimensional sections owing to the three-dimensional nature of the underground structures; the resulting 2-D images can contain significant distortions. In order to overcome the above-mentioned problem, full three-dimensional measurements of the resistivity must be considered. In the full three-dimensional surveys the pole-pole configuration is commonly used and the electrodes are normally arranged in a square or rectangular grid with the same unit electrode spacing in the *x* and *y* direction [14]. The main disadvantage is the time required to gather complete sets of measurements, particularly when typical single-channel resistivity meters are used. Nowadays multichannel automated resistivity meters have been developed reducing the overall time taken to collect such data. However, the time needed has not yet been reduced to an acceptable level to be able to conduct such surveys on a routine basis [10]. So, in many cases, 3-D data sets are constructed from parallel two-dimensional lines with interline spacing equal to the smallest electrode spacing used [33, 10]. If the 3-D survey is carried out with pole-dipole or dipole-dipole array, the distance between the lines can be larger about two or three times the inline unit electrode spacing [33]. Ideally, the data must be collected from a set of survey lines with measurements in the x-direction, followed by another series of lines in the y-direction. The use of measurements in two perpendicular directions helps to reduce any directional bias in the data.

Albeit the development of advanced instrumentation and three-dimensional interpretation techniques, common geophysical practice still relies mainly on two-dimensional approaches, both in view of measurements and interpretations [38]. Parallel two-dimensional images are interpreted using two-dimensional inversion algorithms and the results are combined to create a quasi-three-dimensional (*x, y, z*) image of the subsurface resistivity distribution. This type of result often suffers from artefacts, either due to the fact that three-dimensional responses are attributed to two-dimensional structures or due to the varying level of misfit that individual two-dimensional inversions may reach [39].

Recently, some studies have been published which compare results of combined two-dimensional inversions (quasi-three-dimensional) with the full three-dimensional inversions. Chambers et al. have conducted a 3-D ERI survey over oil-and tar-contaminated soils, with orthogonal sets of collinear pole-dipole arrays, within a grid measuring 95 x 95 m [6]. The survey was motivated by discrepancies between 1-D and 2-D geophysical data and ground. Slater et al. have used cross hole 2-D and 3-D induced polarization and resistivity images to investigate the integrity of permeable reactive barriers [40]. They concluded that 2-D imaging is sufficient over most of the barrier but that 3-D imaging would improve the assessment of the ends of the barrier and might be required to assess the variability in the barrier at a finer scale. Ogilvy et al. have conducted 3-D ERI surveys over an old quarry site used as a landfill because the heterogeneity of the site precluded the use of 2-D arrays [41]. Bentley et al. showed how 3-D geometric effects can contaminate and distort 2-D images [7]. They compare and discuss results from 2-D and 3-D surveys, obtained over heterogeneous remediation site, in relation to field validation and the forward modelling results. The 2D images indicated several features inconsistent with other data collected at the remediation site and with knowledge of the geological and geochemical distributions across the site. They concluded that 3-D surveying may be the most cost-effective surveying method in some field situations. Chambers et al. have used orthogonal sets of dipole-dipole and Wenner 1-D lines to image known targets at an experimental site [42]. They concluded that the 3-D inversions are superior to quasi-3-D images produced from sets of 2-D inversions. Papadopoulos et al. compared results of combined two-dimensional inversions (quasi-three-dimensional) with the full three-dimensional inversions from data collected in archaeological areas [10]. The comparisons were carried out in relation to optimum survey direction using the pole-pole array for synthetic data arising from three-dimensional structures commonly encountered in archaeological sites. Results indicate that a single survey direction is adequate to produce a valid three-dimensional subsurface image when full three-dimensional inversion is used in contrast to the quasi-three-dimensional approach, which would require that two survey directions be used to obtain satisfactory results.

Despite the gathering of resistivity data in parallel tomographies being the most common field practice nowadays, the quality of the quasi-three-dimensional images depends on the degree of noise of the measurements and the complicated nature of the subsurface structure [10]. At heterogeneous sites the 3-D ERI surveys provide the best information of the subsurface.

2.4. Instrumentation and Signal Processing

The equipment needed for electrical resistivity imaging consists of a transmitter, which injects current into the ground, and a receiver which measures the voltage between two points. This voltage is proportional to the injected current. In order to obtain a good signal to noise ratio in the measurements made, it is important to have a high enough current. Both transmitter and receiver, together with the power supply, are usually enclosed in a single instrument.

Traditionally, the transmitter applies a constant voltage, which can go from 50 V to 1500 V, to the two current electrodes placed in the ground. The resulting current, which usually can go up to 5 A, depends on the resistance of the electric circuit formed by the cables, connectors, electrodes, ground and most importantly, the interface between electrode and ground. Depending on the distance between current electrodes, the total resistance can vary typically between 100 Ω to 100 kΩ. To have a higher current as possible care should be taken to put the electrodes deep into the ground, watering the ground around them (with salt water if possible) or even using more than one electrode, connected in parallel, at a given location.

In order to build a detailed map of the resistivity of the ground in a given area, it is necessary to inject the current and measure the voltage in more than one location. It is common to have electrode spacing from 3 m to 10 m. To cover an area of several hundred square meters, hundreds of measurements have to be made. Not only does the voltage between those electrodes has to be measured but also the location where the current is injected as to be changed. Modern systems use switching units which are able to select, at a given time, a pair of current electrodes and a pair of potential electrodes. The transmitter is connected two each pair of current electrodes in sequence. For each of those pairs, the voltage between different combinations of potential electrodes is measured. These systems not only make the process of data gathering more efficient and thus less time consuming, but also allow a greater number of measurements to be made which increases resolution and allows for full 3-D surveys. There are commercial systems that are even capable of measuring the voltage between many pairs of electrodes at the same time (usually 10) which further speeds up the whole procedure.

In order to connect the transmitter, receiver and switch to the hundreds of electrodes used, a multi-core electrical cable is used. They allow for easier storage and set-up since it is not necessary to deal with a multitude of individual conductors. The use of a reel makes it possible to easily lay out the cable on the ground. Those cables have small cylindrical metallic sections along their length, connected to the different cores, to allow easy attachment of the electrodes. 2-D surveys are done using two of these cables placed in a single line with the instrument in the middle. 3-D surveys are done using several cables arranged in parallel lines. In this case it is possible to inject the current using electrodes in one cable and measure the voltage between electrodes connected to a different cable. In standard cables there is one core for each electrode. To avoid crosstalk, each core should be shielded. It is not practical to have too many cores since the weight of the entire cable, which can run for more than 100 m, becomes prohibitive. An alternative is to use two cores to connect to the potential electrodes and two cores to connect to the current electrodes. At each connection point there is a remotely controlled switch which connects, or not, a given electrode to a given core. This requires additional cores for power supply and communication with the switches but reduces substantially the total number of cores. The whole cable is more expensive but it is lighter and can be used with more electrodes.

The currents injected into the ground can be DC, pulsed DC or AC. The first case is the easier one in terms of transmitter complexity but leads to electrode polarization. To avoid this, pulsed DC is typically used. In pulsed DC current signals the current is positive for a given time interval then null, then negative and then null again. The time interval usually ranges from 200 ms to 5 s. This type of signal is useful not only for resistivity measurement but also for chargeability measurement since the decay curves in the measured voltages depend on the chargeability of the ground. AC signals, which sometimes are used, are sine waves whose frequency can be varied typically from under 1 Hz to a few dozen Hz.

The measurement of the voltage between pairs of electrodes is done with a digital acquisition system. This kind of system is based on one or more analogue-to-digital converters (ADCs) and has programmable gain amplifiers with high input impedance for optimum range selection, multiplexer for multi-channel measurement, filters for noise reduction, and data storage for later transfer to a computer. The use of 24-bit ADCs reduces the amount of quantization error which allows lower voltages to be measured. Other sources of noise are thermal noise in the cables, telluric noise due to currents in the ground induced by the changing magnetic field of the Earth, coupling between measurement channels and coupling from the AC power supply.

The acquired signals are then transferred to a computer where they are digitally processed to remove noise and to compute the resistance values and from them the apparent resistivity. 2D/3D inversion software is used to build the resistivity images of the ground.

3. Case Study in Stone Cultural Heritage

3.1. Description of the Site and Panels

Santa Cruz Monastery is a National Monument in Coimbra, Portugal. Founded in 1131 outside the protecting walls of Coimbra, the Santa Cruz Monastery was the most important monastic house during the first times of the Portuguese monarchy. It is located in Coimbra's downtown where the groundwater level is shallow. In its Manueline cloister, of quadrangular planimetry there are four magnificent stone bas-reliefs with scenes from the Passion of Christ created by the sculptor Nicolau Chanterenne. Nowadays only three of them are visible: the *Ecce Homo* (Figure 6), the *Descent from the Cross* (Figure 7) and the *Way of Calvary* (Figure 8) the first plays an engraving of Albrecht Dürer. These bas-reliefs have about 1.60 m width and 2.30 m height. They are located in the walls of the cloister, 1.5 m from the floor.

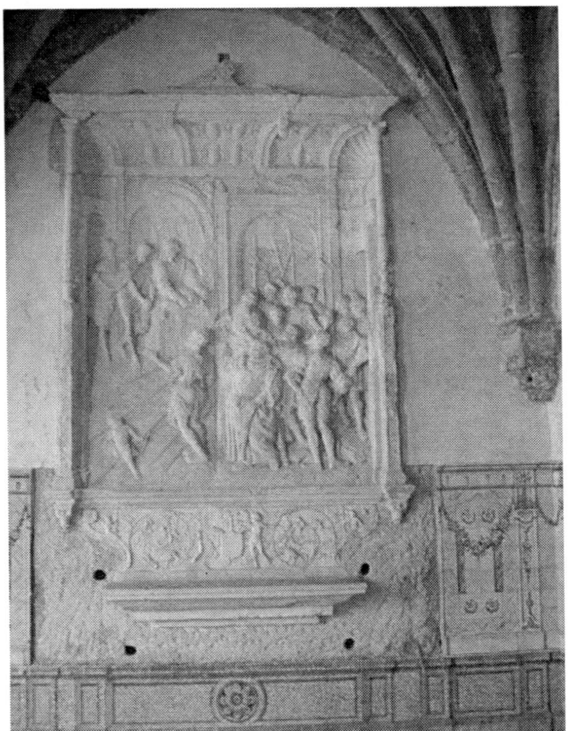

Figure 6. – *Ecce Homo* Retable.

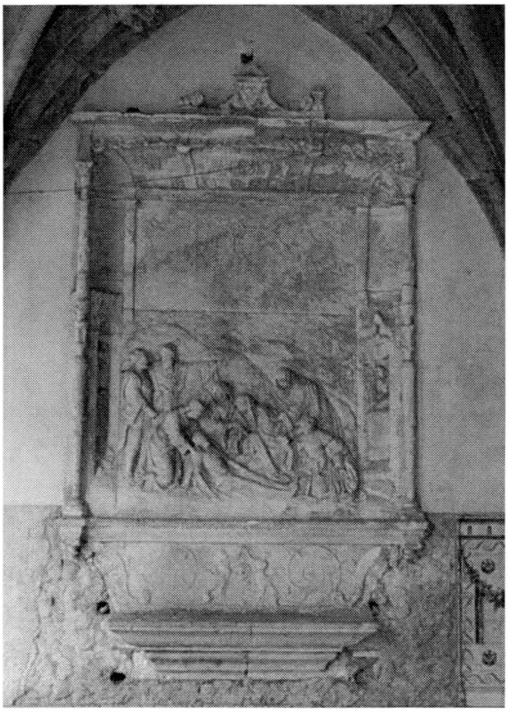

Figure 7. – Descent from the Cross Retable.

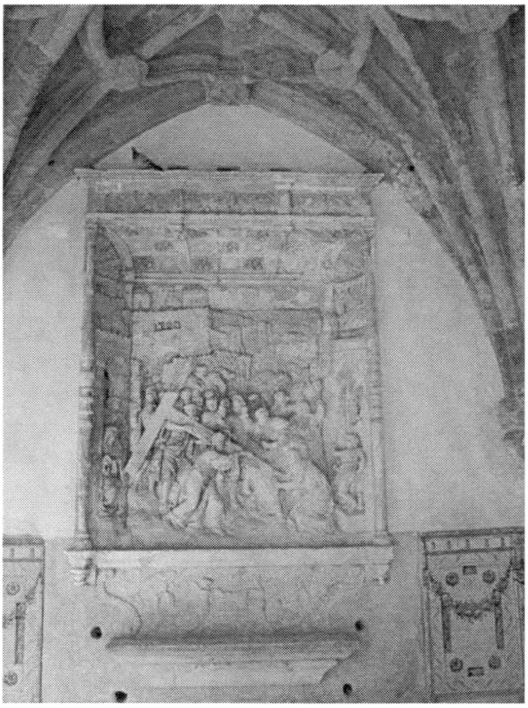

Figure 8. – *Way of Calvary* Retable.

The bas-reliefs were made using one of the most famous natural stones used in Portugal since Roman times, Pedra de Ançã. This type of stone is a light whitish-yellow fine-grained compact and homogeneous limestone belonging to the Jurassic Ançã limestone formation (Coimbra, Portugal). The stone is bioclastic and calciclastic, showing oolitic tendency and containing rather spathized micritic cement. The mineralogical composition is predominately calcitic with a $CaCO_3$ relative weight proportion higher than 96.5%. This lithotype has been widely used as raw material in sculpture and architecture, mainly because it is a very soft light-coloured rock, without any veins. Heritage employing this material can be found all over Portugal, as well as in most parts of Spain, and reaching other places in Europe. It occurs in a large outcrop area, located in the Beira Litoral region, in the Coimbra District, near Cordinhã, Zambujeiro and Ançã. Is part of a thick carbonated formation of Bajocian-Bathonian age (Middle Jurassic), which constitutes a slight synclinal fold [43].

These magnificent bas-reliefs present nowadays severe decay phenomena, clearly revealing that they are not immune to decay factors and pathologies like powdering, saline efflorescences, multiple exfoliation, crusts and blistering. Moisture and salts were identified as the most damaging factors to these bas-reliefs.

3.2. Previous Investigations

A preliminary work was performed in order to characterize the typology of salts present in the retables and also their spatial distribution. This geochemical investigation was carried out using cellulose paste imbibed in deionised water that were applied during one hour, in sampling areas of 5×5 cm^2 regularly distributed within the retables. In each retable twelve sampling points were considered.

After that time period the pastes were removed, transported to laboratory and filtrated. The obtained solution was analysed by ion chromatography and the concentration of sulphates, chlorides and nitrates was determined, using a chromatographer Dionex 2000i/SP with an anion separator column (Dionex AS4A).

Based on the chemical information obtained from the 12 sampling points the estimation of the spatial distribution of concentration of these anions was established using kriging as the interpolation method of the experimental values. The SURFER 7.0 software for Windows was used.

Figures 9 and 10 present the distribution of salts in two of the panels.

The *Descent from the Cross* Retable has a clearly marked area for the presence of chloride and nitrate (Figure 9a and b), which corresponds roughly to the area where there is greater loss of stone material, making its iconographic interpretation difficult.

The *Ecce Homo* Retable distinguishes from earlier since highest concentrations of nitrate and chloride (Figure 10a and b) are located in the highest part of the panel and are almost nonexistent in the lower left corner. The spatial distribution of sulphate in this retable should also be highlighted (Figure 10c): there is an area where its concentration is clearly higher than that of the rest of the retable where sulphates concentration is almost nil. This is a result consistent with the macroscopic observation of the panel.

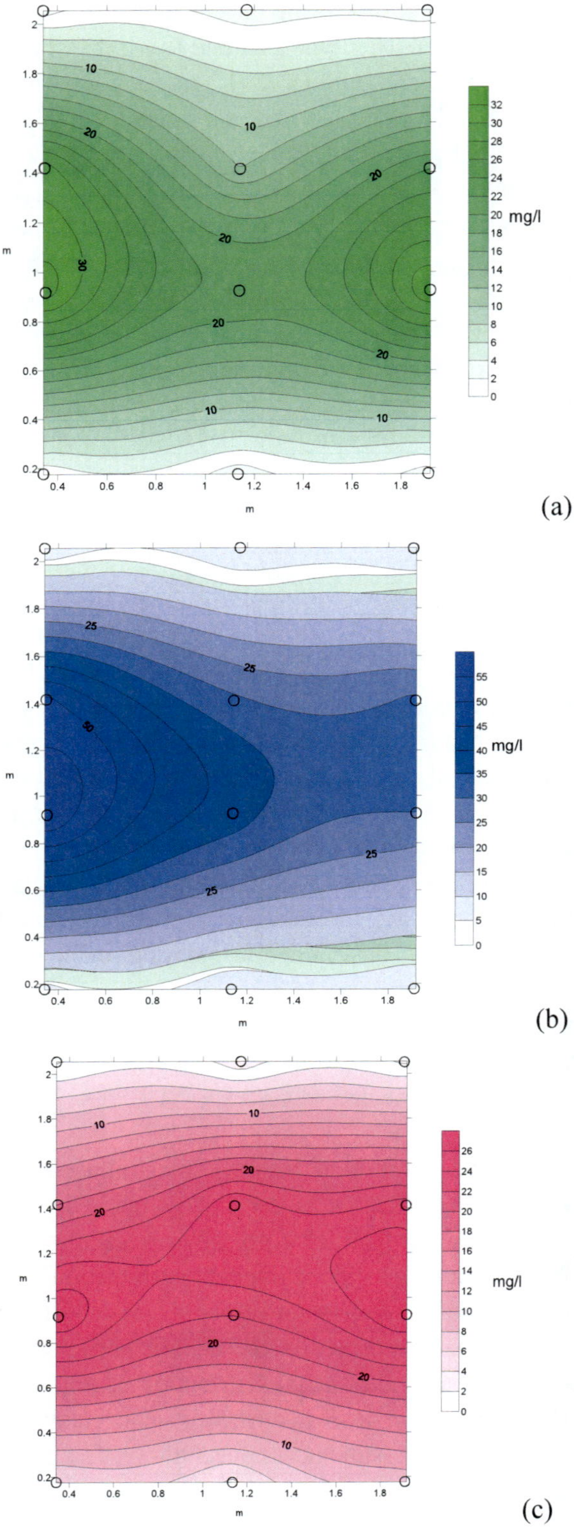

Figure 9. – Estimation of the spatial distribution of salts concentration in *Descent from the Cross* Retable. a) Chlorides; b) Nitrates; c) Sulphates.

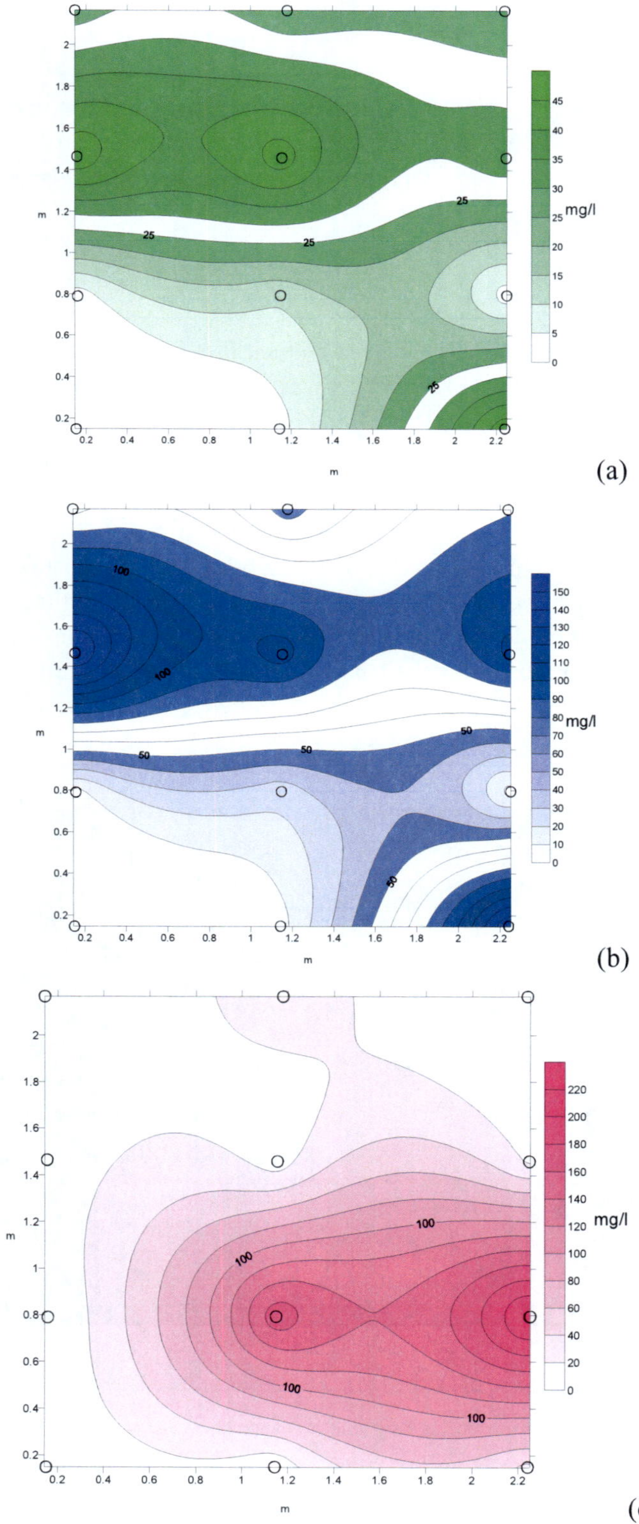

Figure 10. – Estimation of the spatial distribution of salts concentration in *Ecce Homo* Retable. a) Chlorides; b) Nitrates; c) Sulphates.

3.3. 3-D Electric Imaging

The electrical resistivity of porous solids is largely based on the moisture content so, the records of this parameter allow a good estimation of rock moisture. In order to identify the main source of moisture in the panels and walls of the cloister in the Santa Cruz Monastery, 3-D resisitivity surveys were carried out.

Data Acquisition

In order to efficiently inject the current and to measure the voltage, a custom build system was created. It was centred on a laptop which was connected, through an USB interface, to three National Instruments' multifunction input/output boards. One of them, model USB-6218, with a 16-bit ADC, 32-channels and 250 kSamples/s maximum sampling rate, was used to measure the voltages between the potential electrodes in the wall and the reference potential electrode placed on the ground in the centre of the cloister. A separate identical board was used, with the help of a 100 Ω sampling resistor, to measure the current being injected. A third multifunction board, model USB-6251, with 24 digital I/O terminals was used to control a custom made switching box made of relays to connect the 300 V power source to the current electrodes in the wall. The reference current electrode was placed in the centre of the cloister, far away from the potential reference electrode, and about 35 m from the wall.

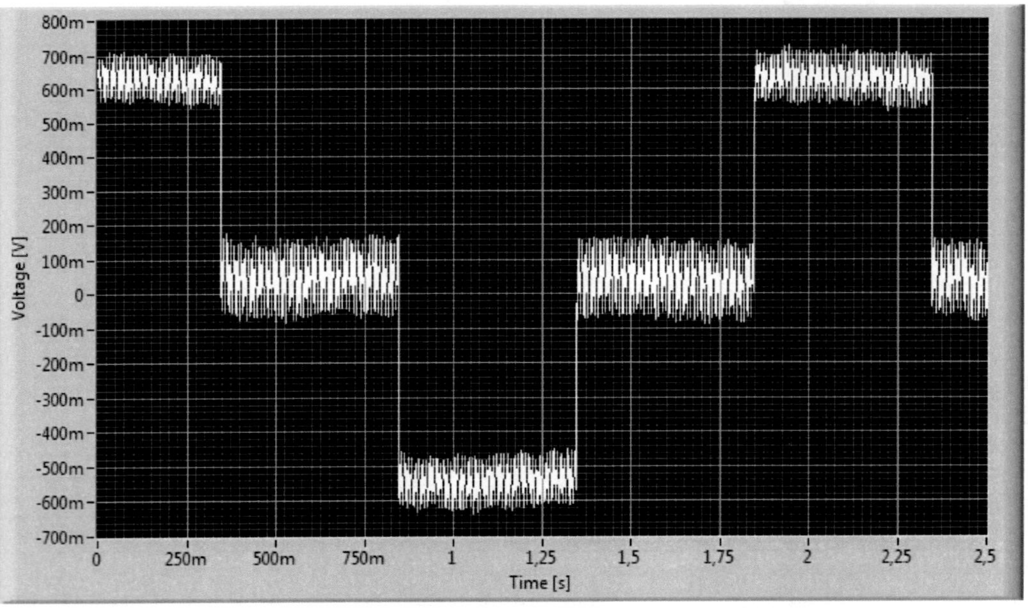

Figure 11. – Illustration of one of the voltage signals measured.

An application was developed in National Instruments' LabVIEW graphical programming language to control the switch box, acquire the data from the potential electrodes and compute the apparent resistivity values. Figure 11 shows an example of one of the voltage waveforms acquired when a pulsed DC current was injected. The noise visible is mainly due to 50 Hz coupling from the power supply. It was digitally removed from the data with a custom made filter which scans the waveform for level transitions at +25% and -25% of the peak-to-peak amplitude, splits the waveform into distinct segments and filters them by doing an average of the data points. Care was taken to set the positive, negative and null current intervals to a length which was multiple of 20 ms (period of a 50 Hz signal). The length chosen was 500 ms. Since no chargeability effects are visible in the waveform (curve decay around the transitions), this interval could have been made shorter. For a given current electrode selected (of the 17 used), all potential electrode voltages (18) were acquired simultaneously during 5 s with a sampling rate of 2 kHz per channel. The whole procedure took less than 2 minutes thanks to the automatic system implemented.

Each level transition, after noise filtering, was used to compute a resistance value. The apparent resistivity is computed from the resistance using the information input into the application about the position of the electrodes. Since there are 9 transitions in each 5 s interval there are 9 values of apparent resistivity values (for each combination of current and potential electrode). Those 9 values were used to compute their average and standard deviation. Figure 12 shows an example.

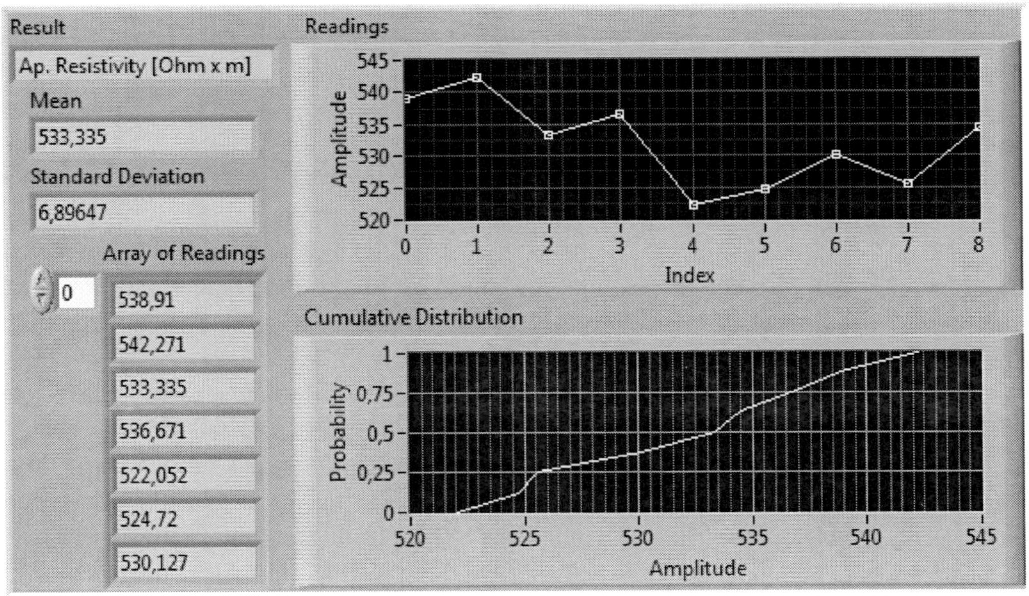

Figure 12. – Illustration of the statistics computed for each apparent resistivity value (mean, standard deviation and cumulative distribution).

A graph with the cumulative probability distribution is visible in the bottom right corner. It was used to check the type of statistical distribution of the apparent resistivity estimates. In a test run where 1000 readings were made (for just one pair of current and potential electrode) it was concluded that it was a normal distribution (not clearly seen with just the 9 measurement shown in the figure). This, together with the value of standard deviation computed, can be used to calculate the confidence interval for the estimated value of apparent resistivity:

$$\bar{x} - t_{1-\delta/2}\frac{s}{\sqrt{n}} < \text{Apparent Resistivity} < \bar{x} + t_{1-\delta/2}\frac{s}{\sqrt{n}},$$

where $\bar{x}$ is the average of the apparent resistivity values, s is the standard deviation, n is the number of measurements and $t_{1-\delta/2}$ is the Student-t distribution percentile for a confidence level of δ.

If the variability of the apparent resistivity values obtained for the entire combination of current and potential electrode pairs is of the same magnitude of the confidence interval length it may signify that the variability observed is due to measurement uncertainty and not to actual change of the resistivity of the media (or wall). It is recommended, in these situations, to look more closely at the possible sources of noise and to increase the value of the injected current in order to improve the signal-to-noise ratio which, in turn, will lead to smaller values of measurement standard deviation and corresponding confidence interval length (lower measurement uncertainty).

Non-polarizable $Cu/CuSO_4$ electrodes were used as current and potential electrodes. They are stable and have a concentration of $CuSO_4$ liquid and solid in order to maintain a constant potential. This is achieved by two chemical reactions. The first one takes place in the supersaturated solution and keeps the ions concentrations from forming or dissolving the copper sulphate. The second one exchanges the electrons across the copper shell with the solution.

A general supporting structure for both potential and current electrodes has been developed (Figure 13). It consists on a light weight rectangular aluminium structure having 5 by 7 equally spaced fixation (0.36 m) in the x and y directions (Figure 13a and c), corresponding to the electrodes position. Special electrode fixation (Figure 13b), over the aluminium structure, has also been developed for every electrode so that good coupling was achieved even for the highly irregular surfaces of the panels (Figure 13c).

These electrode supporting structures have been made so that an electrode fixating telescopic plastic arm with the help of a steal coil would make a constant pressure over the masonry wall independently of the distance. This telescopic arm has amplitude of 20 cm, which is enough to cover the wall surface irregularities over this range. Electrical connections to the electrodes were made inside and at the end of the plastic arm tube. Wiring came out on the back of these tubes so that it would not disturb possible amplitude movements, with possible coupling losses.

The 3-D electrical measurements were carried out using a pole-pole array. As most of the problems found in data acquisition are related to the use of potential electrodes that had been used as current injection, two kinds of electrodes were used; one for current injection and another for potential measurements. These ideas were the basis of a pole-pole array approach that leads to the individualization of two circuits (potential and current) and which facilitates the spread electrode commutation. The electrodes were numbered consecutively from left to right and top to bottom; odd-numbered electrodes were used for potential measurement and even-numbered electrodes used for current injection (Figure 14). This system, with 35 electrodes (18 potential and 17 current) provided 306 measurements in each panel and in a side masonry wall. The measurements over masonry wall were carried out at the same height of the panels.

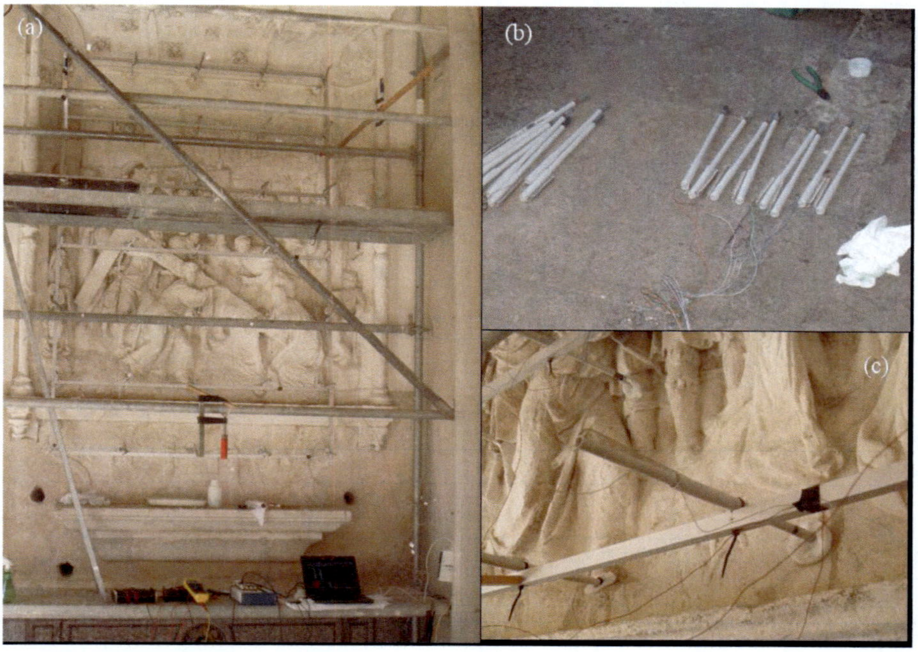

Figure 13. – General supporting structure for 3-D electrical measurements. (a) Light rectangular aluminium structure with 5-by-7 equally spaced fixation joints; (b) special electrode fixation made with telescopic plastic (PVC tube) arm; (c) Detail of electrode fixation over the aluminium structure.

1 P.	2 C.	3 P.	4C.	5 P.
6 C.	7 P.	8 C.	9 P.	10 C.
11 P.	12 C.	13 P.	14 C.	15 P.
16 C.	17 P.	18 C.	19 P.	20 C.
21 P.	22 C.	23 P.	24 C.	25 P.
26 C.	27 P.	28 C.	29 P.	30 C.
31 P.	32 C.	33 P.	34 C	35 P.

Figure 14. – Numbering and relative positioning of the electrodes.

Inversion

The inversion of the resistivity data was carried out using 3-D finite difference inversion program RES3DINV [44]. The resisitvty model is composed by 9 layers with 6x4 voxel which correspond to 24 square cells with a width of 0.38 m and a depth of 0.2 m. The 3-D volume corresponds to 216 voxels with the following dimensions: 1.5 m width, 2.4 m height and 1.8 m depth. The first inversion was made adjusting conveniently the parameters and the anomalous data were rejected (Table 1). The voxels resistivity results used in this work were thus obtained and represented by continuous surfaces, as shown in the figures 16, 17 and 18 with the same colours scale. The obtained inversion values are shown in Table 1.

Table 1. – Inversion parameters.

Name	Number of observation inverted	Number of iterations	RMS error	Voxel Max resistivity	Voxel Min resistivity	Voxel Mean Resistivity
Wall	288	8	12	10925	285	2153
Ecce Homo	265	8	11	1411	31	579
Descent from the Cross	232	7	21	6049	164	2102

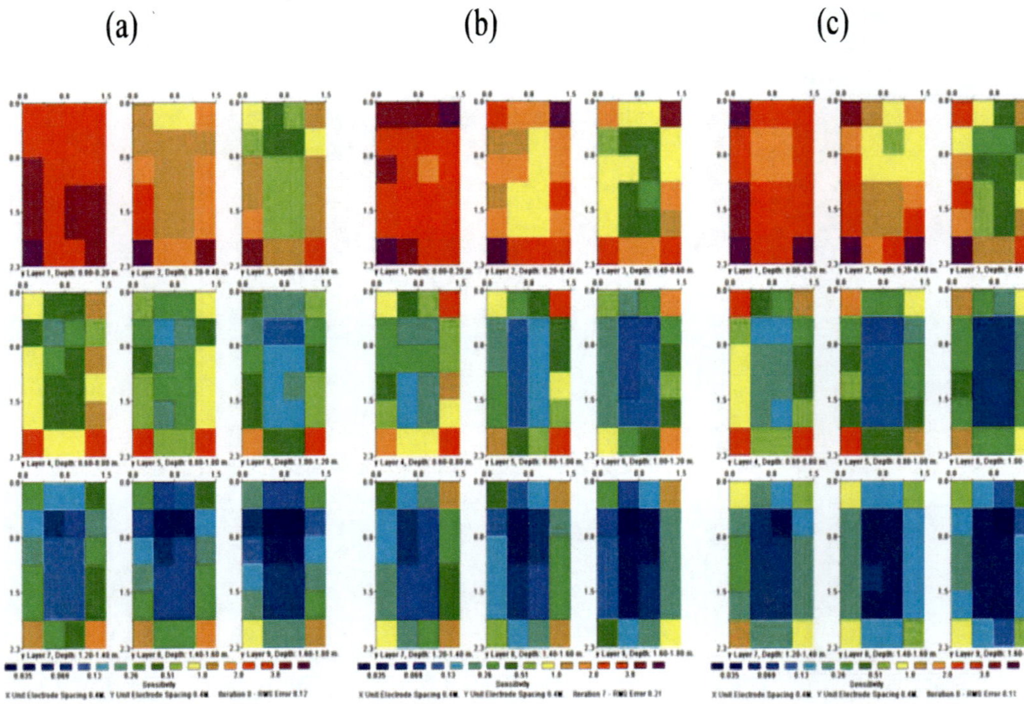

Figure 15. – Layered Voxel Sensitivity values for the resistivity models inverted: (a) Wall; (b) *Descent from the Cross* and (c) *Ecce Homo* panels.

The sensitivity value is a measure of the amount of information about the resistivity of a model block cell (Voxel) in the measured data set. The higher the sensitivity value, more reliable is the model resistivity value. In general, the cells near the surface usually have higher sensitivity values because the sensitivity function has very large values near the electrodes [33]. The average sensitivity value for background wall and *Descent from the Cross* and *Ecce Homo* panels was 1.4, 0.88 and 0.84, respectively. It is shown in Figure 15 the distribution of sensitivity values to the wall, *Descent from the Cross* and *Ecce Homo* panel. Although the models average sensitivity is low, the sensitivity to the surface is high (≈2) which give a guarantee of the models for the surface (corresponding to the panels). The average values found for the sensitivity have the influence of deeper layers (low sensitivity), but it allow also to determine the boundary between the panels and the wall.

3.4. Results and Discussion

The electrical resistivity of porous solids is largely dependent upon the moisture content. The presence of soluble salts as chlorides, sulphates and nitrates also influence the resistivity readings. This last effect is particularly important given the presence of such salts in the stone panels investigated. Moisture and salts are drawn to the edges where water evaporates. Arnold and Zehnder have recorded a vertical zoning of the salts distribution and action near the base of buildings. The salts rise from the ground level and are deposited according to their solubilities. In general, salts of low solubility tend to crystallize at an early stage near the ground surface, like most sulphates; salts of high solubility, like nitrates and chlorides, rise high and often remain in solution, forming wet zones [45].These crystallized salts are concentrated in an area close to the maximum height of the capillary rise of ground moisture. This area is formed at the point where the equilibrium between capillarity and evaporation is reached. Below this area the moisture rises by capillarity. The efflorescences do not appear in this area because the evaporation rate is lower than the rate of replenishment of water by capillary migration and salts are kept in solution. Above this area the moisture varies with environmental conditions. In this area the moisture is sometimes high in order to support the capillary rise and in others is low and only water vapour exists. When the critical moisture is reached, the after front retreats and the evaporation increases the salt concentration and crystallization will start [46]. Thus, smaller quantities of salts are formed in the lower levels of a wall. It is possible that the base of a wall does not contain significant quantities of these salts, even when the process of rising damp occurs for many years.

Inversion results for 3-D surveys over masonry wall, *Descent from the Cross* and *Ecce Homo* bas-relief are shown in Figures 16, 17 and 18, respectively. The resistivity tomograms are shown in Figure 19. These tomograms were constructed with MATLAB using linear interpolation. Background electrical resistivity in the masonry wall is 2000 to 4000 Ω.m as can be seen on top of the sections of Figure 16 and layers 6, 7, 8 and 9 of the Figure 17. As can be seen in sections of the Figure 16, an increase of the resistivity is observed from the base to the top. At the wall base (2.3 m) the resistivity values range from 300 to 500 Ω.m while on the top (0.0 m) they exceed 4000 Ω.m. Low resistivity values observed in the bottom half are related with high level of the moisture. At higher distances from the floor, an increase of resistivity values is observed due to a decrease of moisture content. On the top, the wall is dry.

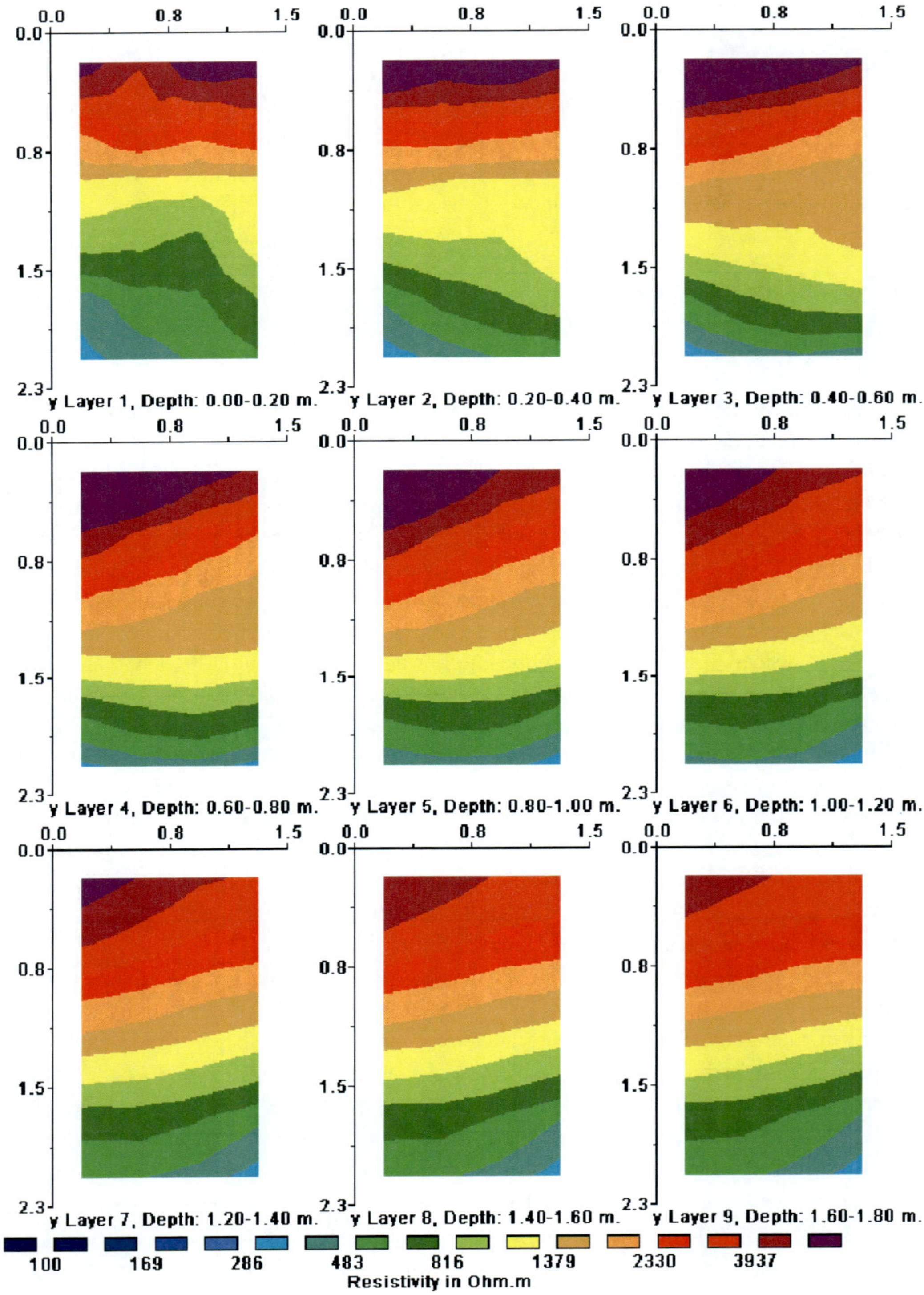

Figure 16. – Resistivity sections in X-Y plane generated from 3D inversion of resistivity survey over masonry wall.

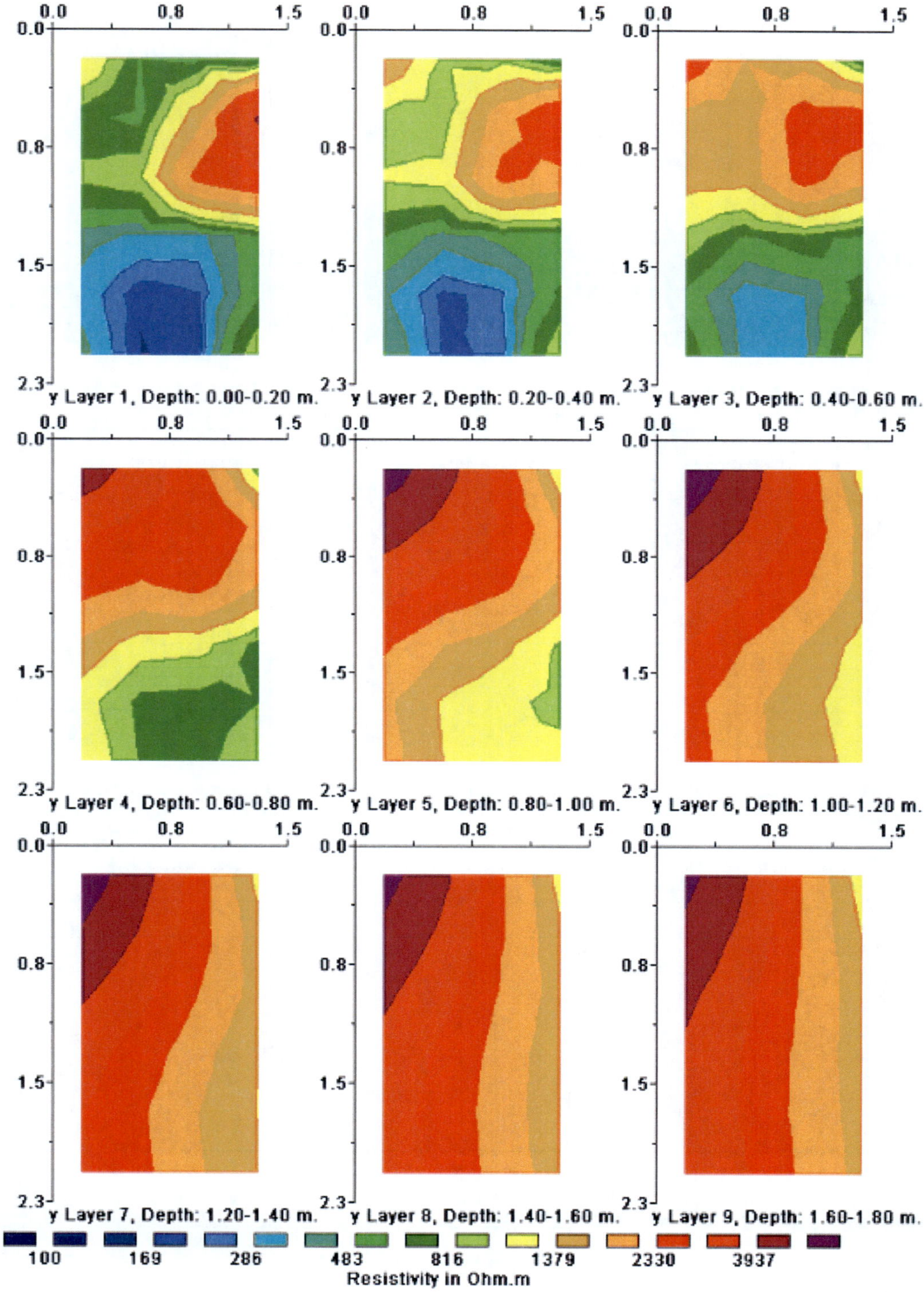

Figure 17. – Resistivity sections in X-Y plane generated from 3D inversion of resistivity survey over *Descent from the Cross* Retable.

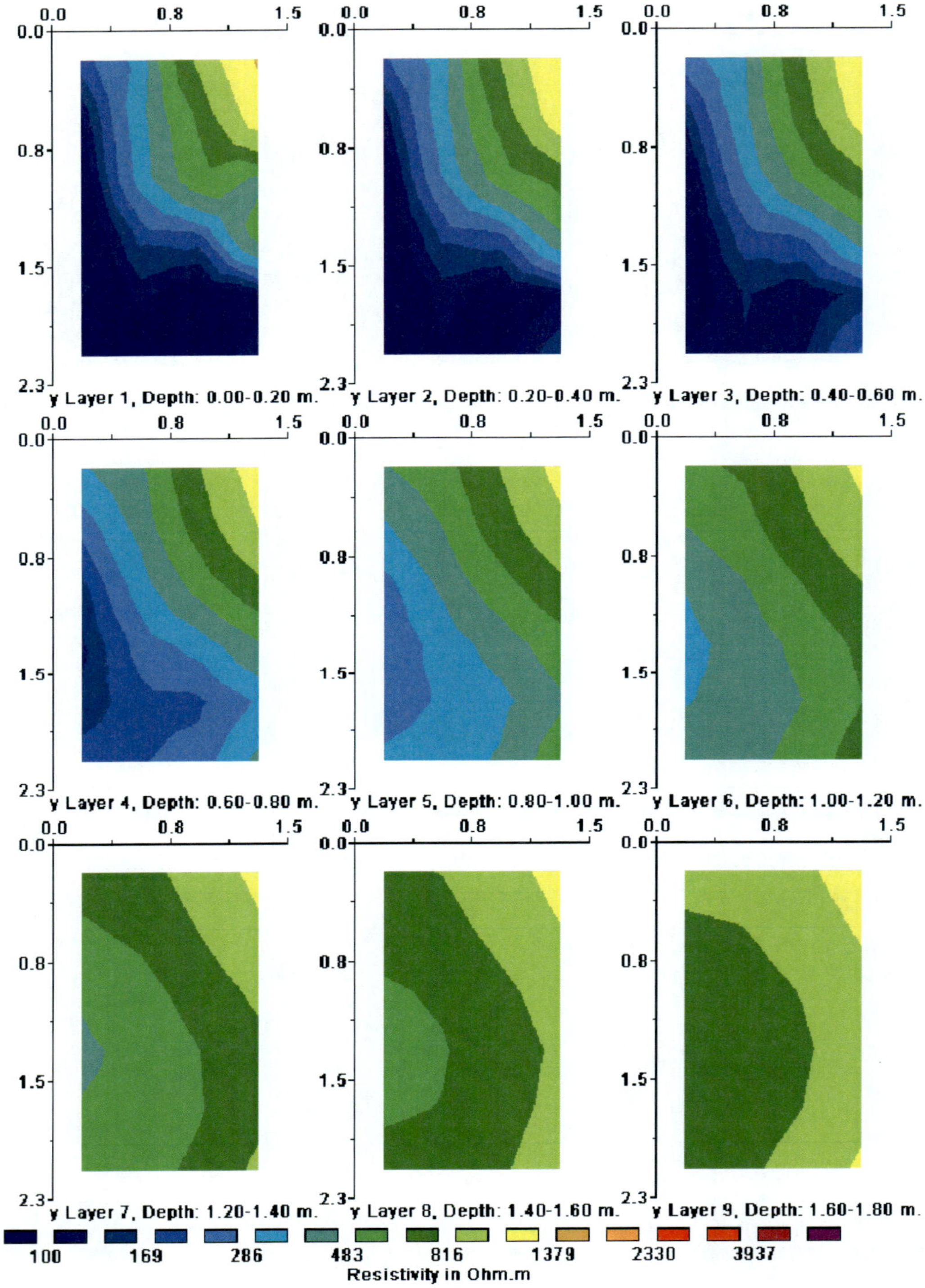

Figure 18. – Resistivity sections in X-Y plane generated from 3D inversion of resistivity survey over *Ecce Homo* Retable.

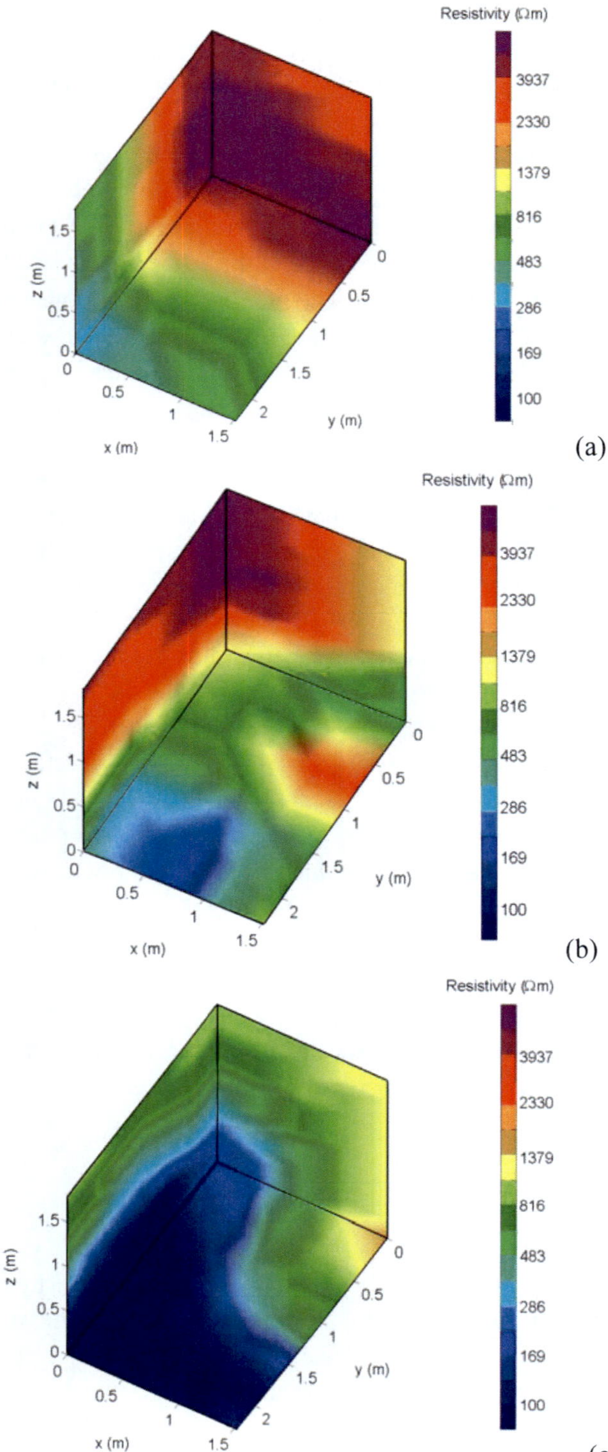

Figure 19. – Resistivity tomograms: (a) Wall; (b) *Descent from the Cross* panel; (c) *Ecce Homo* panel.

3-D resistivity sections of the *Descent from the Cross* panel (Figure 17) reveal the pattern of the moisture distribution either in the panel, either in the wall behind it. These sections also allow estimating the thickness of the panel. To the depth of 0.6 m (layer 1, 2 and 3) is clearly visible a dry zone at the top of the panel (high resistivity values) and a zone with higher moisture content in the bottom half of the panel (low resistivity values). Comparing the resistivity values observed at the top of sections 4 and 5 (2000-4000 Ω.m) with the values observed in sections 6, 7, 8 and 9 (Figure 17) and with the values obtained at the top of the background wall (Figure 16), we can conclude that the sections obtained between 0.6 and 1.8 m (Figure 17) correspond to masonry wall. The resistivity values obtained in the bottom half of the 4 and 5 sections (800-1400 Ω.m) indicate that, for depths between 0.6 and 1.0 m, the bottom half of the wall is also wet. In this panel the highest concentration of salts is roughly in the middle of the panel (Figure 9), above the area where low resistivity values are observed (area with high moisture content, Figure 17). Therefore, the low resistivity values are related to moisture content and not with a higher concentration of salts. The results of 3-D resistivity in the *Descent from the Cross* panel shows that: 1) the wall in the vicinity of the panel is also wet in its bottom half and that the moisture content decreases inside the wall; beyond a depth of 1.0 m the wall is dry (Figure 17) which is due to the existence of a rainscreen venner wall that is located behind the wall; 2) the moisture comes preferentially from the ground, rises along the wall and reaches the stone panel; 3) the thickness of the panel is about 0.6 m.

The 3-D survey over *Ecce Homo* panel (Figure 18) shows that the stone panel and the wall have moisture content much higher than the *Descent from the Cross* panel. Resistivity values lower than 300 Ω.m are observed in almost all the panel (sections 1, 2 and 3, Figure 18) and in the first 40 cm depth of the wall (sections 4 and 5, Figure 18). Even in the deepest areas of the wall (sections 7, 8 and 9, Figure 18) the resistivity values range from 500 to 1100 Ω.m, which are much lower than those obtained in the background wall (2000-4000 Ω.m). This shows that the source of high moisture content is not just the ground. As in the *Descent from the Cross* panel, the higher concentration of crystallized salts (Figure 10) is not coincident with the lowest values of resistivity (Figure 18).

The 3-D resistivity results are in accordance with salts distribution (Figure 9 and 10). The highest moisture content (lowest resistivity values) is located in the bottom half of the panels and of the background wall, below the area where the concentration of crystallized salts is greatest.

3.5. Conclusion

The 3-D electrical resistivity imaging allowed the study of moisture movements in the masonry wall and stone panels and estimates the thickness of the panels (0.6 m). The moisture comes preferentially from the ground, where the groundwater level is near to the floor of the cloister, rises along the walls and reaches the stone panels. The moisture migrates through the panels since the Pedra de Ançã has high porosity and capillarity. During its moving, the water career solubilized salts from the soil of the foundation which are then transported through the walls. When the water reaches the panels rise by capillarity and the salts crystallize above to the maximum height of the rise of moisture and remain deposited there, clogging gradually the pores of the materials thus reducing the permeability to water vapour. As this moisture shows some variability throughout the year, there are cycles of crystallization – deliquescence of salts which leads to the stone decay phenomenon.

During the last decades reference documents, called "Charters" were produced, through which the basic principles which should govern/guide any intervention in the architectural heritage were established, adapted, as expected, to the cultural diversity of each country. Among these documents is the Venice Charter and more recently the Charter of Krakow. According to the Charter of Krakow the "conservation may be achieved through different types of interventions, such as monitoring of the environment, maintenance, repair, renovation and rehabilitation" and is done under the project of restoration that "should be based on a range of appropriate technical options and prepared in a cognitive process of gathering knowledge and understanding of the building or site" [47]. Here we presented a case-study related to the application of a non-destrutive technique to stone Cultural Heritage - the ERI technique. This technique is truly non-destructive and provides highly interesting insights into the moisture distribution in stone structures and masonry walls. Thus, representing a further important instrument of knowledge, introductory to the conservation/restoration practice, permitting a more perceptive and interdisciplinary approach and facilitating the choice of the most efficancy decisions for conservation.

Acknowledgments

This work was financed by the CEPGIST FCT subproject DECASTONE. The work also received support from Instituto de Telecomunicações and from Programa de Financiamento Plurianual da Unidade de Investigação da FCT, financed by European Union FEDER and national budget of Portuguese Republic. The authors also thank CaCO3- Conservação do Património Artístico Lda, for their help in the preliminary filed work and also Direcção Regional de Cultura do Centro for its continued support and facilities.

References

[1] Dahlin, T., 2001. The development of electrical imaging techniques. *Computers and Geosciences* 27: 1019-1029.

[2] Bichler, A., Bobrowsky, P., Best, M., Douma, M., Hunter, J., Calvert, T., Burns, R., 2004. Three-dimensional mapping of a landslide using a multi-geophysical approach: the Quesnel Forks landslide. *Landslides* 1: 29-40.

[3] Konagai, K., Numada, M., Zaferiakos, A., Johansson, J., Sadr, A., Katagiri, T., 2005. An example of landslide-inflicted damage to tunnel in the 2004 Mid-Niigata prefecture earthquake. *Landslides* 2: 159-163.

[4] Drahor, M.G., Göktürkler, G., Berge, M.A., Kurtulmus, T.O., 2006. Application of electrical resistivity tomography technique for investigation of landslides: a case from Turkey. Environ. *Geol.* 50: 147-155.

[5] Schwindt, D., Kneisel, C., 2009. Quasi-3D resistivity imaging – results from geophysical mapping and forward modeling. *Geophysical Research Abstracts* 11:1156.

[6] Chambers, J.E., Ogilvy, R., Meldrum, P., Nissen, J., 1999. 3D resistivity imaging of buried oil-and tar-contaminated waste deposits. *European Journal of Environmental and Engineering Geophysics* 4: 3-15.

[7] Bentley, L.R., Gharibi, M., 2004. Two-and three-dimensional electrical resistivity imaging at a heterogeneous remediation site. *Geophysics* 69: 674-680.

[8] Martinho, E., Almeida, F., 2006. *3D behaviour of contamination in landfill sites using 2D resistivity/IP imaging:* case studies in Portugal.

[9] Almeida, F.; Carminé, P.; Gonçalves, L. and Daniel, L (2001) - *Odd-Even Pole-Pole spread electrode commutation in resistivity - 2D cross borehole and 3D surface imaging* (Porto/Portugal underground tunnelling case studies). Proceedings –Extended Abstracts - 7th Meeting of the Environmental and Engineering Geophysical Society (European Section), Birmingham, England, EGSI01 pp. 50-51.

[10] Papadopoulos, N.G., Tsourlos, P., Tsokas, G.N., Sarris, A., 2006. Two-dimensional and three-dimensional resistivity imaging in archaeological site investigation. *Archaeological Prospection* 13:163-181.

[11] Tsokas, G.N., Stampolidis, A., Mertzanidis, I., 2007. Geophysical exploration in the church of Protaton in Karyes of Mount Athos (Holy Mountain) in Northern Greece. *Archaeological Prospection* 14: 75-86.

[12] Compare, V., Cozzolino, M., Mauriello, P., Patella, D., 2009. Three-dimensional resistivity probability tomography at the prehistoric site of Grotta Reali (Molise, Italy). *Archaeological Prospection* 16: 53-63.

[13] Diamanti, N., Tsokas, G., Tsourlos, P., Vafidis, A., 2005. Integrated interpretation of geophysical data in the archaeological site of Europos (northern Greece). *Archaeological Prospection,* 12: 79-91.

[14] Loke, M.H., Barker, R.D., 1996a. Pratical techniques for 3D resistivity surveys and data inversion. *Geophysical Prospecting* 44: 499-523.

[15] ______ 1996b.Rapid least-squares inversion of apparent resistivity pseudo-sections using quasi-Newton method. Geophysical Prospecting 44:131-152.

[16] Tsokas, G.N., Tsourlos, P.I., Vargemezis, G., Novack, M., 2008. Non-destructive electrical resistivity tomography for indoor investigation: the case of Kapnikarea Church in Athens. *Archaeological Prospection* 15: 47-61.

[17] Linford, N., 2004. From hypocaust to hyperbola: ground-penetrating radar surveys over mainly Roman remains in the UK. *Archaeological Prospection* 11: 237-246.

[18] Piro, S., Goodman, D., Nishimura, Y., 2003. The study and characterization of emperor Traiano's villa (Altopiani di Arcinazzo, Roma) using high-resolution integrated geophysical surveys. *Archaeological Prospection* 10: 1-25.

[19] Vaish. J.N., Sharma, R.S., 2000. *Ground probing radar for foundations and other subsurface features at a historical site.* In Eighth International Conference on Ground Penetrating Radar, Gold Coast, Australia, 308-313.

[20] Perez, V., Canas, J.A., Pujades, L., 1998. *GPR survey to confirm the location of ancient structures under the Valencian Cathedral (Spain).* In Seventh International Conference on Ground Penetrating Radar, Lawrence, USA, 47-52.

[21] Leckebusch, J., 2000. Two and three-dimensional ground-penetrating radar surveys across a medieval choir: a case study in archaeology. *Archaeological Prospection* 7: 189-200.

[22] Colla, C., Maierhofer, C., 2000. *Investigationof historic masonry via radar reflection and tomography.* In Eighth International conference on Ground Penetrating Radar, Gold Coast, Australia, 893-898.

[23] Leucci, G., 2002. Ground – Penetrating Radar survey to map the location of buried structures under two churches. *Archaeological Prospection* 9: 217-228.

[24] Savvaidis, A., Tsokas, G.N., Liritzis, Y., Apostolou, M., 1999. The location and mapping of ancient ruins on the castle of Lefkas (Greece) by resistivity and GPR methods. *Archaeological Prospecting* 6: 63-73.

[25] Tsokas, G., Tsourlos, P., Papadopoulos, N., Manidaki, V., Ioannidou, M., Sarris, A., 2006. Non destrutive ERT survey at the south wall of the Akropolis of Athens. *Extended Abstract of Near Surface 2006*, Helsinki, Finland, B040.

[26] Carrara, E., Carozo, MT., Fedi, M., (2001). Resistivity and radar surveys at the Archaeological site of Ercolano. *Journal of Environmental and Engineering Geophysics* 6: 123-132.

[27] Cosentino, P., Martorana, R., 2001. *The resistivity grid applied to wall structures: first results.* Proceedings of the 7th Meeting of the Environmental and Engineering Geophysical Society, European Section, Birmingham, UK.

[28] Sass, O., 2005. Rock moisture measurements: techniques, results, and implications for weathering. *Earth Surface Processes and Landforms*, 30: 359-374.

[29] Said, N.M., 2004. Moisture measurement guide for building envelope applications. *NRC Canada Res. Rept.*, 190: 1-34.

[30] Larson, P.K. Moisture Measurement in Tirsted Church, *J. Archit. Cons.,* 2004, 10: 22-35.

[31] Sass, O., Viles, H.A., 2006. How wet are these walls? Testing a novel technique for measuring moisture in ruined walls. *Journal of Cultural Heritage*, 7: 257-263.

[32] Viles, H., Sass, O., Mol, L., 2008. *2D resistivity surveys as a tool for investigating moisture in historic masonry walls.* Proceedings of the International Workshop In Situ Monitoring of Monumental Surfaces (SMW08),P439-p444, (Tiano, P. & Pardini, C., edts)

[33] Loke, M.H., 2004. Tutorial notes: 2-D and 3-D electrical imaging surveys. *http://www.geoelectrical.com/downloads.php.*

[34] Dobrin, M.B., Savit, C.H., 1988. *Introduction to Geophysical Prospecting.* McGraw-Hill International Editions, 867 pp.¨

[35] Telford, W.M., Geldart, L.P., Sheriff, R.E. 1990. *Applied Geophysics.* Cambridge University Press, Cambridge, 770 pp.

[36] Sharma, P.V., 1997. *Environmental and Engineering Geophysics.* Cambridge University Press, Cambridge, 475 pp.

[37] Xu, B., Noel, M., 1993. On the completeness of data sets with multielectrode systems for electrical resistivity survey. *Geophysical Prospecting* 41: 791-801.

[38] Chambers, J.E., 2001. *The application of 3D electrical tomography to the investigations of brownfield sites.* PhD thesis, University of Sheffield.

[39] Dahlin, T., Loke, M.H., 1997. *Quasi-3D resistivity imaging-mapping of three dimensional structures using two dimensional DC resistivity techniques.* Proceedings of the 3rd Meeting of the Environmental and Engineering Geophysics. 8-11 September 1997, Aarhus, Denmark; 143-146.

[40] Slater, L., Binley, A., 2003. Evaluation of permeable reactive barrier (PRB) integrity using electrical imaging methods. *Geophysics* 68: 911-921.

[41] Ogilvy, R., Meldrum, P., Chambers, J.E., 1999. Imaging of industrial waste deposits and buried quarry geometry by 3-D resistivity tomography. *European Journal of Environmental and Engineering Geophysics*, 3: 103-113.

[42] Chambers, J.E., Ogilvy, R.D., Kuras, O., Cripps, J.C., Meldrum, P.I., 2002. 3D electrical imaging of known targets at a controlled environmental test site. *Environmental Geology* 41: 690-704.

[43] Dionísio A. *Mineralogical, petrographical and petrophysical characterisation of Ançã limestone (Portugal)*. MscE Thesis, Universidade Técnica de Lisboa, Instituto Superior Técnico 1997, Portugal (in Portuguese).

[44] Loke and Barker, 1996. Pratical techniques for 3D resistivity surveys and data inversion. *Geophys. Prosp.* 44:491-523.

[45] Arnold, A., Zehnder, K., 1990. *Salt weathering on monuments.* Advanced Workshop. Analytical methodologies for the investigation of damaged stones. Pavia, Italy, 58pp.

[46] Amoroso, G.G. and Fassina, V., 1983. *Stone Decay and Conservation. Atmospheric Pollution, Cleaning, Consolidation and Protection*, Elsevier, Amsterdam, p. 453.

[47] Charter of Krakow 2000: Principles for conservation and restoration of built heritage. *Archaologia Polona* 38: 251-256.

In: 3D Imaging: Theory, Technology ... ISBN: 978-1-60876-885-1
Editors: E. H. Duke and S. R. Aguirre, pp.231-234

Chapter 10

RESEARCH ON MEDICAL 3D IMAGING IN THAILAND

Viroj Wiwantikit*
Wiwanitkit House, Bangkhae, Bangkok, Thailand 10160

ABSTRACT

Three-dimensional (3D) imaging is a new technology that can be applied to a broad scope of disciplines, including medicine. The application of 3D imaging research in medicine is a new and interesting topic. This type of research began in developed countries in the West and spread around the world. The status of medical 3D research in developing countries is worthy of investigation. In this brief report, the author summarizes research in medical 3D imaging in Thailand.

INTRODUCTION [1 - 2]

Imaging is a new technology based on the concept that visualization gives more diagnostic information, and further advancements in interpretation include touch or sound. It is a present focus of development in the hi-tech era. Imaging technology has many advantages, including its ability to be applied to a wide range of disciplines. It is appropriate for many kinds of scientific and engineering applications. It can also be applied in medicine. It falls within the scope of radiology, which includes the study of images. Three-dimensional imaging merges medical science and engineering science. Also, with the advent of medical informatics technology, medical 3D imaging has a glorious future. The next step is 4D imaging technology, which will include the dimension of time [3].

Table 1. Possible application of medical 3D imaging

Areas	Details
1. Neurology	Brain mapping, localization and sizing of intracranial lesions, and gamma knife therapy planning
2. Obstetrics	Prenatal diagnosis
3. Oncology	Localization and sizing of intra-abdominal lesions and radiosurgery planning

* Corresponding author: Wiwanitkit House, Bangkhae, Bangkok Thailand 10160

Three-dimensional imaging in medicine is an important new and interesting field of research. There have been several research studies and developments in this area.

This type of research began in developed countries in the West and spread around the world. The status of medical 3D research in developing countries is worthy of investigation. In this brief report, the author summarizes research in medical 3D imaging in Thailand, a developing country in Southeast Asia. The important research studies and events are hereby summarized in this chapter.

THREE-DIMENSIONAL IMAGING RESEARCH IN THAILAND

As already mentioned, 3D imaging research is new in Thailand. Therefore, there are only a few published research papers in this area. The author hereby summarizes the important research in each specific area.

1. Neurology

There have been reports in Thailand that focus on the application of 3D imaging technology for gamma knife therapy planning and localization and sizing of intracranial lesions. The important ones are summarized and presented in Table 2.

Table 2. Important research studies on 3D imaging in neurology in Thailand

Authors	Details
Saekho et al. [4]	Saekho et al. presented a small-flip-angle, three-dimensional tailored radiofrequency pulse that excited thin slices with an adjustable quadratic in-plane spatial variation in this paper [4]. This technique is useful in brain imaging [4].
Suthipongchai et al. [5]	In this work, a retrospective study of 101 patients with hemifacial spasm who underwent magnetic resonance imaging and magnetic resonance angiography (MRA) of the brain was done [5]. Suthipongchai et al. evaluated the magnitude images of the 3D-PC MRA in axial and oblique coronal reconstruction planes blindly from symptomatic information [5]. Suthipongchai et al. conclude that this simple technique is useful for demonstrating the neurovascular contact of the facial nerve [5].

Table 3. Important research studies on 3D imaging in obstetrics in Thailand

Authors	Details
Tantbirojn et al. [7]	Tantbirojn et al. reported on successful prenatal diagnosis of agnathia-otocephaly by 3D ultrasongraphy [7].
Wanitpongpan et al. [8]	Wanitpongpan et al. reported that spatio-temporal image correlation was marginally clinically effective in comparison with simple 2D ultrasongraphy if used by general obstetricians [8].
Wataganara et al. [9]	Wataganara et al. reported on the use of 3D ultrasonography for prenatal diagnosis of achondrogenesis [9].
Patipanawat et al. [10]	Patipanawat et al. performed this work to determine the correlation of measuring fetal upper arm and thigh volume using 3D ultrasonography with weight estimation in large and small fetuses and reported that “Upper arm and thigh

	volumes measured by 3D ultrasound highly correlate with weight estimation in large and small fetuses and can be used as a new modality for estimating fetal weight" [10].

2. Obstetrics

There are some reports focusing on the application of 3D imaging technology for prenatal diagnosis in Thailand. The important ones are summarized and presented in Table 3 above.

3. Oncology

There are some reports focusing on the application of 3D imaging technology for localization and sizing of intra-abdominal lesions and radiosurgery planning in Thailand. The important ones are summarized and presented in Table 4.

Table 4. Important research studies on 3D imaging in oncology in Thailand

Authors	Details
Pattaranutaporn et al. [11]	Pattaranutaporn et al. reported on 3D conformal radiation therapy and periodic irradiation with the deep insipration breath-hold technique for hepatocellular carcinoma [11]. Pattaranutaporn et al. said that "This technique is an effective and safe treatment for palliation in hepatocellular carcinoma especially in locally advanced stages with large or multiple lesions" [11].
Wiwanitkit [12]	Wiwanitkit applied 3D reconstruction technology in estimation of the prostate gland [12].

CONCLUSION

There are only a few publications on 3D imaging research from Thailand. Most papers only cover the use of the technique in diagnosis.

REFERENCES

[1] Seeram, E. 3-D imaging: basic concepts for radiologic technologists. *Radiol Technol.*, 1997, Nov-Dec; 69(2), 127-44.

[2] Stytz, MR; Frieder, O. Three-dimensional medical imaging modalities: an overview. *Crit Rev Biomed Eng.*, 1990, 18(1), 1-25.

[3] Thomas, CF; White, JG. Four-dimensional imaging: the exploration of space and time. *Trends Biotechnol.*, 1998, Apr, 16(4), 175-82.

[4] Saekho, S; Yip, CY; Noll, DC; Boada, FE; Stenger, VA. Fast- three-dimensional tailored radiofrequency pulse for reduced B1 inhomogeneity. Magn Reson Med. 2006 Apr;55(4):719-24. Prenatal three-dimensional ultrasonography in a case of agnathia-otocephaly. *J Obstet Gynaecol Res.*, 2008, Aug, 34(4 Pt 2), 663-5.

[5] Wanitpongpan, P; Kanagawa, T; Kinugasa, Y; Kimura, T. Spatio-temporal image correlation (STIC) used by general obstetricians is marginally clinically effective

compared to 2D fetal echocardiography scanning by experts. *Prenat Diagn.*, 2008, Oct, 28(10), 923-8.

[6] Wataganara, T; Sutanthavibool, A; Limwongse, C. Real-time three dimensional sonographic features of an early third trimester fetus with achondrogenesis. *J Med Assoc Thai.*, 2006, Oct, 89(10), 1762-5.

[7] Patipanawat, S; Komwilaisak, R; Ratanasiri, T; Pattaranutaporn, P; Chansilpa, Y; Ieumwananonthachai, N; Kakanaporn, C; Onnomdee, K; Mungkung, N; Santisiri, R. Three-dimensional conformal radiation therapy and periodic irradiation with the deep insipration breath-hold technique for hepatocellular carcinoma. *J Med Assoc Thai.*, 2001, Dec; 84(12), 1692-700.

[8] Wiwanitkit, V. 3D image construction for normal male prostate. *Sexaul Disabl.*, 2007, 25(3), 147-150.

In: 3D Imaging: Theory, Technology ... ISBN: 978-1-60876-885-1
Editors: E. H. Duke and S. R. Aguirre, pp.235-237

Chapter 11

THREE-DIMENSIONAL IMAGE RECONSTRUCTION IN MEDICAL IMAGING: CONCEPT

Viroj Wiwanitkit
Wiwanitkit House, Bangkhae, Bangkok, Thailand 10160

ABSTRACT

At the present time, the three-dimensional image has become the focus in medical imaging. It is accepted that three-dimensional images provide more information than two-dimensional images. In this brief chapter, the author reviews the concept of three-dimensional image reconstruction in medical imaging.

INTRODUCTION [1 – 6]

An image is a basic tool for understanding. Human beings are familiar with images and use them as a tool for communication. An image can provide many senses to those who view it and can represent thousands of words. In the past, images were created by hand drawing. This lasted for thousands of years. In medicine, images play an important role. Historically, during the Greco-Roman era, hand-drawn images were also used in medicine. Medical drawings from the Renaissance are well known, including the anatomical drawings of Leonardo da Vinci. The development of medical imaging was advanced by the invention of the camera era. With the development of the camera, photography could be generated and used in medicine. Such images were a better represention of reality than hand-drawn ones. Further use of the Xray, a technology based high-energy electromagnetic radiation as opposed to visible light, was developed and became the most useful tool in the medical world until the present day.

All of these medical techniques are two dimensional. Today, the field has advanced to three- and four-dimensional imaging technology. The construction of three- and four-dimensional images is interesting and is the topic of this brief chapter.

Dimension: Many Meanings

"Dimension" is one word that can reflect many meanings or senses. In general, based on the concept of perception, the dimensional perception of human beings can comprise one-, two-, three- or four-dimensional views. A one-dimensional view is a simple line. Length can be measured easily. When lines converge, a two-dimensional view can be obtained: width and length. Area builds upon the two-dimensional view, which implies a flat plane, as in the concept of the Earth as flat that prevailed until the era of circumnavigation. Everything becomes planar in the two-dimensional view. However, this is also used in communication and can provide some sensorial information. In the previous day, two-dimensional image was widely used in medicine, as already noted in this chapter. The disadvantage of the two-dimensional view is lack of depth. One can estimate the contour but cannot estimate the exact shape or volume based on a two-dimensional view.

The three-dimensional view can solve this problem. The three-dimensional view has depth, which reflects volume. When used in medicine, the actual shape of an object can be imagined. For example, the correct volume of a tumor mass can be more precisely determined. The three-dimensional model is also constructed and widely used in medical education, and now it has even advanced to the four-dimensional view. This step is the combination of the basic three-dimensional view with the element of time. The addition of time frame can reflect change and is useful in the observation of movement. This new four-dimensional view is available and applied in medical imaging, especially for some specialties such as cardiology and obstetrics.

How to Create a Three-Dimensional Medical Image: A Concept

Creating a three-dimensional image generally can be done based on plan drawing principles. Plan drawing is a basic tool of engineering. It is also applied in the medical field. Plan drawing and conjunctions of lines with light and shade can reflect the three-dimensional view. However, more complex techniques are available, i.e., the use of the visual image reconstruction technique. This is the application of the available numerical values of a two-dimensional image to create a three-dimensional one. Computational alignment of available two-dimensional images is done stepwise and further used to generate the finalized three-dimensional image. This kind of medical imaging technology is very useful in current medicine. In oncolology and radiotherapy [7–12], it is used for estimation of the size of a tumor for the planning of treatment. The standard referencing tool for visual image reconstruction is referenced in the table below.

Standard tools for visual image reconstruction

Authors	Details
Neumann et al. [13]	Neumann et al. developed an easy-to-handle user interface, namely MeVisTo-Jaw, a visual and force-feedback device to define subvolumes of a patient's volume dataset [13].
Zhou et al. [14]	Zhou et al. developed a computer-aided diagnosis/detection method, a picture archiving and communication system integration tool kit based on digital imaging and communications in medicine secondary capture, structured report and Integrating the Healthcare Enterprise workflow profiles [14].

References

[1] Farman, A. G. Fundamentals of image acquisition and processing in the digital era. *Orthod Craniofac Res.*, 2003, 6, Suppl 1, 17-22.

[2] Williams, L. E. Anniversary paper: nuclear medicine: fifty years and still counting. *Med Phys.*, 2008, Jul; 35(7), 3020-9.

[3] Elke, M. One century of diagnostic imaging in medicine. *Experientia.*, 1995, Jul 14, 51(7), 665-80.

[4] Seeram, E. 3-D imaging: basic concepts for radiologic technologists. *Radiol Technol.*, 1997, Nov-Dec; 69(2), 127-44; quiz 145-8.

[5] Thomas, CF; White, JG. Four-dimensional imaging: the exploration of space and time. *Trends Biotechnol.*, 1998, Apr; 16(4), 175-82.

[6] Potchen, E. J. Prospects for progress in diagnostic imaging. *J Intern Med.*, 2000, Apr; 247(4), 411-24.

[7] Fujino, T; Kobayashi, M; Calderhead, RG. The computer and simulation surgery. Keio *J Med.*, 2001, Mar; 50, Suppl 2, 39-85.

[8] Régis, J; Tamura, M; Wikler, D; Porcheron, D; Levrier, O. Radiosurgery: operative technique, pitfalls and tips. *Prog Neurol Surg.*, 2008, 21, 54-64

[9] Knott, PD; Batra, PS; Citardi, MJ. Computer aided surgery: concepts and applications in rhinology. *Otolaryngol Clin North Am.*, 2006, Jun; 39(3), 503-22, ix.

[10] Verlaan, JJ; van de Kraats, EB; Dhert, WJ; Oner, FC. The role of 3-D rotational x-ray imaging in spinal trauma. *Injury*, 2005, Jul; 36, Suppl 2, B98-103.

[11] Feuvret, L; Noël, G; Nauraye, C; Garcia, P; J-Mazeron, J. Conformal index and radiotherapy. *Cancer Radiother.*, 2004, Apr; 8(2), 108-19.

[12] Rassweiler, J; Frede, T. Robotics, telesurgery and telementoring--their position in modern urological laparoscopy. *Arch Esp Urol.*, 2002, Jul-Aug; 55(6), 610-28.

[13] Neumann, P; Siebert, D; Faulkner, G; Krauss, M; Schulz, A; Lwowsky, C; Tolxdorff, T. Virtual 3D cutting for bone segment extraction in maxillofacial surgery planning. *Stud Health Technol Inform.*, 1999, 62, 235-41.

[14] Zhou, Z; Liu, BJ; Le, AH. CAD-PACS integration tool kit based on DICOM secondary capture, structured report and IHE workflow profiles. *Comput Med Imaging Graph.*, 2007, Jun-Jul; 31(4-5), 346-52.

In: 3D Imaging: Theory, Technology... ISBN 978-1-60876-885-1
Editors: E. H. Duke and S. R. Aguirre, pp. 239-274

Chapter 12

Personalized Noninvasive Imaging of Three-Dimensional Volumetric Cardiac Electrophysiology

Linwei Wang and Pengcheng Shi
Golisano College of Computing and Information Sciences
Rochester Institute of Technology, Rochester, NY, USA

Abstract

Three-dimensionally distributed electrical functioning is the trigger of mechanical contraction of the heart. Disturbance of this electrical flow predisposes the heart to mechanical catastrophe that hinders sufficient blood supply to the body. Because this electrical dysfunction is amenable to proper intervention, a detailed understanding of subject-specific cardiac electrophysiological conditions is of great medical interest. In current clinical practice, body surface potential recording is the standard tool for observing cardiac electrical dysfunctions. However, successful treatments require a more detailed imaging of these dysfunctions, which is normally done by laborious and invasive catheter mapping. The prospect to obtain this imaging in a less destructive and safer manner is the main motivation of our work.

We have developed a system approach to pursue personalized noninvasive imaging of cardiac electrical activity and tissue property of the 3D muscle of the heart wall for individual subjects. Under the guidance of existing scientific knowledge of the cardiac electrophysiological system, we extract the subject-specific cardiac electrical information from noninvasive body surface potential mapping and tomographic imaging data. In this way, *a priori* knowledge of cardiac system leads the physiologically meaningful interpretation of personal data; at the same time, subject-specific information contained in the data identifies parameters in individual systems that differ from prior knowledge. In this framework, we first developed a coupled meshfree-BE (boundary element) modeling approach to represent existing physiological knowledge of the cardiac electrophysiological system on personalized heart-torso structures. Through a state space system approach and sequential data assimilation techniques, we then developed statistical model-data coupling algorithms for quantitative reconstruction of volumetric transmembrane potential dynamics and tissue property of 3D myocardium from body surface potential recoding of individual subjects.

Phantom experiments and real-data human studies demonstrate the potential of our framework in providing intuitive 3D visualization and quantitative understanding of volumetric cardiac electrophysiology and latent threats in the heart for individual subjects. This technique could aid in personalized diagnose, treatment planning, and fundamentally, prevention of fatal cardiac arrhythmia and cardiac arrest.

1. Introduction

Myocytes, cells of the heart muscle, excite electrically as cell membrane conductance to various ionic specie changes locally; the resulting membrane current creates electrical potential difference across the membrane (transmembrane potential); the same membrane current also gives rise to local changes in intracellular ionic concentration, which in turn trigger local subcellular mechanical events and lead to a tight coupling of electrical and mechanical functions in the heart. Because of this tight electromechanical coupling, a coordinated contraction of the heart can only be achieved when the inciting electrical functioning is properly coordinated: electrical dysfunction commonly predisposes the heart to mechanical catastrophe that hinders a sufficient supply of blood flow to meet the body's needs. At the same time, most electrical dysfunctions are amenable to proper intervention if the responsible *substrate* is detected and repaired in advance. Spatiotemporally distributed electrophysiological details of the 3D heart wall, such as transmembrane potential (TMP) and tissue property, are of fundamental medical interest for improving diagnosis, treatment and prevention of cardiac dysfunctions.

However, while modern medical imaging modalities, such as computed tomography (CT) and magnetic resonance imaging (MRI), are able to provide noninvasive structural and kinematic observations of the 3D heart wall, currently there is no modality for noninvasive electrophysiological imaging of the 3D myocardium. Instead, noninvasive observations of cardiac electrical activity are commonly provided by electrical potential mapping on the body surface, such as the standard 12-lead electrocardiogram (ECG). This body surface potential (BSP) difference is a result of the quasi-static electromagnetic field on the torso: during the electrical functioning of the heart, the membrane current distributed inside the three-dimensional heart wall serves as local *source* currents that produce *Ohmic* currents throughout the passive volume conductor of the torso [1]; these Ohmic currents reflect as electrical potential difference that can be measured between any two points within the torso, including on the body surface. These measurements are limited in spatial resolution and remote from the heart. Moreover, as defined by the quasi-static electromagnetic theory [2], BSP is produced by the integration of electrical events throughout the entire myocardium but not the internal 3D-distributed details.

In consequence, successful treatment of cardiac electrical dysfunctions still requires a detailed *imaging* of these dysfunctions. In current clinical practice, this is widely done by invasive and laborious endocardial catheter mapping: in this procedure, cardiac electrophysiologists place one or more catheters within the patient's heart, pace the heart to induce electrical dysfunctions, and record electrical signals produced in the cavitary of the heart. This procedure is complicated and expensive. Moreover, it irritates the myocardium and frequently triggers fatal cardiac arrhythmia that could lead to sudden death.

Great effort, therefore, has been put to develop a technique capable of *imaging* spatiotemporally distributed electrical functioning of the heart in a less destructive and safer manner [3, 4, 5, 1]. Moreover, because phenomenal electrical functioning is largely determined by the inherent electrophysiological property of myocardial tissue, the prospect of quantifying subject-specific tissue property of the heart using noninvasive observations is another important motivation for our effort. In this chapter, we present a framework that uses BSP mapping and tomographic imaging data for noninvasive imaging of subject-specific cardiac electrophysiology, including volumetric TMP dynamics and electrophysiological tissue property of the 3D myocardium; these two reconstructed quantities allow us to further identify and analyze the latent substrate that is responsible for electrical dysfunctions in the heart of individual subjects.

In section 2., we review the inverse problem of electrocardiography and introduce the basic structure of our framework. We continue to describe the two major components of our framework, *system modeling* and *information recovery*, in section 3. and 4., respectively. In section 5., we present an example of the application of our framework in identification and electrical analysis of arrythmogenic substrate that exists after myocardial infarction. Section 6. concludes this chapter with a brief discussion.

2. Framework Overview: A System Approach

The inverse problem of electrocardiography (IECG) aims at quantitation of electrophysiological information in the heart from BSP data of individual subjects. Because BSP alone is not sufficient for determining unique 3D distribution of electrical sources inside the myocardium [6], most IECG efforts are confined to constructing simplified physical models of cardiac sources [3] or TMP on heart surfaces [4]. To estimate unique TMP dynamics inside the 3D myocardium, prior physiological knowledge of volumetric TMP activity is needed to constrain the solution space [5]: this knowledge is usually described by physiological models of general population and inevitably differs from patient-specific conditions; at the same time, personal tomographic imaging and BSP mapping data are always corrupted by noise. Deterministic model-based optimization [5] does not address these uncertainties of prior physiological models and input personal data.

In our framework, we approach this classical IECG problem from a system perspective. To understand the patho-physiological condition of individual living systems, there are two major information sources available. On one side, *in situ* observations of each individual provide subject-specific information about the normal or diseased functions for the organism of the particular individual. These observations are commonly created using sophisticated physical mechanisms; therefore they reflect the underlying physiological functions in an indirect, incomplete, sparse and noisy manner. As a result, without appropriate guidance or constraints, understanding of these observations is likely to fall short of physiological plausibility. On the other side, prior knowledge of system physiology, acquired by scientists, physiologists and biologists over the years, comprehensively describes the structural, functional and interactive behaviors of the intact organism across different temporal and spatial scales. This scientific knowledge, nevertheless, is obtained from the general population and essentially differs from any subject-specific condition.

We therefore propose a system approach that pursues a statistical combination of these two sources of information for personalized patho-physiology: fundamentally, it extracts subject-specific information from external observations of an individual system under the guidance of existing scientific knowledge of that system. In this way, *a priori* knowledge

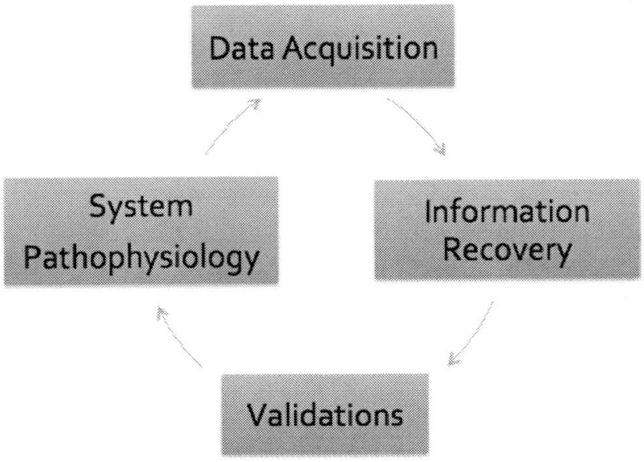

Figure 1. Overview of the framework structure.

of system physiology leads the physiologically meaningful interpretation of personal data; at the same time subject-specific information in the data identifies parameters / structures in the individual's living system that differ from the general population. Based on this perspective, we develop a physiological-model-constrained statistical framework that reconstruct subject-specific electrical functioning and tissue property inside the 3D heart wall by statistically coupling scientific knowledge of the cardiac electrophysiological system for the general population and subject-specific information in personal data with regard to their respective uncertainties.

Accordingly, our framework can be broken into several major components as shown in the diagram of Figure 1. On one hand, different observational data from individual subjects needs to be properly acquired and processed. On the other hand, prior scientific knowledge of the physiology / pathology about the cardiac electrophysiological system needs to be incorporated on personalized heart and torso structures. With these two sources of information, an appropriate strategy of information recovery has to be developed to couple them for reconstructing subject-specific electrical activity and electrophysiological property inside the 3D myocardium; from these two estimates, a suitable method is needed for the imaging, quantitative identification and electrical analysis of the substrate that is responsible for cardiac electrical dysfunctions. The performance of this framework should be validated and evaluated through sufficient experiments; these experiments could also further provide feedback for the methodological revision and improvement of the framework. A brief description of each major component is provided in the following.

1. **Data Acquisition and System Physiology.**

   Body surface potential recording and tomographic image, such as MRI, are the primary input data for this framework; the acquisition of these is usually accomplished in collaboration with experimental laboratories and hospitals.

   At the same time, computational modeling provides a powerful vehicle to incorporate and represent the existing physiological knowledge of the cardiac electrical system. In this framework, we model the cardiac electrophysiological system on heart-torso structures personalized from input tomographic images, including 1), system dynamics in terms of the spatiotemporal dynamics of volumetric transmembrane potential (TMP) for the general population in normal conditions; and 2), system observation process in terms of the physical relationship between TMP inside the 3D myocardium and BSP. We develop a novel coupled meshfree-BE (boundary element) platform for this purpose, where the 3D heart wall is represented by a cloud of unconnected points (meshfree points) and the torso is represented by boundary element on the body surface. This platform allows for the investigation of volumetric electrical conduction inside the 3D myocardium; at the same time it simplifies the complexity of the torso structure and discards excessive variables that describe electrical potential distribution throughout the volume conductor and are of no interest to the problem.

2. **Information Recovery**

   - Statistical Model-Data Coupling: Fundamental of Personalized Cardiac Electrophysiology.

     The premise of a successful coupling of prior knowledge represented in the mathematical models, and subject-specific information encoded in personal data, is to acknowledge the fact that both the prior physiological knowledge and individual observations have uncertainties: the knowledge represented in general models is different from subject-specific conditions, while the individual BSP measurements and tomographic images are always corrupted by noise. To allow uncertainties to exist in both information sources, we develop a statistical approach to transform the physiological system into stochastic state space representation. Sequential data assimilation method is adopted to combine personal BSP recordings with model predictions to produce estimates of subject-specific cardiac electrophysiological information.

   - System Identification: Simultaneous Reconstruction of Myocardial TMP and Tissue Property.

     When prior physiological models guide a physiologically meaningful understanding of personal data, it is also vital to use the subject-specific information in the data to identify the model parameters and/or structures that are altered from those for the general population in normal conditions. Furthermore, these model parameters usually correspond to critical electrophysiological properties in the heart; a noninvasive quantitation of them is therefore valuable for assessing the arrhythmia susceptibility of individual subjects. Based on the system perspective, we approach the problem as system identification, and develop a dual estimator for simultaneous reconstruction of myocardial TMP and tissue property from BSP observations.

In comparison to the existing IECG effort, our framework exhibits the following strengths:

1. In addition to the phenomenal electrical functioning of the heart, our framework is also able to provide quantitative description of the inherent electrophysiological property of the 3D myocardial tissue. The understanding of these two different aspects

of personalized cardiac electrophysiology enables further investigation of latent substrate in the heart of each individual, and therefore the assessment of individual arrhythmia susceptibility.

2. Because of the system perspective, we are able to utilize the computational modeling as a powerful tool to quantitatively and comprehensively represent existing prior knowledge of cardiac electrophysiology for the general population, and therefore incorporate it to guide the interpretation of personal data.

3. Centered on a statistical approach, our framework performs the model-data coupling with explicitly-quatified model and data uncertainties. It addresses the issue that, prior knowledge represented in general models essentially differs from individual conditions, and personal data are always corrupted by measurement noise.

3. System Physiology

The first step of our framework is to use mathematical models as a vehicle for quantitative description of the prior knowledge of cardiac electrophysiology, in other words, to model the cardiac electrophysiological system on personalized heart-torso structures, including 1) the general volumetric TMP activity and 2) the physical mechanism that governs the relationship between volumetric TMP and BSP observations. A proper numeric model is first needed to represent the heart-torso structures from tomographic images of individual subjects. On the personalized heart structure, the general spatial and temporal TMP dynamics throughout the heart wall is modeled to impose physiologically meaningful constraints on the subsequent cardiac electrophysiological reconstruction. This model takes into account the anisotropic conductivity of the 3D heart wall determined by its fiber structure, as well as the heterogeneity of TMP shape and inhomogeneity of tissue conductivity throughout the heart wall. At the same time, the relationship between TMP and BSP on personalized heart-torso structure is established according to the governing physical mechanism. This *forward* modeling of TMP-to-BSP mapping is the premise for the inverse problem of personalized noninvasive imaging of cardiac electrophysiology. In the following, we briefly review the volumetric TMP activity model (for more details refer to [7, 8]); we focus on the personalization of heart-torso structures and the forward electrocardiographic modeling of TMP-to-BSP mapping. With a view towards this inverse problem of electrophysiological reconstruction, our approach aims to balance the modeling accuracy with the reconstructibility and computational feasibility of the inverse problem.

3.1. Background

Common descriptions of TMP-to-BSP mapping are based on biodomain theory, where any point in the myocardium is considered to be in either the intra- or extra-cellular space [9]. Mostly, it is simplified to a boundary element (BE) formulation where conductive anisotropy and inhomogeneity are ignored in both spaces [10, 11]. This *surface method* simplifies the complex structure of torso and heart volume, and involves fewer unknown variables. When applied to IECG problem, however, BE formulation only considers TMP activity on heart surfaces. Alternatively, the finite element (FE) formulation takes into account electrical anisotropy in both spaces, and describes the 3D torso structure using volumetric element. Accordingly, this *volume method* enables the investigation of volumetric electrical conduction within the myocardial mass [12]. However, it increases the problem size by involving a large amount of unknown variables, such as myocardial extracellular potential which is of no interest to the IECG problem, but is usually high-dimensional because of the fine spatial resolution needed to represent the heart.

It is desirable to combine the advantages of both BE and FE formulations, so that the investigation of volumetric electrical conduction is allowed while irrelevant variables are not involved. In [13, 14, 15], this is done by dividing the heart into several discrete dipoles, the sum of which is used to approximate the overall cardiac electrical sources. In this framework, we present a novel coupled meshfree-BE platform that combines the advantages of the *volume* and *surface method*. In order to allow the investigation of volumetric myocardial TMP dynamics, meshfree points are used to detail anatomical structure, as well as electrical anisotropy and heterogeneity, of the 3D myocardium. Additionally, we replace the multiple dipole simplification used in [13, 14, 15] with the meshfree-based approximation of the integration of cardiac sources throughout the heart wall. At the same time, to avoid irrelevant unknown variables, the torso is assumed to be an isotropic and homogeneous volume conductor represented with boundary elements on the body surface. In this way, our approach emphasizes the accuracy of geometrical modeling and relaxes unnecessary restrictions on conductive anisotropy or inhomogeneity of different torso tissues. This combination of meshfree and BE representation stresses the anisotropy of active current conduction but neglects that for passive currents. This allows for the examination of volumetric TMP inside the 3D myocardium while staying away from unwanted model complexity caused by irrelevant variables.

3.2. Personalized Heart-Torso Structures

Using *in-vivo* volumetric data derived from thorax and cardiac structural images of individual subjects, personalized information on the heart-torso structures can be incorporated into the cardiac electrophysiological system. As mentioned above, we develop a coupled meshfree-BE platform to personalize the heart-torso model. The objective is to capture the primary modeling factors of the cardiac electrophysiological imaging problem, while relaxing excessive restrictions for the sake of computational efficiency.

3.2.1. Heart Representation

To be able to consider three-dimensionally distributed TMP dynamics inside the myocardium, it is necessary to detail the anatomical structure of the 3D myocardium, as well as its electrical anisotropy and heterogeneity. Myocardial anisotropy and heterogeneity are not only closely related to normal/abnormal spatiotemporal evolution of myocardial TMP [15], but also affect potential distributions on the body surface [16]. In order to describe these attributes, the meshfree strategy is used to represent 3D myocardial mass by a cloud of unstructured nodes (meshfree points) without any explicit connectivity[7, 8]. This meshfree representation excels in describing 3D myocardial fiber structure, dealing with geometry discontinuity and reducing the computational challenge of re-meshing during myocardial deformation.

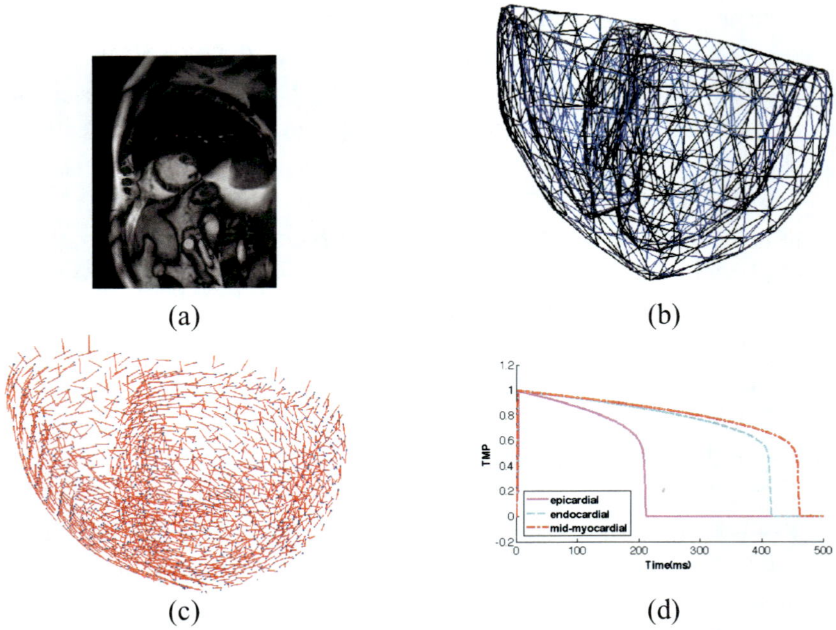

Figure 2. (a) Representative short-axis cardiac MRI slice of a specific subject. (b) MRI-derived triangulated heart surfaces (epicardium and both endocardia). (c) Patient's 3D ventricular myocardium represented by 3339 meshfree points (blue dot) with the associated 3D fiber structure (red line) of the patient. (d) Different TMP shapes in epi-, endo-, mid-myocardial tissues due to transmural heterogeneity of the myocardium.

Given a set of short-axis structural image slices from apex to base of the heart, such as the MRI in Figure 2 (a), 2D contours of epicardium and endocardia are extracted by hand tracing these images slice by slice; from these contours triangulated surface meshes for epicardium and endocardia are then built. These initial surfaces are faceted because of the independent segmentation among slices and the relatively low inter-slice image spacing. A two-stage Gaussian surface smoothing algorithm [17] is applied to keep surface size and shape-feature during surface smoothing. A cloud of meshfree points with predefined density (specified according to application requirements) is then dropped within the surface meshes (Figure 2 (b)) to represent the 3D volume of the myocardium (Figure 2 (c)).

With regard to the electrophysiological property, due to the lack of knowledge on the distribution of electrical conductivity in different myocardial regions, we do not consider myocardial conductive inhomogeneity in this framework. In future work, it can be incorporated by using different values of the diffusion tensor on different meshfree points. The conductive anisotropy and transmural heterogeneity of the entire 3D myocardium is taken into account. Transmural electrical heterogeneity is considered by associating different TMP shapes [18] with meshfree points distributed in the epi-, endo- and mid-myocardial regions (Figure 2 (d)). Myocardial conductive anisotropy is determined by the detailed 3D ventricular fiber structures, which, in our framework, are mapped from the standard ventricular fibrous structure mathematical model established in experimental studies [19]. The procedure is briefly described below.

1. Fiber structures on epicardium and endocardia of the personalized heart model are mapped from the reference fiber structure after registering the corresponding surfaces of the personalized and reference heart model.

2. Since ventricular fibers are spirally arranged and fiber orientations change from epi- to endo-cardium in a counterclockwise manner [20], fiber orientations on the meshfree points within the myocardial mass are interpolated from surface fiber structures.

    - On the heart surfaces, fiber orientations are calculated in the local coordinate system of each point defined by its normal and circumferential directions.
    - For each meshfree point, if the difference of the surface's normal between its closest endo- and epi-cardial points is smaller than a pre-defined value ($15° - 30°$ in the current study [21]), the local fiber direction is interpolated from the corresponding endo- and epi-cardial points. In this study, linear interpolation is used according to the distances of the meshfree point to the corresponding closest endo- and epi-cardial points. A coordinate transform is then performed to calculate global fiber directions of these meshfree points.
    - Fiber orientations on the remaining meshfree points are then calculated by meshfree interpolation [22] from their neighbors.

This method shares similarity with the work of [21]. The reason for mapping fiber orientations on heart surfaces only and then interpolating them to meshfree points (as opposed to mapping fiber orientations on all meshfree points from reference model) is that it is quite challenging to register 3D myocardial masses of two different hearts due to their significant geometrical difference. Figure 2 (c) exemplifies the 3D fiber structure of a human heart constructed with the procedure described above. In the future, more realistic subject-specific 3D fiber structures could be reconstructed from diffusion tensor MRI data.

3.2.2. Torso Representation

In the presence of a 3D heart model with detailed geometrical structures and electrical properties, the torso representation needs to be efficient enough without sacrificing physiological plausibility. Regarding the impact of torso modeling on forward and inverse electrocardiographic problems, the consensus has been reached that geometry is the leading factor compared to material property [23, 24]. As documented in the literature, the anisotropic effect on BSP distributions is dominated by the material property of myocardial tissues [25], and conductive inhomogeneity among different torso tissues (*e.g.,* lungs, skeletal muscle, spine, sternum, etc.) has a negligible impact on BSP pattern [26]. To reduce model complexity, it is reasonable to emphasize the accuracy of geometrical modeling while relaxing unnecessary restrictions on tissue anisotropy or inhomogeneity. Therefore, the boundary element method (BEM) provides an appropriate option for efficient torso representation in our study.

It is time-consuming and impractical to create a torso model from thorax structural images (Figure 3 (a)) in the same way the model of the heart is constructed. In comparison, heart structures have larger population variability in shape, orientation and position, which also have larger impact on both the forward and inverse electrocardiographic problem [27].

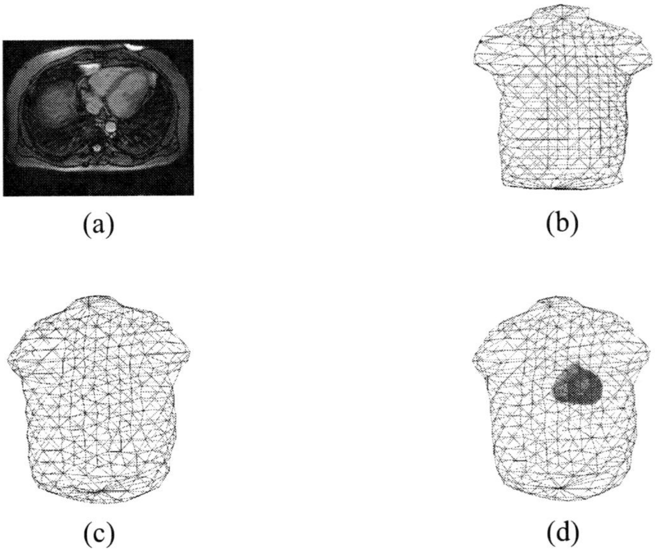

Figure 3. (a) Exemplary thorax MRI slice of a specific patient. (b) Reference torso model in BE representation. (c) Patient-specific torso model customized to patient's MRIs (BE representation). (d) Combined heart-torso model of the specific patient on the coupled meshfree-BE platform. The ventricles are represented with a cloud of meshfree points, and the torso is described by triangulated body surface.

Torso structures, on the other hand, typically have similar topological features. Therefore, it would be beneficial to personalize a torso model by deforming a reference model to match the imaging data of specific subjects [27]. In this study, we adopt the method of host mesh customization presented in [27]:

1. The reference torso model (Figure 3 (b)) is embedded in a larger and coarser host mesh.

2. The local coordinate of each vertex on the body surface in the host mesh is calculated according to the finite element method. These local coordinates are assumed to be constant.

3. A few landmarks (control point pairs) are picked out from both the reference and subject-specific thorax structural images.

4. The host mesh is deformed by minimizing the relative mean squared distances between control point pairs.

5. Because we assume constant local coordinates, the embedded torso model implicitly follows the deformation of the host mesh and transforms into a personalized model (Figure 3 (c)).

In this way, subject-specific torso structure is efficiently reconstructed with only a few parameters.

3.2.3. Combined Heart-Torso Model

Figure 3 (d) illustrates the combined heart-torso model on the coupled meshfree-BE platform. The torso is assumed to be a homogeneous volume conductor and is represented as a triangulated body surface. The 3D ventricular mass is described by a cloud of meshfree points. In practical IECG studies, the number of meshfree points usually ranges from 1500 to 3000 for a physiologically plausible yet computationally feasible representation of the 3D myocardium. In comparison, the triangulated body surface usually only consists of 300 to 1000 vertices; as we observe in our experiments [28, 29], the BE representation has a low impact on the accuracy of TMP-to-BSP mapping models. The spatial resolution of the heart-torso representation is determined by the limited spatial resolution of the input BSP and tomographic imaging data, as well as the available computational resources.

3.3. Volumetric Myocardial TMP Activity Model

This nonlinear dynamic model includes the general knowledge of the spatiotemporal TMP evolution throughout the 3D myocardial mass. It is briefly presented here for an integrated understanding of the cardiac electrophysiological system and sufficient background for the information recovery strategy developed in subsequent chapters. For details refer to [7, 8].

Complexity of models for cardiac electrical activity ranges from macroscopic-level two-variable equations [30] to the cellular-level Luo-Rudy model [31] with an excess of fifteen variables. Among them, the family of two-variable diffusion-reaction systems [30, 32, 33], pioneered by the FitzHugh-Nagumo (FHN) models [30], is favored in IECG studies for its ability to balance model plausibility with the solvability and computational feasibility of the inverse problem:

$$\begin{cases} \frac{\partial u}{\partial t} = \nabla \cdot (\mathbf{D}_d \nabla u) + f_1(u, v) \\ \frac{\partial v}{\partial t} = f_2(u, v) \end{cases} \tag{1}$$

where u stands for TMP and v for recovery current. $\mathbf{D}_d$ is diffusion tensor and diffusion term $\nabla \cdot (\mathbf{D}_d \nabla u)$ accounts for the intercellular coupling of electrical propagation. Variations of $f_1(u, v)$ and $f_2(u, v)$ produce different TMP shapes. The associated boundary condition $\frac{\partial u}{\partial \vec{n}} = 0$ assumes no active current leaving heart surfaces ($\vec{n}$ is the outward normal vector of boundary surfaces).

The meshfree method [22] is utilized to spatially discretize (1) on personalized ventricles, giving volumetric TMP activity model over the entire ventricular mass [7, 8]:

$$\begin{cases} \frac{\partial \mathbf{U}}{\partial t} = -\mathbf{M}^{-1}\mathbf{K}\mathbf{U} + f_1(\mathbf{U}, \mathbf{V}) \\ \frac{\partial \mathbf{V}}{\partial t} = f_2(\mathbf{U}, \mathbf{V}) \end{cases} \tag{2}$$

where $\mathbf{U}$ and $\mathbf{V}$ are vectors composed of u and v from all meshfree points. Matrices $\mathbf{M}$ and $\mathbf{K}$ are constructed based on the meshfree method and encode 3D myocardial structure as well as its conductive anisotropy. Parameters in $f_1(\mathbf{U}, \mathbf{V})$ and $f_2(\mathbf{U}, \mathbf{V})$ usually represent important electrophysiological properties of the heart; they can be used to reflect transmural electrical heterogeneity of the 3D myocardium.

By imposing this model to constraint the noninvasive imaging of cardiac electrophysiology, we include prior knowledge not only from temporal TMP shapes as [34, 35, 36], but also from spatial volumetric TMP evolution affected by myocardial anisotropy and heterogeneity. With this physiologically meaningful guidance, it becomes feasible to obtain unique solutions of volumetric electrophysiological details inside the 3D myocardium from given BSP data.

3.4. TMP-to-BSP Mapping Model

3.4.1. Basic Assumption and Formulation

As described by quasi-static approximation of Maxwell's equations, electrical potential difference within the torso's volume conductor is generated by cardiac electrical sources [2]. Within the myocardium volume Ω_h, the bidomain theory [9] defines the distribution of extracellular potentials ϕ_e as a result of the gradients of TMP:

$$\begin{aligned} \nabla \cdot ((\mathbf{D}_i(\mathbf{r}) + \mathbf{D}_e(\mathbf{r}))\nabla\phi_e(\mathbf{r})) &= \nabla \cdot (\mathbf{D}_k(\mathbf{r})\nabla\phi_e(\mathbf{r})) \\ &= \nabla \cdot (-\mathbf{D}_i(\mathbf{r})\nabla u(\mathbf{r})) \qquad \forall \mathbf{r} \in \Omega_h \end{aligned} \tag{3}$$

where $\mathbf{r}$ stands for the spatial coordinate. $\mathbf{D}_i$ and $\mathbf{D}_e$ are effective intracellular and extracellular conductivity tensors, and their summation, $\mathbf{D}_k$, is termed as the bulk conductivity tensor. In the region $\Omega_{t/h}$ bounded by the heart's surfaces and body surface, potential ϕ_t is calculated assuming that no other active electrical source exists within the torso:

$$\nabla \cdot (\mathbf{D}_t(\mathbf{r})\nabla\phi_t(\mathbf{r})) = 0 \qquad \forall \mathbf{r} \in \Omega_{t/h} \tag{4}$$

where $\mathbf{D}_t$ is the torso's conductivity tensor.

Because anisotropic ratio of $\mathbf{D}_k$ is a magnitude smaller than that of $\mathbf{D}_i$, we only retain the anisotropy of $\mathbf{D}_i$ to reduce model complexity. This assumption is an analogue to the oblique dipole model that considers anisotropic tissue properties for the genesis of impressive primary current but not for passive or secondary current [37]. Furthermore, since conductive inhomogeneity among torso tissues is reported as having little impact on BSP patterns, we propose the use of the homogeneous torso model in TMP reconstruction to reduce the problem size. To justify this assumption, this study compares two formulations with different levels of simplification on (3) and (4).

• Formulation 1 ($F1$) assumes Ω_h and $\Omega_{t/h}$ as two compartments in the volume conductor of torso, with different conductivity $\sigma_k \neq \sigma_t$. It reduces (3) and (4) into a Poisson's equation (5) and a homogeneous Laplace equation (6) respectively:

$$\sigma_k \nabla^2 \phi_e(\mathbf{r}) = \nabla \cdot (-\mathbf{D}_i(\mathbf{r})\nabla u(\mathbf{r})) \qquad \forall \mathbf{r} \in \Omega_h \tag{5}$$

$$\sigma_t \nabla^2 \phi_t(\mathbf{r}) = 0 \qquad \forall \mathbf{r} \in \Omega_{t/h} \tag{6}$$

The potential and current is continuous on heart surfaces Γ_h:

$$\phi_e(\mathbf{r}) = \phi_t(\mathbf{r}) \qquad \forall (\mathbf{r}) \in \Gamma_h \tag{7}$$

$$\sigma_k \frac{\partial \phi_e(\mathbf{r})}{\partial \vec{n}} + \mathbf{D}_i(\mathbf{r})\frac{\partial u(\mathbf{r})}{\partial \vec{n}} = \sigma_t \frac{\partial \phi_t(\mathbf{r})}{\partial \vec{n}} \qquad \forall (\mathbf{r}) \in \Gamma_h \tag{8}$$

and no current leaves torso surface Γ_t:

$$\frac{\partial \phi_t(\mathbf{r})}{\partial \vec{n}} = 0 \qquad \forall \mathbf{r} \in \Gamma_t \tag{9}$$

where $\vec{n}$ stands for the outward normal of a surface.

• Formulation 2 ($F2$) simplifies the torso Ω_t into a homogeneous volume conductor ($\sigma_k = \sigma_t = \sigma$) and unifies (3, 4) into a Poisson's equation describing distribution of potential ϕ within Ω_t :

$$\sigma\nabla^2\phi(\mathbf{r}) = \nabla\cdot(-\mathbf{D}_i(\mathbf{r})\nabla u(\mathbf{r})) \qquad \forall\mathbf{r}\in\Omega_t \tag{10}$$

where Ω_t includes $\Omega_{t/h}$ and Ω_h but without interface between them. The boundary condition on the body surface (9) still applies.

3.4.2. TMP-to-BSP Modeling

• $F1$: By the *direct method* solution to Poisson's equation [38], equation (5) is reformulated into:

$$\begin{aligned} c(\xi)\phi_e(\xi) \; &+ \int_{\Gamma_h}\phi_e(\mathbf{r})q^*(\xi,\mathbf{r})\,\mathrm{d}\Gamma_h - \int_{\Gamma_h}(\frac{\partial\phi_e(\mathbf{r})}{\partial\vec{n}})\phi^*(\xi,\mathbf{r})\,\mathrm{d}\Gamma_h \\ &= \int_{\Omega_h}\frac{(\nabla\cdot(\mathbf{D}_i(\mathbf{r})\nabla u(\mathbf{r})))\phi^*(\xi,\mathbf{r})}{\sigma_k}\,\mathrm{d}\Omega_h \end{aligned} \tag{11}$$

where $c(\xi)$ is related to the surface smoothness of any point ξ on Γ_h:

$$c(\xi) = \begin{cases} \frac{1}{2} & \text{if } \Gamma_h \text{ is smooth at } \xi \\ \frac{\theta}{4\pi} & \text{else.} \end{cases} \tag{12}$$

with θ as the internal solid angle. $\phi^*(\xi,\mathbf{r})$ and $q^*(\xi,\mathbf{r})$ are the so-called fundamental solution and its normal derivative. In 3D conditions, $\phi^*(\xi,\mathbf{r})$ is defined as $\phi^*(\xi,\mathbf{r}) = \frac{1}{4\pi|\xi-\mathbf{r}|}$ where $|\xi-\mathbf{r}|$ is the Eulerian distance between ξ and $\mathbf{r}$. The volume integral on the right hand side (rhs) of (11) is commonly approximated as a summation of several current dipoles [14, 15]. Instead, we introduce the meshfree strategy [22] into (11) for a simpler yet more direct approximation. By Green's theorem and integral by parts, the rhs of (11) is written as:

$$\frac{1}{4\pi\sigma_k}(\int_{\Gamma_h}\frac{\mathbf{D}_i(\mathbf{r})}{|\xi-\mathbf{r}|}\frac{\partial u(\mathbf{r})}{\partial\vec{n}}\,\mathrm{d}\Gamma_h - \int_{\Omega_h}\nabla\frac{1}{|\xi-\mathbf{r}|}\cdot(\mathbf{D}_i(\mathbf{r})\nabla u(\mathbf{r})))\,\mathrm{d}\Omega_h \tag{13}$$

where boundary condition (8) transforms the first term into:

$$\frac{1}{4\pi\sigma_k}\int_{\Gamma_h}\frac{1}{|\xi-\mathbf{r}|}(\sigma_t\frac{\partial\phi_t(\mathbf{r})}{\partial\vec{n}} - \sigma_k\frac{\partial\phi_e(\mathbf{r})}{\partial\vec{n}})\,\mathrm{d}\Omega_h \tag{14}$$

By eliminating the equivalent terms on the left hand side (lhs) and rhs, equation (11) is simplified into:

$$\begin{aligned} c(\xi)\phi_e(\xi) \; &+ \int_{\Gamma_h}\phi_e(\mathbf{r})q^*(\xi,\mathbf{r})\,\mathrm{d}\Gamma_h - \int_{\Gamma_h}\frac{\sigma_t}{\sigma_k}\phi^*(\xi,\mathbf{r})\frac{\partial\phi_t(\mathbf{r})}{\partial\vec{n}}\,\mathrm{d}\Gamma_h \\ &= -\frac{1}{4\pi\sigma_k}\int_{\Omega_h}\nabla\frac{1}{|\xi-\mathbf{r}|}\cdot(\mathbf{D}_i(\mathbf{r})\nabla u(\mathbf{r}))\,\mathrm{d}\Omega_h \end{aligned} \tag{15}$$

The boundary integral on the lhs of (15) is discretized as the sum of integrals on each single BE calculated by Gaussian quadrature [38]. At the same time, by the meshfree method, the volume integral on the rhs of (15) is discretized by Gaussian quadrature over the whole myocardium [22]:

$$
\begin{aligned}
c(\xi)\phi_e(\xi) &+ \sum_{i=1}^{N_h^e} \int_{\Gamma_h^e} \phi_e(\mathbf{r}) q^*(\xi,\mathbf{r})\,\mathrm{d}\Gamma_h^e - \sum_{i=1}^{N_h^e} \int_{\Gamma_h^e} \frac{\sigma_t}{\sigma_k} \phi^*(\xi,\mathbf{r}) \frac{\partial \phi_t(\mathbf{r})}{\partial \vec{n}}\,\mathrm{d}\Gamma_h^e \\
= c(\xi)\phi_e(\xi) &+ \sum_{i=1}^{N_h^e} \sum_{j=1}^{n_g} \phi_{e_j}(\mathbf{r}) q^*(\xi,\mathbf{r}_j) - \sum_{i=1}^{N_h^e} \sum_{j=1}^{n_g} \frac{\sigma_t}{\sigma_k} \phi^*(\xi,\mathbf{r}_j) \frac{\partial \phi_{t_j}(\mathbf{r})}{\partial \vec{n}} \\
= & -\frac{1}{4\pi\sigma_k} \sum_{k=1}^{N_g} \nabla \frac{1}{|\xi - \mathbf{r}_k|} \cdot (\mathbf{D}_{i_k}(\mathbf{r}) \nabla u_k(\mathbf{r})) \qquad (16)
\end{aligned}
$$

where N_h^e is the number of triangular elements Γ_h^e in Γ_h, and n_g is the number of Gauss nodes used in Γ_h^e. N_g is the total amount of Gauss nodes used inside the myocardium. Lower subscripts j, k represent the index of Gauss nodes.

By the BEM, variables on any point in Γ_h^e are interpolated from all the vertices of Γ_h^e; by the meshfree method, variables for each point within Ω_h are interpolated from all the meshfree points. Shape functions used for interpolations are constructed by the BEM [38] and meshfree method [22] respectively. Letting vectors $\mathbf{\Phi}_e$ and $\mathbf{Q}_{et}$ consist of ϕ_e and $\frac{\partial \phi_t}{\partial \vec{n}}$ from all N_h vertices, we get a compact matrix formulation of (16):

$$
\mathbf{L}_h \mathbf{\Phi}_e + \mathbf{P}_h \mathbf{Q}_{et} = \mathbf{B}\mathbf{U} \qquad (17)
$$

where $\mathbf{L}_h$ and $\mathbf{P}_h$ ($N_h \times N_h$) are constructed from the boundary integral and $\mathbf{B}$ ($N_h \times M$) from the meshfree method. Similarly, we could write (6) into a boundary integral formulation as:

$$
c(\xi)\phi_t(\xi) + \int_{\Gamma_{h/t}} \phi_t(\mathbf{r}) q^*(\xi,\mathbf{r})\,\mathrm{d}\Gamma_{h/t} = \int_{\Gamma_{h/t}} (\frac{\partial \phi_t(\mathbf{r})}{\partial \vec{n}}) \phi^*(\xi,\mathbf{r})\,\mathrm{d}\Gamma_{h/t} \qquad (18)
$$

where $\Gamma_{h/t}$ includes Γ_h and Γ_t. The outward normal direction of Γ_h in $\Gamma_{h/t}$ is, nevertheless, opposite to that of Γ_h used in solving (5). Letting $\mathbf{\Phi}_{te}$ and $\mathbf{Q}_{te}$ consist of ϕ_t and $\frac{\partial \phi_t}{\partial \vec{n}}$ from N_h vertices on Γ_h, and $\mathbf{\Phi}$ and $\mathbf{Q}$ of those from N vertices on Γ_t, we get the matrix formulation of (18) as:

$$
\mathbf{L}_t \mathbf{\Phi}_t + \mathbf{P}_t \mathbf{Q}_t = \mathbf{0} \qquad (19)
$$

where $\mathbf{\Phi}_t = (\mathbf{\Phi}_{te}^T\, \mathbf{\Phi}^T)^T$ and $\mathbf{Q}_t = (\mathbf{Q}_{te}^T\, \mathbf{Q}^T)^T$. At the same time, the boundary condition (7) defines:

$$
\mathbf{\Phi}_{te} = \mathbf{\Phi}_e \qquad (20)
$$

$$
\mathbf{Q}_{te} = -\mathbf{Q}_{et} \qquad (21)
$$

The minus sign in (21), as mentioned above, is a result of the opposite outward normal direction for the boundaries of Ω_h and $\Omega_{h/t}$. Coupling (17) and (19) on Γ_h by (20, 21), we obtain the relationship between $\mathbf{U}$ and $\mathbf{\Phi}$ after matrix reassembling:

$$
((\begin{array}{cc} \mathbf{L}_h & \mathbf{0} \end{array}) + (\begin{array}{cc} \mathbf{P}_h & \mathbf{0} \end{array}) \mathbf{P}_t^{-1} \mathbf{L}_t) \begin{pmatrix} \mathbf{\Phi}_e \\ \mathbf{\Phi} \end{pmatrix} = \mathbf{B}\mathbf{U} \qquad (22)
$$

The variable $\mathbf{\Phi}_e$ involved in this formulation (22) is of no interest to the problem of cardiac electrophysiological reconstruction, yet its high dimensionality largely increases the computational requirement and numerical difficulty of this model.

• $F2$: Following the same line, the *direct method* solution [38] reformulates equation (10) into:

$$c(\xi)\phi(\xi) + \int_{\Gamma_t} \phi(\mathbf{r}) q^*(\xi, \mathbf{r})\, \mathrm{d}\Gamma_t - \int_{\Gamma_t} (\frac{\partial \phi(\mathbf{r})}{\partial \vec{n}}) \phi^*(\xi, \mathbf{r})\, \mathrm{d}\Gamma_t$$
$$= \frac{1}{4\pi\sigma} (\int_{\Gamma_t} \frac{\mathbf{D}_i(\mathbf{r})}{|\xi - \mathbf{r}|} \frac{\partial u(\mathbf{r})}{\partial \vec{n}}\, \mathrm{d}\Gamma_t - \int_{\Omega_t} \nabla \frac{1}{|\xi - \mathbf{r}|} \cdot (\mathbf{D}_i(\mathbf{r}) \nabla u(\mathbf{r})))\, \mathrm{d}\Omega_t \tag{23}$$

By boundary condition (9) and the assumption of no active source current leaving Γ_t, the 3rd terms on the lhs and the 1st term on the rhs of (23) are removed. Similarly by the BEM and meshfree method, equation (23) links $\mathbf{U}$ with $\mathbf{\Phi}$ as:

$$\mathbf{L\Phi} = \mathbf{BU} \tag{24}$$

where $\mathbf{L}$ ($N \times N$) is constructed from the boundary integral and $\mathbf{B}$ ($N \times M$) from the meshfree method. The solutions of $\mathbf{\Phi}$ to (24) given $\mathbf{U}$ are underdetermined up to a constant factor. For the sake of a unique solution, an additional constraint $\mathbf{A\Phi} = 0$ is applied by defining the potential integral over $\mathbf{\Gamma}_t$ as zero ($\int_{\Gamma_t} \phi(\mathbf{r})\, \mathrm{d}\Gamma_t = 0$) [39]. Augmenting $\mathbf{L}$ into $\mathbf{L}_a$ with $\mathbf{A}$ and $\mathbf{B}$ into $\mathbf{B}_a$ with the corresponding all-zero row, we rearrange (24) into:

$$\mathbf{L}_a \mathbf{\Phi} = \mathbf{B}_a \mathbf{U} \tag{25}$$

Given $\mathbf{U}$ at a specific time instant, $\mathbf{\Phi}$ could be calculated by solving the linear system of (25). To avoid this additional computation during TMP reconstruction, the minimal norm method is applied to get a linear TMP-to-BSP model:

$$\mathbf{\Phi} = (\mathbf{L}_a^T \mathbf{L}_a)^{-1} \mathbf{L}_a^T \mathbf{B}_a \mathbf{U} = \mathbf{HU} \tag{26}$$

where the transfer matrix $\mathbf{H}$ encodes all the anatomical and conductivity information in personalized heart-torso structures.

Compared to $F1$, $F2$ focuses only on the two vectors (TMP and BSP) that are of direct interest to TMP reconstruction. This reduces the computational requirement in this large-scale modeling and reconstruction problem, while preserving the most significant factors such as the relative heart-torso position and 3D myocardial anisotropy.

4. Information Recovery

After incorporating prior physiological knowledge through modeling the cardiac electrophysiological system, and collecting noninvasive BSP and structural imaging data from individual subjects, the next step is to develop an appropriate model-data coupling strategy so that the general knowledge can be used as a guidance to extract subject-specific information out of observational data. A statistical approach is necessary to acknowledge the fact that 1) prior physiological knowledge represented in the system's models is developed for the general population and therefore essentially differs from individual conditions under study; and 2) in practice, BSP recording and medical imaging data are inevitably corrupted by noise. Based on the system perspective, we approach the IECG problem as to estimate the latent state dynamics (volumetric TMP dynamics) and system parameters (electrophysiological property of the myocardium) of the cardiac electrophysiological system of each individual from his / her BSP recordings, given the condition that personal data are noisy and the scientific knowledge about the system is imperfect. To implement this idea, we take the state space system approach that reformulates the cardiac electrophysiological system into a stochastic state space representation to take into account model and data errors; nonlinear data assimilation is then developed to estimate volumetric myocardial TMP dynamics and to identify myocardial tissue property from input BSP sequence.

4.1. Stochastic State Space Interpretation

In constraining personalized TMP imaging, general physiological models (2, 26) introduce errors because the information they represent is different from subject-specific conditions, usually in terms of parameter variations among the population and imprecise model structures in pathological conditions. Additional modeling errors also arise from the personalization of heart-torso structures from tomographic images. Furthermore, data errors always exist in input structural images and BSP recordings. To explicitly allow the existence of these uncertainties, the physiological system is reformulated into a state space representation.

With the state vector $\mathbf{X}(t) = \left(\mathbf{U}(t)^T \mathbf{V}(t)^T\right)^T$, the volumetric myocardial TMP activity model (2) is rearranged into the state equation with an additive stochastic component $\omega(t)$ accounting for model uncertainty:

$$\begin{aligned} \frac{\partial \mathbf{X}(t)}{\partial t} &= \begin{pmatrix} -\mathbf{M}^{-1}\mathbf{K} & \mathbf{0} \\ \mathbf{0} & \mathbf{0} \end{pmatrix} \mathbf{X}(t) + \begin{pmatrix} f_1(\mathbf{X}(t)) \\ f_2(\mathbf{X}(t)) \end{pmatrix} + \omega(t) \\ &= F(\mathbf{X}(t)) + \omega(t) \end{aligned} \quad (27)$$

Accordingly, with the measurement vector $\mathbf{Y}(t) = \mathbf{\Phi}(t)$, the TMP-to-BSP model (26) becomes the measurement equation with another additive noise $\nu(t)$ representing model and data errors:

$$\mathbf{Y}(t) = \begin{pmatrix} \mathbf{H} & \mathbf{0} \end{pmatrix} \mathbf{X}(t) + \nu(t) = \tilde{\mathbf{H}}\mathbf{X}(t) + \nu(t) \quad (28)$$

Because BSP data are collected by discrete sampling, the continuous state space system (27,28) is discretized in the time domain:

$$\mathbf{X}_k = F_d(\mathbf{X}_{k-1}, \mathbf{\Psi}_{k-1}) + \omega_k \quad (29)$$

$$\mathbf{Y}_k = \tilde{\mathbf{H}}\mathbf{X}_k + \nu_k \quad (30)$$

where the ordinary differential equation of (27) is discretized by a fourth-order Runge-Kutta solver [40]; this requires high temporal resolution, with automatically and adaptively selected time steps. The discretization is embedded in TMP reconstruction and no explicit formulation is derived for $\mathbf{F}_d$.$\mathbf{\Psi}$ is a general representation of unknown parameters from all meshfree points; the specific parameter of interest will be selected in different applications. Since our reconstruction is performed on personal BSP observation averaged through one or several cardiac cycles, myocardial tissue property is not expected to display rapid change during each investigation. Accordingly we describe $\mathbf{\Psi}$ as spatially inhomogeneous but temporally invariant (short-term) with random disturbance ω_{Ψ_k}:

$$\mathbf{\Psi}_k = \mathbf{\Psi}_{k-1} + \omega_{\Psi_k} \tag{31}$$

For consistency, throughout this chapter, the dimension of TMP vector $\mathbf{U}$ and parameter vector $\mathbf{\Psi}$, namely the number of meshfree points inside the myocardium, is denoted as M; the dimension of BSP vector $\mathbf{\Phi}$, namely the number of vertices on the body surface, is denoted as N.

4.2. Dual Estimation of TMP and Tissue Property

Data assimilation interprets the latent state of a system by combining the information in imprecise system models and observations. Sequential data assimilation, such as a filtering technique, is performed in an iterative manner in the time domain. In each iteration, the previous estimates and system models are used to calculate the predictions of the unknowns; these predictions are then updated to the final estimates given available data [41].

The primary challenges for developing a proper filtering algorithm for the current problem arise from two aspects. On one hand, the nonlinear TMP activity model (2) does not allow easy local linearization or temporal discretization. It makes the widely-used Kalman filter (KF) or extended KF [41] unsuitable because these filters are designed for linear or locally-linearized models with explicit discretized formulations. On the other hand, the problem domain (the heart-torso structure) is of large scale and intricate structure, and the unknown TMP is of high dimension (1500-3000 elements). The alternative Monte Carlo (MC) methods [42], though excellent in dealing with model nonlinearities, become impractical in this study because they require intensive computation.

Various *partial* MC methods [43, 44] have been presented as a combination of the above approaches. In general, prediction of the probabilistic distributions of interest is performed in a MC manner: the distributions are discretely approximated and transformed through state space models using ensemble (a set of samples). The posterior estimates are then obtained in the context of linear KF update rules. While random sampling is the common way to determine ensemble members, such as in the ensemble Kalman filter (EnKF) [43], a deterministic alternative (unscented transform (UT)) [45] was presented for this purpose in the unscented Kalman filter (UKF) [44]. Able to represent the distributions with a minimal ensemble set [45], this deterministic mechanism is of great value to alleviate the computational burden of volumetric TMP imaging.

4.2.1. Volumetric Myocardial TMP Estimation Algorithm

With the objective to combine the advantages of the UT and KF update, we develop a sequential TMP estimation algorithm to iterate in a two-step prediction-correction manner. Regarding the nature of the state model (29) as described above, prediction of probabilistic distributions of $\mathbf{X}_k$ at each iteration is performed in a MC manner and the ensemble is selected in a deterministic way according to the UT. On the other hand, because of the linear measurement model (30), prediction of probabilistic distributions of $\mathbf{Y}_k$ conditioned on $\mathbf{X}_k$ and the estimation of $\mathbf{X}_k$ given available data is executed following the KF update rules.

The UT provides large flexibility in approximating different probabilistic distributions. As an example, the second-order scaled UT is designed for Gaussian probabilistic distributions [45]. Applying it to our problem, we obtain the ensemble set $\{\mathcal{X}_{k-1,i}\}_{i=0}^{4M}$ (sigma point set) for $\mathbf{X}_{k-1}$ at the k-th iteration:

$$
\begin{aligned}
\mathcal{X}_{k-1,0} &= \hat{\mathbf{X}}_{k-1} \\
\mathcal{X}_{k-1,i} &= \hat{\mathbf{X}}_{k-1} + (\sqrt{(n+\lambda)\hat{\mathbf{P}}_{x_{k-1}}})_i \qquad i = 1 \ldots 2M \\
\mathcal{X}_{k-1,i+n} &= \hat{\mathbf{X}}_{k-1} - (\sqrt{(n+\lambda)\hat{\mathbf{P}}_{x_{k-1}}})_i \qquad i = 1 \ldots 2M
\end{aligned} \tag{32}
$$

$$
\begin{aligned}
W_0^m &= \lambda/(2M+\lambda) \\
W_0^c &= \lambda/(2M+\lambda) + (1-\alpha^2+\beta) \\
W_i^m &= W_i^c = 1/2(2M+\lambda) \qquad i = 1 \ldots 4M
\end{aligned} \tag{33}
$$

with

$$
\lambda = \alpha^2(2M+\kappa) - 2M \tag{34}
$$

where $2M$ is the dimension of $\mathbf{X}$. W_i^m and W_i^c are weights for computing sample means and sample covariances respectively. $\hat{\mathbf{X}}_{k-1}$ and $\hat{\mathbf{P}}_{x_{k-1}}$ are the estimated mean and covariance of $\mathbf{X}_{k-1}$ from the previous iteration. Parameter α controls the breadth of sigma point distributions. It is small valued ($0 \leq \alpha \leq 1$) to avoid sampling non-local effects caused by strong nonlinearity of the state model (29) [45]. Parameter κ is set to be ≥ 0 to guarantee the positive semi-definiteness of covariance matrices. Its specific value, nevertheless, is not critical as observed in our experiments. Parameter $\beta \geq 0$ tunes the higher order information of the distribution. Since in this chapter, the underlying distribution is assumed to be Gaussian, β is defaulted to the optimum value 2 and empirically adjusted to reduce estimation errrors.

Prediction of the state vector $\mathbf{X}_k$ (e.g. mean $\bar{\mathbf{X}}_k^-$ and covariance $\mathbf{P}_{x_k}^-$) is then computed by the UT [45]: each ensemble member $\mathcal{X}_{k-1,i}$ is transformed through the deterministic state model (27) into a new variable $\mathcal{X}_{k|k-1,i}$. Predicted mean of $\mathbf{X}_k$, $\bar{\mathbf{X}}_k^-$, is calculated from the weighted sample mean of this new ensemble set and the covariance, $\mathbf{P}_{x_k}^-$, from the weighted sample covariance added by the covariance of model errors $\mathbf{Q}_{\omega_k}$. Prediction of the observation vector $\mathbf{Y}_k$, and correction of $\bar{\mathbf{X}}_k^-$ and $\mathbf{P}_{x_k}^-$ given new observations are performed in the ordinary KF update context. With initialization of $\hat{\mathbf{X}}_0$ and $\hat{\mathbf{P}}_{x_0}$, TMP estimation is performed in an iterative manner following the algorithm in Figure 10.

By putting the UT into the KF context, our TMP estimation algorithm takes advantages of the merits of both techniques:

1. Based on the MC method, the UT is able to fully preserve the nonlinearity of volumetric myocardial TMP activity model (29) and provides higher order accuracy on the TMP estimates. In addition, any numeric solver to (27) can be embedded within the filtering process and the nontrivial computation of Jacobian matrices required in EKF [41] is avoided.

2. Since the MC method is embedded in a KF context, and the minimal ensemble is selected in a deterministic manner, the algorithm is computational feasible and practicable in the presence of a high-dimensional and large-scale system.

3. The UT provides large flexibility in approximating different probabilistic distributions, so uncertainty beyond additive Gaussianity is better tolerated than in standard KF-type methods.

4.2.2. Parameter Identification Algorithm

The parameter estimator is developed following the same line as the TMP estimator, but the filtering algorithm needs to be adapted to the nonlinear and indirect relationship between $\mathbf{\Psi}$ and BSP. This is can be done by using the standard UKF flow, namely, applying the unscented transform [45] not only on the state equation (29) but also the measurement equation (30): at iteration k with previous estimates $\hat{\mathbf{\Psi}}_{k-1}$ and $\hat{\mathbf{P}}_{\Psi_{k-1}}$, an ensemble set $\{\ominus_{k-1,i}\}_{i=1}^{l}$ is generated from $\hat{\mathbf{\Psi}}_{k-1}$ and $\hat{\mathbf{P}}_{\Psi_{k-1}}$ according to the unscented transform [45]; each ensemble member is passed through the system models (2) and (26) with the latest TMP estimates $\hat{\mathbf{U}}_{k-1}$ to generate the predicted ensemble sets of BSP $\{\mathcal{Y}_{k,i}^{\Psi}\}_{i=0}^{l}$; statistics of $\mathbf{\Psi}_k$ and $\mathbf{Y}_k$ are predicted from these ensemble, and are used to produce final estimates of $\hat{\mathbf{\Psi}}_k$ and $\hat{\mathbf{P}}_{\Psi_k}$ by KF update rules. The flow of parameter estimation algorithm at one iteration is shown in Figure 11.

4.2.3. Dual Estimation of TMP and Tissue Property

Simultaneous estimation of TMP and tissue property is done by coupling the parameter estimator with the TMP estimator sequentially in time for each iteration (dual estimation). As shown in Figure 12, at iteration k with the latest TMP estimates ($\hat{\mathbf{U}}_{k-1}$ and $\hat{\mathbf{P}}_{u_{k-1}}$) and parameter estimates ($\hat{\mathbf{\Psi}}_{k-1}$ and $\hat{\mathbf{P}}_{\Psi_{k-1}}$), first the parameter estimator utilizes $\hat{\mathbf{U}}_{k-1}$ to update $\mathbf{\Psi}_k$ as shown in Figure 11; the updated $\hat{\mathbf{\Psi}}_k$ is then used in the TMP estimator for computing $\hat{\mathbf{U}}_k$ and $\hat{\mathbf{P}}_{u_k}$ as shown in Figure 10. Initializing $\mathbf{U}_0$ ($\hat{\mathbf{U}}_0$ and $\hat{\mathbf{P}}_{u_0}$) and $\mathbf{\Psi}_0$ ($\hat{\mathbf{\Psi}}_0$ and $\hat{\mathbf{P}}_{\Psi_0}$), we continue this iteration at each BSP sampling instant in one cardiac cycle; in the end we acquire the reconstruction of the entire TMP sequence in this cardiac cycle and myocardial tissue property from the final estimates of $\mathbf{\Psi}$.

To improve computational efficiency, the frequency of parameter estimation can be reduced. For example, the parameter estimator can be evoked after every m iterations of TMP estimation, or only when the discrepancy between model-generated and patient's BSP is over predefined thresholds. Figure 12 illustrates the schematic of this dual-estimator.

4.3. Identification and Analysis of Electrophysiological Substrates

The reconstructed subject-specific details of TMP dynamics and electrophysiological property inside the 3D heart wall provides information of not only the phenomenal electrical functioning but also the inherent myocardial viability of the heart; this further enables investigation on the relationship between these two quantities and analysis of the arrhythmia susceptibility for individual subjects. On one hand, physiological parameters calculated from TMP activity implies the existence of substrates: the late activation time and reduced TMP duration constitute the characteristics for infarcted tissues; the activation origin beside normal pacemakers points to the ectopic foci; and the asynchronized activation of the ventricles indicate the blocks in bundle branches. On the other hand, tissue property offers a more direct picture of the pathophysiological conditions of the myocardium: areas with abnormally faster or lower conduction indicate the existence of accessory pathways or infarct; tissues with lower or no excitability are usually ischemic or infarcted. Furthermore, the correlation of the abnormal manifestation between electrical function and tissue property is critical for understanding the arrhythmogenic mechanism of electrophysiological substrate: for instance, it is observed in [46] that after myocardial infarction, the border zone between normal and injured tissues exhibits normal electrical functions; it is, therefore, not the extent of injured tissues, but the complex structure and composition of infarct border zone that work in concert to provoke arrhythmia. From our reconstructed results of subject-specific electrical functioning and tissue property, we can further get an in-depth examination of the pathological condition of individual's heart.

5. Application Example: Substrate Imaging in Post Myocardial Infarction

The presence of infarcted tissues after MI creates substrates responsible for fatal cardiac arrhythmia; location and extent of this infarct could be identified by various existing techniques including invasive electrical mapping [47, 48], noninvasive medical imaging [49, 50] and computational reconstruction from BSPM data [51, 52]. Nevertheless, since it is the border zone between infarcted and healthy tissues that constitutes the latent arrhythmogenic substrate, a more detailed imaging of 3D structure and tissue heterogeneity of infarct border zone is of greater medical interest. We apply our framework to the imaging and electrical analysis of post-MI arrhythmogenic substrates, aiming for a more accurate assessment of infarct location and extent, and moreover, a detailed 3D imaging of the tissue property and electrical behavior of the border zone in the heart of individual subjects.

At the current stage, we consider tissue excitability of the myocardium; it is represented by parameter a in TMP activity model (2); accordingly Ψ consists of a from all meshfree points inside the myocardium. With increasing severity of ischemia and infarction, temporal shape of TMP is typically characterized with changes such as progressively reduced potential duration and delayed activation time until no electrical activation can be stimulated in necrotic tissues [53]. This loss of myocardial viability is also reflected as decreased tissue excitability (increasing value of a).

5.1. Initialization

As we observed in experiments, in order to prevent the divergence or error of simultaneous estimation of TMP and tissue excitability, it is desirable to initialize this estimation with subject-specific information regarding the diseased condition of the heart. To obtain this information without using personalized prior knowledge, we first perform TMP estimation under constraints of normally-parameterized models (2, 26) as described in Figure 10. Difference, specifically the change in activation time (AT) and TMP duration (PD), between this initial TMP estimates and simulated normal TMP provides preliminary approximation of local TMP abnormality of specific subjects; this could provide *refined* initialization for simultaneous estimation of TMP and tissue excitability.

In brief, AT and PD are calculated from TMP shapes as illustrated in Figure 4 (a); the order of these two parameters among all meshfree points are then indexed by normalized iAT and iPD (points with earliest activation and longest TMP duration are indexed at $iAT = 0$ and $iPD = 0$, respectively). Differences of iAT and iPD between TMP estimates and simulated normal TMP, dAT and dPD, measure the degree of local TMP abnormality as $M_i = (dAT + dPD)/2$; a higher value of M_i corresponds to a higher level of electrical malfunction. The shape of distribution curve of M_i from all meshfree points, after sorted, in general exhibits a notable change that implies a proper threshold value for differentiating points with abnormal TMP functioning (Figure 4 (b)). Parameter a on points with M_i valued above this threshold are assigned with large value 0.3 for impaired excitability, while the others are standardly-valued from $0.14 - 0.17$ according to TMP heterogeneity across the heart wall. This vector of $\mathbf{\Psi}_0$, with $\mathbf{U}_0$ determined by locations of *normal* earliest ventricular activation, is used to initialize dual $\mathbf{U}$ and $\mathbf{\Psi}$ estimation.

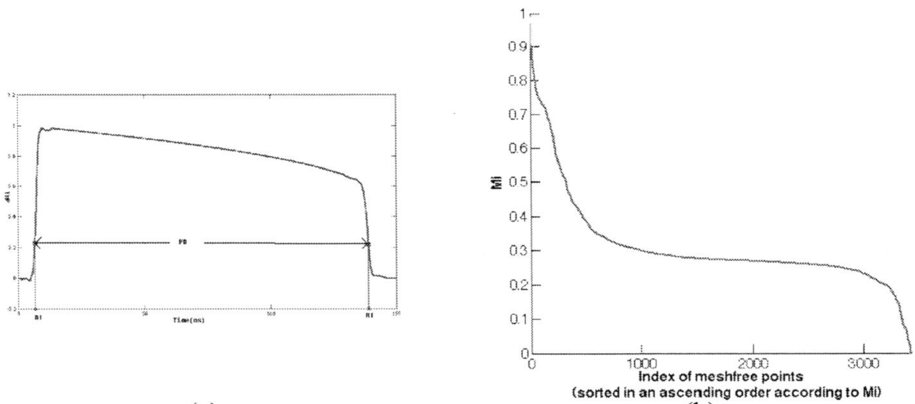

(a) (b)

Figure 4. (a) Calculation of AT and PD from temporal TMP shape. AT is determined by the largest positive derivative; repolarization time RT is determined by the moment TMP value returns below that at AT; $PD = RT - AT$. (b) Typical distribution curve of M_i, after sorted. Notable distinction in its shape is observed around $M_i \approx 0.4$, a proper threshold for differentiating points with local TMP abnormality.

5.2. Substrate Imaging and Quantitative Evaluation

Relationship between electrical malfunction and tissue injury of the myocardium is critical for understanding the mechanisms of arrythmogenic substrate [46]. To investigate this correlation, we localize the abnormality in our estimated TMP dynamics and tissue excitability for 3D superimposed imaging throughout the heart wall of individual subjects.

Using the metrics defined in the *initialization* stage, here we measure TMP abnormality by iAT and iPD of the TMP estimates as well as dAT and dPD as $iComb =$

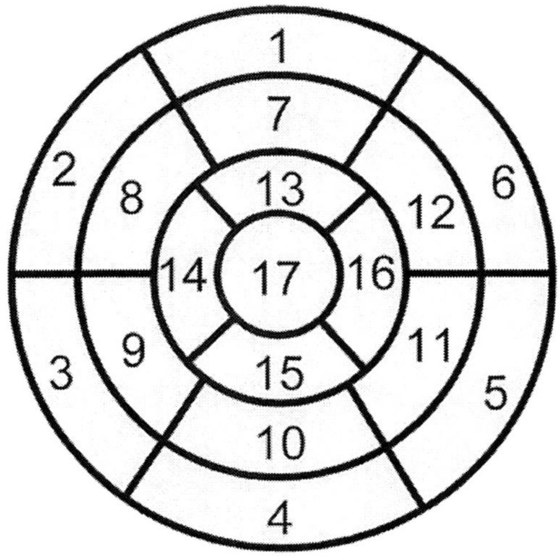

Figure 5. Standard 17-segment division of LV wall (polor map). Segments $1-6$ lie in the basal layer, $7-12$ in the middle layer, $13-16$ in the apical layer and 17 is the apex. At each layer, the segment labeling moves from anterior, septal, inferior to lateral part of the LV.

$(iAT + iPD + dAT + dPD)/4$; the thresholding method used in *initialization* is employed for distinguishing points with abnormally late AT and short PD. At the same time, abnormally high value of tissue excitability directly reflect myocardial inviability, where increasing severity of injury is represented by $a > 0.25$ until the total loss of viability in necrotic tissues with $a > 0.5$ [33]. These two regions of abnormal TMP functions and tissue excitability are superimposed for the imaging of border zone structure and electrical behavior. Furthermore, as an initial attempt to visualize interdigitating infarcted and normal tissues in the border zone, we apply thresholding on the estimated tissue excitability and image the 3D infarct structure on the border zone.

At the same time, according to our knowledge, there is no existing effort that presents similar imaging of volumetric TMP dynamics, tissue excitability distribution, or post-MI substrate. For comparison with gold standard and existing works, we calculate the commonly used metrics for infarct evaluation, including infarct center and extent. Using the standard 17-segment division of LV (Figure 5) [54], we identify segments that cover infarcted tissues and calculate infarct extent (EP) by dividing the number of infarcted meshfree points by the total number of meshfree points. Infarct centroid (CE) is localized as the segment that contains the center of infarcted meshfree points weighted by excitability estimates. Segment overlap (SO) with gold standard measures the percentage of correct identification in our results.

5.3. Experiments

5.3.1. Experimental Data and Data Processing

We apply our framework on 4 sets of MRI and BSP data collected from patients who had acute MI [55]. Cardiac MRI of each patient contains 10 slices from apex to base of the heart,

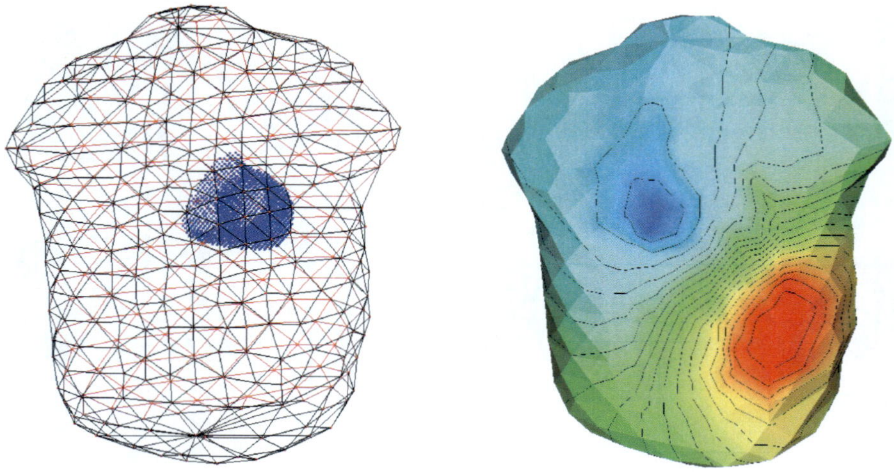

(a) (b)

Figure 6. (a) Personalized heart-torso model in case 2, where the ventricles are represented with 1373 meshfree points and the torso by triangulated body surface with 370 vertices. (b) Exemplary input BSPM at 24ms of ventricular activation in case 2, the color bar encoding BSP magnitude.

with 8mm inter-slice spacing and 1.33mm/pixel in-plane resolution. Heart-torso structure for each case is personalized from input MRI as described in section 3.; case 2 is illustrated in Figure 6 (a) as an example. BSP is recorded by 123 electrodes with known anatomical locations and interpolated to 370 apexes on the body surface. The complete BSP sequence at each electrode consists of a single averaged PQRST complex sampled at 2k Hz, out of which QRST interval for *ventricular* electrical activity is selected as framework inputs. Figure 6 (b) exemplifies a BSP map at $24ms$ of ventricular activation in case 2.

There are no gold standards of volumetric TMP activity or excitability available. Instead, we are provided with reference interpretation of the infarct from cardiologists who examined the gadolinium enhanced images of the heart for each patient. This evaluation, based on the standard 17-segment division of LV (Figure 5) [54], identifies the percentage of infarcted myocardial mass (EP), the segment of infarct centroid (CE), and all infarcted segments as well. This gold standard of quantitative infarct evaluation is listed in Table 1, and the corresponding infarct visualization is provided in Figure 7. As shown, the infarct occupies different parts of the heart in each case: in case 1, infarct collects in septal-anterior part of basal LV and septal part of middle LV, with center in the middle septal-anterior layer; in case 2, infarct collects in septal-inferior part of basal-middle LV with center in the middle layer; in case 3, infarct is distributed in inferior part of basal-middle LV and lateral part of middle-apical LV, with center in middle lateral-inferior layer; in case 4, infarct is separated into two masses at inferior apical-middle LV and anterior-basal LV, with centers in inferior-septal middle layer and anterior-basal layer, respectively. There are also existing efforts of infarct evaluation on the same data sets. We will validate our framework with the gold standard and compare its performance with existing best results [51, 52, 56].

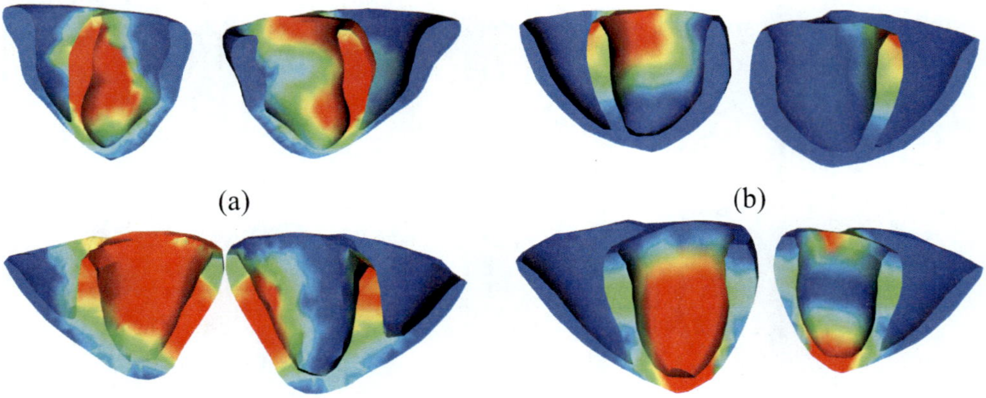

(a) (b)

(c) (d)

Figure 7. Gold standard of infarct (color-highlighted) in four cases. (a) Case 1: infarct collects in septal-anterior part of basal LV and septal part of middle LV. (b) Case 2: infarct collects in septal-inferior part of basal-middle LV. (c) Case 3: infarct is distributed in inferior part of basal-middle LV and lateral part of middle-apical LV. (d) Case 4: infarct is separated into two masses at inferior apical-middle LV and anterior-basal LV, respectively.

5.3.2. Personalized Cardiac Electrophysiological Imaging

In case 1, compared to the normal TMP dynamics simulated in the patient's heart, our volumetric TMP imaging result displays notable activation delay and block in septal-anterior part of basal LV and septal part of middle LV. This electrical dysfunction is localized by black contour in Figure 9 (a) and superimposed with color-encoded excitability estimates where higher value corresponds to lower excitability. In our volumetric TMP imaging result in case 2 (Figure 8 (b)), septal-inferior part of basal-middle LV exhibits distinct conduction delay compared to normal TMP dynamics simulated in the patient's heart (Figure 8 (a)). Figure 9 (b) illustrates the superimposed TMP and excitability abnormality. In case 3, our results show that the conduction abnormality collect in the inferior part of basal-middle LV and lateral part of middle-apical LV (Figure 9 (c)). In case 4, as shown in Figure 9 (d), local TMP abnormality is identified at anterior-basal LV and a small portion of septal-middle LV. In the above experiments, all of our identified infarct locations are in accordance with gold standards.

Furthermore, similar to the observation in [46], regions with electrical malfunctioning do not completely overlap with injured tissues: instead, while abnormal electrical functions mostly occurs within infarct zone, border zone between infarct and healthy tissues exhibits normal electrical functions. The extent of infarct, therefore, is not the most important measure for myocardial arrhythmia susceptibility. It is the complex structure and composite of infarct border zone that work in concert to provoke arrhythmia. In order to explore the information revealed in our results regarding electrophysiological substrate in infarct border zone, we are currently developing more sophisticated classification methods for differentiating between diseased and healthy electrical behavior and property of the myocardium based on our TMP and excitability estimates. The outcome would enable investigation of arrhythmia susceptibility for individual subjects.

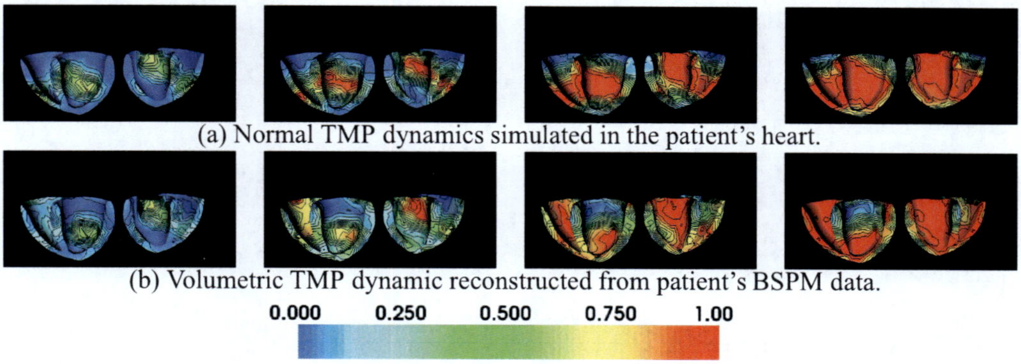

Figure 8. Volumetric myocardial TMP imaging during ventricular activation in case 2; color encodes normalized TMP value. Each column represent a time sequence at $3.8ms$, $8.0ms$, $12.3ms$ and $16.7ms$ after the onset of ventricular activation. In comparison, septal-inferior part of basal-middle LV exhibits distinct conduction delay in (b).

5.3.3. Quantitative Validation and Comparison

Table 1 compares our quantitative infarct evaluation with gold standards. In case 1, we correctly identify all infarcted segments but *overestimate* the infarct extent down to the apex (false positive at segment 17) and localize CE 1 segment away from gold standards. In case 2, we precisely identify the 4 infarcted segments and correctly localize CE. In case 3, we correctly localizes CE and highlights 5 out of 9 infarcted segments, *underestimating* the infarct extent in inferior LV. Among the two separate infarct mass in case 4, our results only identify the anterior-basal part and a small portion in inferior-middle LV. In summary, our framework is able to provide close localization of CE and to identify infarct coverage with high precision SO (low false positive identifications). Because calculation of EP in gold standards is not based on 3D meshfree point cloud (volumetric representation of the myocardium) as our method does, the reason for the discrepancy of EP between our results and gold standards remains unclear.

As implied in the results, the compactness (EP versus number of affected segments) of infarct affects the performance of our framework: the best performance occurs in case 2 that has the most compact infarct (spreading 4 segments and 30% extent); the lowest accuracy arises in case 4 that has the least massive and compact infarct (spreading 6 segments with 2 separate masses and only 14% extent); the framework produces similar in-between performances in the other two cases with moderate infarct.

Table 2 compares the current results with existing best results. In brief, Dawoud *et al* solved the problem by epicardial potential imaging from BSP [51], Farina *et al* estimated the site and size of spherical infarct models [52], and Mneimneh *et al* produced the best results using simple ECG signal analysis [56]. In both case 3 and 4, our results are comparable to the best results and substantially improved over the other two reconstruction results. Note that all the other three approaches used case 1 and 2 as training cases, while our framework has not required any training. In the future, proper training or learning is a possible strategy for improving the performance of our framework.

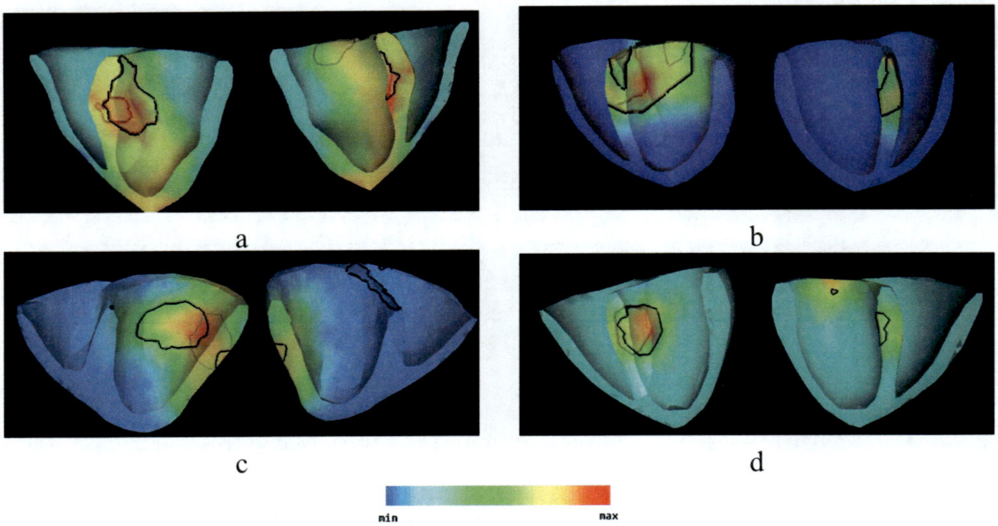

Figure 9. Superimposed imaging of local abnormality of TMP dynamics and tissue excitability inside the 3D myocardium ((a)-(d): case 1 - 4). Black contour encircles region of abnormal TMP functions; color encodes tissue excitability, higher value of which corresponds to lower excitability. Half-transparent visualization is used for better observation across the heart wall.

5.3.4. Discussion

Electrical Analysis of Arrhythmogenic Substrate

It has been recognized that regional myocardial geometry, function, and tissue heterogeneity along infarct border zone are critical variables for understanding post-MI arrhythmogenic substrate, while the definition and mechanism of border zone is still not well established [46, 57]. At current stage, we focus on proposing a novel approach to noninvasively image subject-specific electrophysiological behavior and property around infarct border zone, based on which to enable further electrical analysis of the associated arrhythmogenic substrate.

First, our assessment of the reconstructed subject-specific TMP dynamics and myocardial tissue property is currently in a preliminary stage: thresholding method is used on estimated tissue excitability for differentiating between healthy and infarcted tissues; abnormal electrical behavior is detected according to literature study of ventricular ischemia and infarction [53, 58]. We are now exploring a more sophisticated approach for classifying and interpreting the pathophysiological condition of myocardial TMP dynamics and tissue property, based on pattern recognition and machine learning techniques.

Second, our initial attempt shows the potential of our framework to reveal subject-specific interdigitating infarcted and healthy tissue in infarct border zone. On one hand, the validity of this result needs much further investigation, such as how the interdigitating structure is affected by the resolution of meshfree representation (spatial sampling) of the myocardium. On the other hand, future research will focus on a more in-depth analysis of the pathophysiological implication of our border zone imaging result. For instance, with

Table 1. Comparison of MI evaluation results with gold standard. EP is the percentage of infarcted ventricular mass. CE is the segment that contains infarct centroid. SO measures the percentage of correct identification compared to gold standard. A set of $segments$ that contains infarct are also identified. In each case, the column of *Reference* lists the gold standard and the column of *Results* lists our current results.

	case 1		case 2	
	Referennce	Results	Referennce	Results
EP	31%	17%	30%	20%
CE	8	9	3/4/9/10	9
SO	N/A	97%	N/A	100%
segments	1-3,8-9 13-15	1-3,8-9 13-15,17	3,4,9,10	3,4,9,10
	case 3		case 4	
	Referennce	Results	Referennce	Results
EP	52%	30%	15%	11%
CE	10/11	11	15	9
SO	N/A	100%	N/A	100%
segments	3-5,9-12 15-16	5,10-12 16	1,9-11 15,17	1,9

the subject-specific border zone structure and tissue heterogeneity, we could perform cardiac electrophysiological simulation under different electrical stimuli and investigate under which scenario fatal cardiac arrhythmia will be provoked in that subject's heart. This type of study is of much medical interest for assessing the arrhythmia susceptibility and planning appropriate treatment for individual subjects.

Parameter Estimation

Cardiac electrical conduction depends on both active membrane properties of cardiac cells (*e.g.*, excitability) and passive properties determined by myocardial architectural features (*e.g.*, conductivity) [59]. Infarcted tissues could reflect abnormality in either or both electrophysiological properties. In this chapter, we focus on tissue excitability because its mechanism to MI is better understood [53]. Based on the same framework, nevertheless, imaging of other important electrophysiological properties is also feasible. For example, the diffusion tensor $\mathbf{D}$ in (2) is usually assumed as d diag$\{4, 1, 1\}$ with d proportional to electrical conductivity; therefore imaging of electrical conductivity in the heart can be achieved by the dual estimation of d and TMP. This, however, raises an additional computational issue because updating the distribution of d in the 3D myocardium requires an updating of the TMP activity model (2) embedded in the estimation process. Future study will also investigate whether it is possible, and if so, how to separately estimate several different myocardial tissue properties using BSPM data.

Table 2. Comparison of MI evaluation with existing results in case 3 and 4. EPD is the percentage discrepancy between EP as estimated and as determined from gold standard. CED is the distance between CE as estimated and as determined from gold standard, defined as the number of segment boundaries crossed along the shortest path connecting the estimated and true centroids.

	Our results		Mneimneh		Dawoud		Farina	
	case 3	case 4	case 3	case 4	case 3	case 4	case 3	case 4
EPD	18%	4%	25%	2%	17%	26%	43%	14%
CED	0	1	0	1	1	2	1	1
SO	100%	100%	90%	25%	56%	30%	40%	17%

Beside *dual estimation*, simultaneous reconstruction of TMP and model parameters can also be done by *joint estimation*. In this strategy, TMP and unknown model parameter are concatenated into a single state vector; a state estimator is then applied to the augmented state space system. Compared to dual estimation, this strategy is easier at implementation; however the increase in degree of freedom in the augmented system leads to an unstable estimation, especially at the presence of nonlinear dynamic models [60]. A comparison of the performance of these two estimation strategy in this problem deserves future investigation.

6. Conclusion

Personalized quantitative reconstruction of cardiac electrophysiological information from remote, noninvasive BSP recordings has raised wide interest because of its significant clinical relevance in preventative diagnosis and treatment of cardiac arrhythmia. Based on a system perspective, we develop a physiological model-constrained statistical framework for personalized noninvasive imaging of volumetric cardiac electrophysiology. The fundamental concept is to quantify subject-specific living systems by combining *a priori* physiological knowledge of the general population and observations of each individual in accordance to their respective uncertainties, where

1. Prior knowledge of system physiology is used as general constraints to guide physiologically meaningful understanding of personal data.

2. Subject-specific information in personal data identifies the parameters in the individual system that differ from the prior knowledge.

3. Multiple complementary data are integrated to enhance the available subject-specific information, and therefore to improve the specificity of the system estimation and identification.

4. These two sources of information, general knowledge of system physiology and subject-specific observations, are coupled in a statistical (Bayesian) context so as to allow for the existent of uncertainties in both sources.

Our current experiments have exhibited promising clinical potential of our framework; future development will be focusing on the following aspects:

Modeling of System Patho-Physiology and Biology

Models in the cardiac electrophysiological system could be adjusted to varying complexity and differing specialization in accordance to the applications under study. Moreover, hierarchical modeling of the system could be introduced so that knowledge of a wider category of cardiac diseases could be included into the system. Based on the multiple-model estimation theory [61], the hierarchical model-set could increase the flexibility of the constraints on the estimation, and improve the applicability of the paradigm in more complicated pathological conditions. Furthermore, while the current framework focuses on utilizing the existing knowledge of cardiac physiology, the biological knowledge of the cardiac system could be considered in the future. It would push the development of the framework to a molecular/genomic level of understanding of personalized cardiac electrophysiology, and fundamentally the genomic personalized biomedicine.

Personalized Cardiac Electromechanics

Because of the tight electromechanical coupling of the heart, it is of great clinical interest to pursue the personalized understanding of cardiac electromechanical function, as well as myocardial electrical and mechanical properties. By combining our framework with the existing research effort in cardiac mechanics assessment, we could develop an integrated paradigm for understanding personalized cardiac electromechanics using noninvasive tomographic imaging and electrical mapping data, or more fundamentally, a wide variety of cardiac observations of the same individual.

Online Clinical Practice with Distributed Computing

Expensive computation is a major concern in our framework. For the fundamental purpose of clinical practice of personalized cardiac electrophysiology, it is necessary to investigate the employment of distributed computing techniques so as to achieve real-time application of the framework in clinical practice.

A priori prediction

Ensemble generation

- Sigma points $\mathcal{X}_{k-1,i}$(i=0...4M)

$$\{\mathcal{X}_{k-1,i}\}_0^{2M} = \left(\hat{\mathbf{X}}_{k-1} \quad \hat{\mathbf{X}}_{k-1} \pm \sqrt{(2M+\lambda)\hat{\mathbf{P}}_{x_{k-1}}}\right)$$

- Weights W_i $\quad W_0^m = \lambda/(2M+\lambda)$

$$W_0^c = \lambda/(2M+\lambda) + (1-\alpha^2+\beta)$$

$$W_i^m = W_i^c = 1/(2(2M+\lambda)) \qquad i = 1\ldots 4M$$

Prediction

- Dynamic propagation: $\mathcal{X}_{k|k-1,i} = \tilde{F}_d(\mathcal{X}_{k-1,i})$
- Statistics prediction: $\bar{\mathbf{X}}_k^- = \sum_{i=0}^{4M} W_i^m \mathcal{X}_{k|k-1,i}$

$$\mathbf{P}_{x_k}^- = \sum_{i=0}^{4M} W_i^c(\mathcal{X}_{k|k-1,i} - \bar{\mathbf{X}}_k^-)(\mathcal{X}_{k|k-1,i} - \bar{\mathbf{X}}_k^-)^T + \mathbf{Q}_{\omega_k}$$

$\Downarrow$

A posteriori correction

- Kalman gain $\quad \mathbf{G}_k = \mathbf{P}_{x_k}^- \tilde{\mathbf{H}}^T(\tilde{\mathbf{H}}\mathbf{P}_{x_k}^- \tilde{\mathbf{H}}^T + \mathbf{R}_{\nu_k})^{-1}$
- Mean estimation $\quad \hat{\mathbf{X}}_k = \bar{\mathbf{X}}_k^- + \mathbf{G}_k(\mathbf{Y}_k^o - \tilde{\mathbf{H}}\bar{\mathbf{X}}_k^-)$
- Covariance update $\quad \hat{\mathbf{P}}_{x_k} = (\mathbf{I} - \mathbf{G}_k\tilde{\mathbf{H}})\mathbf{P}_{x_k}^-$

Figure 10. TMP esitmation algorithm at iteration from instant $k-1$ to k. The $2n+1$ sigma point set for n-dimensional vector [45] is used as an example of selecting sigma points. Notations: M: dimension of TMP vector. W: weights for each sigma points, the superscript m and c representing weights for calculating mean and covariance respectively. λ, α and β: parameters used to tune the distribution of sigma points. $\{\cdot\}^-$: prior predictions of $\{\cdot\}$. $\hat{\{\cdot\}}$: posterior estimates of $\{\cdot\}$. $\mathbf{Q}_{\omega_k}$ and $\mathbf{R}_{\nu_k}$: pre-specified covariance matrices for ω_k and ν_k.

A priori prediction

Ensemble generation

- Sigma points $\ominus_{k-1,i}$(i=0...2M)

$$\{\ominus_{k-1,i}\}_0^{2M} = \left(\hat{\mathbf{\Psi}}_{k-1} \quad \hat{\mathbf{\Psi}}_{k-1} \pm \sqrt{(M+\lambda)\hat{\mathbf{P}}_{\Psi_{k-1}}}\right)$$

- Weights W_i $\qquad W_0^m = \lambda/(M+\lambda)$

$$W_0^c = \lambda/(M+\lambda) + (1-\alpha^2+\beta)$$

$$W_i^m = W_i^c = 1/(2(M+\lambda)) \qquad i = 1\dots 2M$$

Prediction

•Dynamic propagation: $\mathcal{U}^{\Psi}_{k|k-1,i} = \tilde{F}_d(\hat{\mathbf{U}}_{k-1}, \ominus_{k-1,i})$

•Measurement propagation: $\mathcal{Y}^{\Psi}_{k|k-1,i} = \mathbf{H}\mathcal{U}^{\Psi}_{k|k-1,i}$

•Statistics prediction: $\mathbf{P}^{-}_{\Psi_k} = \hat{\mathbf{P}}_{\Psi_{k-1}} + \mathbf{Q}_{\omega^{\Psi}_k}$

$$\bar{\mathbf{Y}}^{\Psi-}_k = \sum_{i=0}^{2M} W_i^m \mathcal{Y}^{\Psi}_{k|k-1,i}$$

$$\mathbf{P}^{\Psi}_{y_k} = \sum_{i=0}^{2M} W_i^c (\mathcal{Y}^{\Psi}_{k|k-1,i} - \bar{\mathbf{Y}}^{\Psi-}_k)(\mathcal{Y}^{\Psi}_{k|k-1,i} - \bar{\mathbf{Y}}^{\Psi-}_k)^T + \mathbf{R}_{\nu_k}$$

$$\mathbf{P}_{\Psi_k y_k} = \sum_{i=0}^{2M} W_i^c (\ominus_{k-1,i} - \hat{\mathbf{\Psi}}_{k-1})(\mathcal{Y}^{\Psi}_{k|k-1,i} - \bar{\mathbf{Y}}^{\Psi-}_k)^T$$

⇓

A posteriori correction

•Kalman gain $\quad \mathbf{G}^{\Psi}_k = \mathbf{P}_{\Psi_k y_k} \mathbf{P}^{\Psi-1}_{y_k}$

•Mean estimation $\quad \hat{\mathbf{\Psi}}_k = \hat{\mathbf{\Psi}}_{k-1} + \mathbf{G}^{\Psi}_k (\mathbf{Y}^o_k - \bar{\mathbf{Y}}^{\Psi-}_k)$

•Covariance update $\quad \hat{\mathbf{P}}_{\Psi_k} = \mathbf{P}^{-}_{\Psi_k} - \mathbf{G}^{\Psi}_k \mathbf{P}^{\Psi}_{y_k} \mathbf{G}^{\Psi T}_k$

Figure 11. Flow of parameter estimation algorithm from time instant $k-1$ to k. $\mathbf{Q}_{\omega^{\Psi}_k}$: pre-specified covariance matrix for ω^{Ψ}_k. For detailed notations refer to Figure 10.

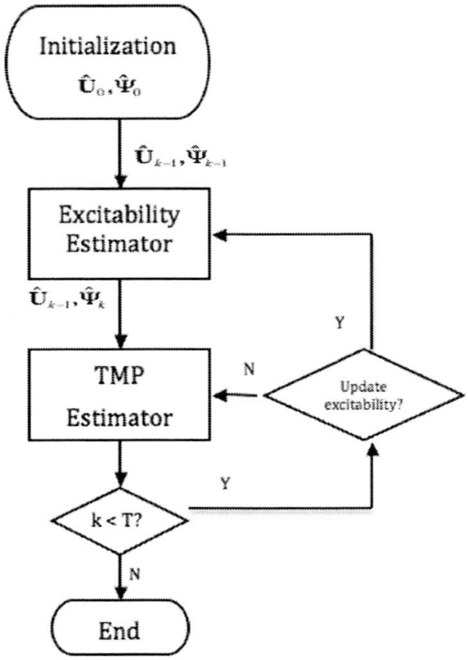

Figure 12. Dual estimator of TMP dynamics and tissue property. T: total number of estimation steps.

References

[1] F. Greensite. Heart surface electrocardiographic inverse solutions. In B. He, editor, *Modeling and Imaging of Bioelectrical Activity*, pages 119–156. Kluwer Academic / Plenum Publishers, 2004.

[2] R. Plonsey. *Bioelectric phenonmena*. McGraw Hill, New York, 1969.

[3] H. S. Oster, B. Taccardi, R. L. Lux, P. R. Ershler, and Y. Rudy. Noninvasive electrocardiographic imaging: reconstruction of epicardial potentials, electrograms, and isochrones and localization of single and multiple electrocardiac events. *Circulation*, 96:1012–1024, 1997.

[4] F. Greensite. The mathematical basis for imaging cardiac electrical function. *Critical Reviews in Biomedical Engineering*, 22:347–399, 1994.

[5] B. He et al. Noninvasive imaging of cardiac transmembrane potentials within three-dimdensional myocardium by means of a realistic geometry aniostropic heart model. *IEEE Transactions on Biomedical Engineering*, 50:1190–1202, 2003.

[6] Y. Yamashita. Theoretical studies on the inverse problem of electrocardiography and the uniqueness of the solution. *IEEE Transactions on Biomedical Engineering*, 29(11):719–725, 1982.

[7] H. Zhang and P. Shi. A meshfree method for solving cardiac electrical propagation. In *Proc. IEEE Engineering in Medicine and Biology Science*, pages 349 – 352, 2005.

[8] H. Zhang, P. Shi, and P. J. Hunter. A meshfree method for simulating myocardial electrical activity. Technical report, Bioengineering Institute University of Auckland, New Zealand, Auckland, New Zealand, July 2008.

[9] C. S. Henriquez. Simulating the electrical behaviour of cardiac tissue using the bidomain model. *Critical Reviews in Biomedical Engineering*, 21:1–77, 1993.

[10] G. Fischer, B. Tilg, P. Wach, G. Lafter, and W. Rucker. Analytical validation of the bem-application of the bem to the electrocardiographic forward and inverse problem. *Computer Methods and Programs in Biomedicine*, 55:99–106, 1998.

[11] C. Bradley and A. Pullan. Application of the bem in biopotential problems. *Engineering Analysis with Boundary Elements*, 26:391–403, 2002.

[12] G. Fischer, B. Tilg, R. Modre, G. J. M. Huiskamp, J. Fetzer, W. Rucker, and P. Wach. A bidomain model based bem-fem coupling formulation for anisotropic cardiac tissue. *Annals of Biomedical Engineering*, 28:1229–1243, 2000.

[13] R. H. Clayton and A. V. Holden. Computational framework for simulating the mechanisms and ecg of re-entrant ventricular fibrillation. *Physical Measurements*, 23:707–726, 2002.

[14] A. C. L. Barnard, I. M. Duck, and M. L. Lynn. The application of electromagentic theroy to electrocardiology. *Biophysical Journal*, 7:443–462, 1967.

[15] D. Wei, O. Okazaki, K. Harumi, E. Harasawa, and H. Hosaka. Comparative simulation of excitation and body surface electrocardiogram with isotropic and anisotropic computer heart models. *IEEE Transactions on Biomedical Engineering*, 42(4):343–357, 1995.

[16] A. Rabinovitch, I. Aviram, N. Gulko, and E. Ovsyshcher. A model for the propagation of action potentials in non-uniformly excitable media. *Journal of Theoretical Biology*, 196:141–154, 1999.

[17] G. Taubin. Curve and surface smoothing without shrinkage. In *Proc. International Conference on Computer Vision*, pages 825–857, 1995.

[18] G. X. Yan, W. Shimizu, and C. Antzelevitch. Charactertistics and distribution of m cells in arterially perfused canine left ventricular wedge preparations. *Circulation*, 98:1921–1927, 1998.

[19] M. Nash. *Mechanics and Material Properties of the Heart using an Anatomically Accurate Mathematical Model*. PhD thesis, Univ. of Auckland, New Zealand, May 1998.

[20] P. M. F. Nielsen, I. J. Le Grice, B. H. Smaill, and P. J. Hunter. Mathematical model of geometry and fibrous structure of the heart. *American Journal of Physiology*, 260:H1365–H1378, 1991.

[21] M. Seger. *Modeling the electrical function of the human heart*. PhD thesis, Univ. for Health Sciences, Medical Informatics and Technology, Austria, 2006.

[22] G.R. Liu. *Meshfree Methods*. CRC Press, Boca Raton, FL, 2003.

[23] C. P. Brandley, A. J. Pullan, and P. J. Hunter. Effects of material properties and geometry on electrocardiographic forward simulations. *Annals of Biomedical Engineering*, 28:721–741, 2000.

[24] L. K. Cheng, J. M. Bodley, and A. J. Pullan. The effect of experimental and modeling errors on the electrocardiographic inverse problem. *IEEE Transactions on Biomedical Engineering*, 50(1):23–32, 2003.

[25] S. Rush, J.A. Abildskov, and R.McFee. Risistivity of body tissues at low frequencies. *Circulation Research*, 12:40–50, 1963.

[26] C. Ramanathan and Y. Rudy. Electrocardiographic imaging: effect of torso inhomogeneities on noninvasive reconstruction of epicardial potentials, electrograms, and isochrones. *Journal of Cardiovascular Electrophysiology*, 12:241–252, 2001.

[27] L. Cheng. *Non-invasive Electrical Imaging of the Heartl*. PhD thesis, Univ. of Auckland, New Zealand, 2001.

[28] L. Wang, H. Zhang, Ken C.L. Wong, and P. Shi. Coupled meshfree-bem platform for electrocardiographic simulation: Modeling and validations. In *Proc. International Workshop on Medical Imaging and Augmented Reality*, volume 1, pages 98–107, 2008.

[29] L. Wang, H. Zhang, K. Wong, H. Liu, and P. Shi. Electrocardiographic simulation on personalized heart-torso structures using coupled meshfree-bem platform. *International Journal of Functional Informatics and Personalized Medicine*, Under review, 2009.

[30] R. Fitzhugh. Impulses and physiological states in theoretical models of nerve membrance. *Biophysical Journal*, 1:445–466, 1961.

[31] C. Luo and Y. Rudy. A dynamic model of the cardiac ventricular action potential: Simulations of ionic currents and concentration changes. *Circulation Research*, 74:1071–1096, 1994.

[32] J. M. Rogers and A. D. McCulloch. A collocation-galerkin finite element model of cardiac action potential propagation. *IEEE Transactions on Biomedical Engineering*, 41(8):743–757, 1994.

[33] R. R. Aliev and A. V. Panfilov. A simple two-variable model of cardiac excitation. *Chaos, Solitions & Fractals*, 7(3):293–301, 1996.

[34] G. Huiskamp and F. Greensite. A new method for myocardial activation imaging. *IEEE Transactions on Biomedical Engineering*, 44(6):446, 1997.

[35] A. J. Pullan, L. K. Cheng, M. P. Nash, C. P. Bradley, and D. J. Paterson. Noninvasive electrical imaging of the heart: theory and model development. *Annals of Biomedical Engineering*, 29:817–836, 2001.

[36] R. Modre, B. Tilg, G. Fischer, and P. Wach. Noninvasive myocardial activation time imaging: a novel inverse algorithm applied to clinical ecg mapping data. *IEEE Transactions on Biomedical Engineering*, 49:1153–1161, 2002.

[37] P. Colli-Franzone, L. Guerri, C. Viganotti, E. Macchi, S. Baruffi, S. Spaggiari, and B. Taccardi. Potential fields generated by oblique dipole layers modelling excitation wavefronts in the anisotropic myocardium. *Circulation Research*, 51:330–346, 1982.

[38] C. A. Brebbia, J. C. F. Telles, and L. C. Wrobel. *Boundary element techniques: theory and applications in engineering*. Springer-Verlag, 1984.

[39] A. Heringa, D. F. Stegeman, G. J. H. Uijen, and J. P. C. de Weerd. Solution method of electrical filed problems in physiology. *IEEE Transactions on Biomedical Engineering*, 29(1):34–42, 1982.

[40] J. Butcher. *Numerical Methods for Ordinary Differential Equations*. Wiley, 2008.

[41] B. D. Anderson and J. B. Moore. *Optimal Filtering*. Prentice-Hall, New Jersey, 1979.

[42] B. Ristic. *Beyond the Kalman Filter: Particle Filters for Tracking Applications*. Artech House, Boston,MA, 2004.

[43] G. Evensenl. *Data assimilation: the Ensemble Kalman filter*. Springer-Verlag, 2006.

[44] S. J. Julier and J. K. Uhlmann. A new extension of the kalman filter to nonlinear systems. In *International Symposium on Aerospace/Defense Sensing, Simulation, and Controls*, pages 182–193, 1997.

[45] S.J. Julier. The scaled unscented transform. *International Journal for Numerical Methods in Engineering*, 47:1445–1462, 2000.

[46] H. Ashikaga et al. Electromechanical analysis of infarct border zone in chronic myocardial infarction. *American Journal of Physiology - Heart and Circulatory Physiology*, 289:H1099–H1105, 2005.

[47] M. A. Fallert et al. Myocardial electrical impedance mapping of ischemic sheep hearts and healing aneurysms. *Circulation*, 87:199–207, 1993.

[48] M. Volkmer et al. Substrate mapping vs. tachycardia mapping using carto in patients with coronary artery disease and ventricular tachycardia: impact on outcome of catheter ablation. *Europace*, 8:968–976, 2006.

[49] H. Ashikaga et al. Magnetic resonance-based anatomical analysis of scar-related ventricular tachycardia. implications for catheter ablation. *Circulation*, 101:939–947, 2007.

[50] A. Schmidt et al. Infarct tissue heterogeneity by magnetic resonance imaging identifies enhanced cardiac arrhythmia susceptibility in patient's with left ventricular dysfunction. *Circulation*, 115:2006–2014, 2007.

[51] F. D. Dawoud. Using inverse electrocardiography to image myocardial infarction. In *Proc. Computers in Cardiology*, pages 177–180, 2007.

[52] D. Farina. Model-based approach to the localization of infarction. In *Proc. Computers in Cardiology*, pages 173–176, 2007.

[53] W. T Miller and D. B Geselowitz. Simulation sutdies of the electrocardiogram. ii. ischemia and infarction. *Circulation Research*, 43:315–323, 1978.

[54] M. D. Cerqueira, N. J. Weissman, V. Dilsizian, A. K. Jacobs, S. Kaul, W. K. Laskey, D. J. Pennell, J. A. Rumberger, T. Ryan, and M. S. Verani. Standardized myocardial segmentation and nomenclature for tomographic imaging of the heart. *Circulation*, 105:539–542, 2002.

[55] A. L. Goldberger et al. Physiobank, physiotoolkit, and physionet components of a new research resource for complex physiological signals. *Criculation*, 101:e215–e220, 2000.

[56] M. A. Mneimneh and R. J. Povinelli. Rps/gmm approach toward the localization of myocardial infarction. In *Proc. Computers in Cardiology*, pages 185–188, 2007.

[57] B. M. Jackson, L. M. Parish, J. H. Gorman, et al. Borderzone geometry after acute myocardial infarction: a three-dimension contrast enhanced echocardiographic study. *Ann Thorac Surg*, 80:2250–2256, 2005.

[58] M. C. Maclachlan, J. Sundnes, and G. T. Lines. Simulation of st segment changes during subendocardial ischemia using a realistic 3d cardiac geometry. *IEEE Transactions on Biomedical Engineering*, 52(5):799–807, 2005.

[59] N. S. Peters and A. L. Wit. Myocardial architecture and ventridular arrhythmogenesis. *Circulation*, 97:1746–1754, 1998.

[60] H.V. Gupta H. Moradkhani, S. Sorooshian and P.R. Houser. Dual state-parameter estimation of hydrological models using ensemble kalman filter. *Advances in Water Resources*, 28:135–147, 2005.

[61] X. R. Li and Y. Bar-Shalom. Multiple-model estimation with variable structure. *IEEE Transactions on Automatic Control*, 41(4):478–493, 1996.

In: 3D Imaging: Theory, Technology... ISBN: 978-1-60876-885-1
Editors: E. H. Duke and S. R. Aguirre, pp.275-292

Chapter 13

3D Euclidean Reconstruction of Structured Scenes from Uncalibrated Images

Guanghui Wang and Q. M. Jonathan Wu
Department of Electrical and Computer Engineering, University of Windsor,
Windsor, Ontario, Canada, N9B 3P4

Abstract

In this chapter, we will focus on the problem of 3D Euclidean reconstruction of structured scenes from uncalibrated images based on the property of vanishing points. Firstly, under the assumption of three-parameter-camera model with varying parameters, we prove that the camera projection matrix can be uniquely determined from three mutually orthogonal vanishing points under an arbitrary preassigned world coordinate system. Secondly, when multiple images of an object are present, we prove that a set of global consistent projection matrices can be recovered if an arbitrary reference point in space is observed across the views. In addition, we present some techniques to take geometric measurement from a single image, by which we can recover the 3D structure of the entire scene with several architectures. Compared with previous stereovision technique which is fully rely on the feature matches, the proposed method computes projection matrices from the vanishing points of parallel lines. Thus the bottleneck problem of feature matching is avoided, and more accurate, robust and realistic results are expected. Extensive experiments on synthetic and real world images validate the effectiveness of the proposed method. The proposed method is applicable to reconstruct photo-realistic and accurate model of structured scenes, especially those containing three dominate directions and some planar surfaces.

1 Introduction

Three Dimensional Reconstruction from uncalibrated images is a central problem in computer vision community. Examples and applications of this task include robot navigation, obstacle recognition, augmented reality, architectural surveying, forensic science etc. The classical method for solving such a problem is to reconstruct the metric structure of the scene from two or more images using stereovision techniques [12][9]. However, this is a hard task due to the problem of seeking correspondences between different views. In addition to this, the error introduced by matching and calibration propagates along the computational chain and causes a loss of accuracy in the final results. In recent years, researchers have focused on using geometric constraints arising from the scenes to optimize the reconstruction, especially for architecture scenes [28][24]. Such constraints may be expressed in terms of parallelism, orthogonality, coplanarity and other special inter-relationship of features and camera constraints.

For a wide variety of man-made objects, we can usually obtain three vanishing points that correspond to three mutually orthogonal directions in space [1]. There are many techniques for accurately and automatically detecting the vanishing points from images [1][15][21]. The vanishing points play an important role in the Euclidean reconstruction and is widely studied in literature. Caprile and Torre [5] proposed a method for camera calibration from the vanishing points computed from the projected edges of a cuboid. Following this idea, several approaches that make use of vanishing points and lines have been proposed for either cameras calibration or scene reconstruction [14][25]. Most of the methods assume a simplified camera model of three parameters. Wilczkowiak *et.al.* [28] expanded the idea for general parallelepided structures, and used the constraints of parallelepipeds for camera calibration. Grossmanna and Victor [10] proposed to explore some geometrical regularity to recover a least-square estimates of 3D points from one or more images a scene. Pu and Vosselman [17] proposed to automatically extract building features from terrestrial laser scanned data and then reconstruct 3D city models. Košechá and Zhang [13] proposed to extract dominant rectangular structures from a single view based on a higher-level information. Müller *et.al.* [16] proposed to combine the procedural modeling pipeline of shape grammars with image analysis to derive a meaningful hierarchical facade subdivision, and derive 3D models of high visual quality from single facade images of arbitrary resolutions. Saxena *et.al.* [18] proposed to use Markov Random Field to model the depths and estimate detailed 3D structure from a single still image of an unstructured environment.

Criminisi *et.al.* [7] proposed to compute 3D affine measurement from a single image based on the vanishing line of a reference plane and the vertical vanishing point. A similar technique is studied in [23] and there are some available in Photogrammetry as well[22]. Most of these methods are based on a single view and only part of the structure or some metrical quantities can be inferred with the prior knowledge of geometrical scene constraints.

When multiple images are present, Werner and Zisserman [27] present a coarse-to-fine strategy to reconstruct buildings. The planar model of the principal scene planes is generated by plane sweeping and used as a basis to estimate more details around the plane. Baillard and Zisserman [3] use inter-image homographies to validate and estimate the plane models. Bartoli and Sturm [4] describe the geometric relationships between points and planes as multi-coplanarity constraints, and a maximum likelihood estimator that incorporates the constraints and structures is used in a bundle adjustment manner. Wang *et.al.* [24] refined the space plane homographies recursively by combining the point and line correspondences. Most of these methods rely on the initial matching or a relatively good projective or metric reconstruction of points and lines, which may not be available in some situations. Some commercial systems, such as Facade [8] and Photobuilder [6] can produce very realistic results, but these systems usually require a lot of human interactions.

Most previous studies on vanishing points is mainly focused on camera calibration or stratify the reconstruction from perspective to Affine or metric. To the best of our knowledge, the most similar study in the literature was proposed by Cipolla *et.al.* [6]. Where three orthogonal vanishing points were used directly to estimate the projection matrices. However, the estimation is not unique as indicated in the chapter and the authors did not propose how to deal with the ambiguity.

In this chapter, we will target on man-made structures that typically contain three orthogonal principal directions. Assuming the cameras are of three parameters, we propose to recover the camera projection matrices directly from a set of three orthogonal vanishing points, thus avoiding the bottleneck problem of image matching and the instability in computing the fundamental matrix caused by the critical configuration of the scenes or cameras. Part of this chapter was previously published in [25][26].

The chapter is organized as follows: In section 2, some preliminaries on projection matrix and camera calibration are reviewed. The proposed method to recover the projection matrix from vanishing points is elaborated in section 3. Section 4 presents the techniques for geometric measurement and reconstruction. Some test results with synthetic and real images are presented in section 5 and 6 respectively. Finally, the conclusion is discussed in section 7.

2 Camera Matrix and Calibration

In order to facilitate our discussions in the subsequent sections, some preliminaries on projection matrix and camera calibration are presented here. Readers can refer to [12] and [25] for more details.

2.1 Camera projection matrix

Under perspective projection, a 3D point $\mathbf{x} \in \mathbb{R}^3$ in space is projected to an image point $\mathbf{m} \in \mathbb{R}^2$ via a rank-3 projection matrix $\mathbf{P} \in \mathbb{R}^{3\times 4}$ as

$$s\tilde{\mathbf{m}} = \mathbf{P}\tilde{\mathbf{x}} = \mathbf{K}[\mathbf{R}, \mathbf{t}]\tilde{\mathbf{x}} = [\mathbf{p}_1, \mathbf{p}_2, \mathbf{p}_3, \mathbf{p}_4]\tilde{\mathbf{x}} \tag{1}$$

where, $\tilde{\mathbf{x}} = [\mathbf{x}^{\mathrm{T}}, 1]^{\mathrm{T}}$ and $\tilde{\mathbf{m}} = [\mathbf{m}^{\mathrm{T}}, 1]^{\mathrm{T}}$ are the homogeneous forms of points $\mathbf{x}$ and $\mathbf{m}$ respectively, $\mathbf{R}$ and $\mathbf{t}$ are the rotation matrix and translation vector from the world system to the camera system, s is a non-zero scalar, $\mathbf{K}$ is the camera calibration matrix in form of

$$\mathbf{K} = \begin{bmatrix} f_u & \varsigma & u_0 \\ 0 & f_v & v_0 \\ 0 & 0 & 1 \end{bmatrix} \tag{2}$$

where, f_u and f_v represent the camera's focal length corresponding to the u and v axes of camera coordinates; $[u_0, v_0]^{\mathrm{T}}$ is the coordinates of the camera's principal point; $\varsigma = f_u \cot\theta$ refers to the skew factor, with θ the included angle of the u and v axes. For most CCD cameras, we assume square pixels (i.e. $\varsigma = 0$ and $f_u = f_v$), so that the camera becomes a simplified one with only three intrinsic parameters. There are also two other kinds of assumptions for three-parameter-camera. One is to assume the principal point at origin. The other is to assume rectangle pixels with known aspect ratio $\gamma = f_v/f_u$.

Lemma 1 *The first three columns of the projection matrix correspond to the vanishing points of the X, Y and Z axes of the world system respectively, and the last column of the projection matrix is the image of the world origin.*

Proof: In the normalized world coordinate system, the direction of X, Y and Z axes are $\tilde{\mathbf{x}}_w = [1,0,0,0]^{\mathrm{T}}$, $\tilde{\mathbf{y}}_w = [0,1,0,0]^{\mathrm{T}}$ and $\tilde{\mathbf{z}}_w = [0,0,1,0]^{\mathrm{T}}$ respectively, and the homogeneous vector of the world origin is $\tilde{\mathbf{o}}_w = [0,0,0,1]^{\mathrm{T}}$. Then from eq.(1), we have:

$$\begin{aligned} s_x\tilde{\mathbf{v}}_x &= \mathbf{P}\tilde{\mathbf{x}}_w = [\mathbf{p}_1,\mathbf{p}_2,\mathbf{p}_3,\mathbf{p}_4][1,0,0,0]^{\mathrm{T}} = \mathbf{p}_1 \\ s_y\tilde{\mathbf{v}}_y &= \mathbf{P}\tilde{\mathbf{y}}_w = [\mathbf{p}_1,\mathbf{p}_2,\mathbf{p}_3,\mathbf{p}_4][0,1,0,0]^{\mathrm{T}} = \mathbf{p}_2 \\ s_z\tilde{\mathbf{v}}_z &= \mathbf{P}\tilde{\mathbf{z}}_w = [\mathbf{p}_1,\mathbf{p}_2,\mathbf{p}_3,\mathbf{p}_4][0,0,1,0]^{\mathrm{T}} = \mathbf{p}_3 \\ s_o\tilde{\mathbf{v}}_o &= \mathbf{P}\tilde{\mathbf{o}}_w = [\mathbf{p}_1,\mathbf{p}_2,\mathbf{p}_3,\mathbf{p}_4][0,0,0,1]^{\mathrm{T}} = \mathbf{p}_4 \end{aligned}$$

Thus the four columns of the projection matrix are defined by $\mathbf{v}_x, \mathbf{v}_y, \mathbf{v}_z$ and $\mathbf{v}_o$ up to nonzero scalars. □

Lemma 2 *Given a point $\mathbf{m}$ in an image, its back-projection is a ray in space passing through the camera center and the point $\mathbf{m}$, which can be expressed as $\mathbf{L}_b = \{\boldsymbol{x} | s\tilde{\boldsymbol{m}} = \boldsymbol{P}\tilde{\boldsymbol{x}}, \boldsymbol{x} \in \mathbb{R}^3\}$.*

Lemma 3 *Given a line $\mathbf{l}$ in an image, its back-projection spans a plane in space passing through the camera center and the line $\mathbf{l}$, which is defined as $\Pi = \mathbf{P}^T\mathbf{l}$.*

2.2 The image of the absolute conic and camera calibration

The absolute conic $\mathbf{C}_\infty = \mathbf{I} = diag(1,1,1)$ is a conic on the plane at infinity, which is a conic composed of purely imaginary points on the infinite plane. Under perspective projection, we can easily obtain the image of the absolute conic (IAC) as $\omega = \mathbf{K}^{-\mathrm{T}}\mathbf{K}^{-1}$, which is an invisible imaginary point conic in an image. The dual image of the absolute conic (DIAC) is referred as $\omega^* = \omega^{-1} = \mathbf{K}\mathbf{K}^{\mathrm{T}}$, which is a dual conic of ω.

It is clear that both the IAC and the DIAC depend only on the camera calibration matrix $\mathbf{K}$. If the value of the matrix ω or ω^* is known, then the intrinsic parameters of the camera $\mathbf{K}$ can be recovered directly by Cholesky decomposition. Thus we often refer to camera calibration as the computation of the IAC or the DIAC.

Lemma 4 *The camera can be calibrated linearly from a set of three orthogonal vanishing points under the three-parameter-assumption.*

with five degrees of freedom, since it is defined up to scale. It can be verified that a pair of orthogonal vanishing points (say $\mathbf{v}_1, \mathbf{v}_2$) are conjugate with respect to the IAC, i.e. $\mathbf{v}_1^{\mathrm{T}}\omega\mathbf{v}_2 = 0$. Thus a set of three orthogonal vanishing points can provide three linearly independent constraints to ω.

Under square-pixel assumption, it is easy to verify that $\omega_{12} = \omega_{21} = 0$ and $\omega_{11} - \omega_{22} = 0$. For the assumption of known principal points, we may move the image center to the principal point and obtain that $\omega_{13} = \omega_{31} = 0$ and $\omega_{23} = \omega_{32} = 0$. When the camera is of rectangle-pixel with known aspect ratio γ, it is easy to verify that $\omega_{12} = \omega_{21} = 0$ and $\omega_{11} = \gamma^2\omega_{22}$. Hence the three-parameter-assumption provides two additional linear constrains on the IAC and the camera can be calibrated linearly.

3 Recovery of Projection Matrix

From Lemma 1, we know that $\mathbf{P} = [s_x\tilde{\mathbf{v}}_x, s_y\tilde{\mathbf{v}}_y, s_z\tilde{\mathbf{v}}_z, s_o\tilde{\mathbf{v}}_o]$, where $\tilde{\mathbf{v}}_x$, $\tilde{\mathbf{v}}_y$, $\tilde{\mathbf{v}}_z$ are the homogeneous form of the three vanishing points, $\tilde{\mathbf{v}}_o$ is the image of the world origin, s_x, s_y, s_z, s_o are four unknown scalars. In the following, we will show how to determine these unknowns in a specific world coordinate system.

3.1 Projection matrix of a single view

Proposition 5 *Given a set of three orthogonal vanishing points $\mathbf{v}_x$, $\mathbf{v}_y$ and $\mathbf{v}_z$ under a certain world system, the scalars s_x, s_y and s_z can be uniquely determined if the camera is assumed to be a three-parameter-model.*

Instead of proving the proposition directly, we will give an analysis on how to compute these scalars in the following. Let $\mathbf{M} = [s_x\tilde{\mathbf{v}}_x, s_y\tilde{\mathbf{v}}_y, s_z\tilde{\mathbf{v}}_z] = [\tilde{\mathbf{v}}_x, \tilde{\mathbf{v}}_y, \tilde{\mathbf{v}}_z]diag(s_x, s_y, s_z)$ be the first three columns of the projection matrix, and let $\mathbf{C} = \mathbf{M}\mathbf{M}^{\mathrm{T}}$, then we have

$$\mathbf{C} = \mathbf{M}\mathbf{M}^{\mathrm{T}} = [\tilde{\mathbf{v}}_x, \tilde{\mathbf{v}}_y, \tilde{\mathbf{v}}_z]\begin{bmatrix} s_x^2 & & \\ & s_y^2 & \\ & & s_z^2 \end{bmatrix}[\tilde{\mathbf{v}}_x, \tilde{\mathbf{v}}_y, \tilde{\mathbf{v}}_z]^{\mathrm{T}} \tag{3}$$

On the other hand, we know that $\mathbf{M} = \mathbf{K}\mathbf{R}$ from eq.(1). Thus

$$\mathbf{C} = \mathbf{M}\mathbf{M}^{\mathrm{T}} = \mathbf{K}\mathbf{R}\mathbf{R}^{\mathrm{T}}\mathbf{K}^{\mathrm{T}} = \mathbf{K}\mathbf{K}^{\mathrm{T}} = \omega^* \tag{4}$$

where ω^* is the dual of the IAC which can be obtained from the three vanishing points via Lemma 2. So the three scalars can be obtained by incorporating eq.(3) and eq.(4).

$$\begin{bmatrix} s_x^2 & & \\ & s_y^2 & \\ & & s_z^2 \end{bmatrix} = [\tilde{\mathbf{v}}_x, \tilde{\mathbf{v}}_y, \tilde{\mathbf{v}}_z]^{-1}\omega^*[\tilde{\mathbf{v}}_x, \tilde{\mathbf{v}}_y, \tilde{\mathbf{v}}_z]^{-\mathrm{T}} \tag{5}$$

However, the computed scalars are not unique, since $-s_x$, $-s_y$ and $-s_z$ hold true for eq.(5). Thus there are eight solutions that correspond to different selections of the signs in world coordinate axes. This ambiguity can be solved practically in a systematic manner as follows.

Result 6 *The signs of the scalars s_x, s_y and s_z correspond to the directions of X, Y and Z axes of the world coordinate system respectively.*

The result is obvious. Suppose point $\mathbf{m} = [u, v]^{\mathrm{T}}$ is the image of a space point $\mathbf{x} = [X, Y, Z]^{\mathrm{T}}$, then from eq.(1) and Lemma 1 we have

$$s\begin{bmatrix} u \\ v \\ 1 \end{bmatrix} = [s_x\tilde{\mathbf{v}}_x, s_y\tilde{\mathbf{v}}_y, s_z\tilde{\mathbf{v}}_z, s_o\tilde{\mathbf{v}}_o]\begin{bmatrix} X \\ Y \\ Z \\ 1 \end{bmatrix} \tag{6}$$

It is easy to verify that the same image point can be obtained if we reverse the sign of $\{X, s_x\}$, $\{Y, s_y\}$ or $\{Z, s_z\}$ simultaneously. In practice, we usually adopt the right-handed system in practice. Suppose $\{X, Y, Z\}$ is a correct selection of the world system, then

$\{-X, -Y, Z\}$, $\{-X, Y, -Z\}$ and $\{X, -Y, -Z\}$ also satisfy the right-handed rule and result the same vanishing points of the image, since the vanishing point of an axis is irrelevant to its direction. Among the four selections of the world system, only two of them can ensure that the reconstructed object lies in front of the camera. One can also verify that the vector directed towards the front of the camera along the principal axis may be computed from $\mathbf{v} = \det(\mathbf{M})\mathbf{m}^3$, where $\mathbf{M}$ represents the first three columns of the projection matrix, $\mathbf{m}^3$ is the third row of $\mathbf{M}$. Thus we have the following result.

Result 7 *The sign ambiguity of the three scalars in (5) can be reduced from eight to four if right-handed world system is assumed. The ambiguity can be further reduced to two if we assume that the object lies in front of the camera.*

Result 8 *Suppose the last column of the projection matrix $\mathbf{p}_4$ is known, then the signs of the scalars may be uniquely determined in practice for a given object under certain world coordinate system.*

In Result 8, we assume $\mathbf{p}_4$ is known. Actually, from eq.(1) and Lemma 1 we have that $\mathbf{p}_4 = \mathbf{Kt} = s_o\tilde{\mathbf{v}}_o$, which corresponds to the translation vector of the camera to the world origin. Since there is no absolute measurement about the scene geometry, the projection matrix is only defined up to scale, thus the value of s_o may be set freely. In practice, we may choose s_o such that $(\mathbf{p}_4)_3 = 1$, which means the third element of the translation vector $(\mathbf{t})_3 = 1$.

The ambiguity is reduced to two from Result 7. Suppose the two projection matrices are $\mathbf{P}_1$ and $\mathbf{P}_2$. Under a given world frame, we can arbitrary choose a space point $\mathbf{S}_a = [X_a, 0, 0]^{\mathrm{T}}$ on the positive direction of X axis, suppose its corresponding image point is $\mathbf{m}_a$, then from $s\tilde{\mathbf{m}}_a = \mathbf{P}_1[X_a, 0, 0, 1]^{\mathrm{T}}$, we can obtain the estimate of X_a. A unique solution of the projection matrix $\mathbf{P}$ can be determined from the sign of X_a. If X_a is positive, then $\mathbf{P} = \mathbf{P}_1$, otherwise, $\mathbf{P} = \mathbf{P}_2$.

3.2 Projection matrices of multiple views

We have now proven the uniqueness of the first three columns of the projection matrix under a given world system. For a single view, the scalar of the last column of the projection matrix can be chosen freely. Nevertheless, when we have multiple views of the scene, the scalars corresponding to the projection matrices of these views must be consistent so as to obtain a global reconstruction consistently.

Proposition 9 *Given an arbitrary reference point in space which can be observed across multiple views, a consistent set of scalars associated with the translation terms of the projection matrices of these views can be uniquely determined.*

Proof: Without loss of generality, suppose we have two views, $\mathbf{S}_c = [X_c, Y_c, Z_c]^{\mathrm{T}}$ is an arbitrary reference point in space, with $\mathbf{m}_{c1}$ and $\mathbf{m}_{c2}$ the observed images of the reference point in the two views. Let $\mathbf{P}_1 = [\mathbf{M}_1, s_{o1}\tilde{\mathbf{v}}_{o1}]$, $\mathbf{P}_2 = [\mathbf{M}_2, s_{o2}\tilde{\mathbf{v}}_{o2}]$ be the two projection matrices, where $\mathbf{M}_i (i = 1, 2)$ have been determined in the previous section, $\tilde{\mathbf{v}}_{o1}$ and $\tilde{\mathbf{v}}_{o2}$ are the images of the world origin in the two views. Then from

$$\begin{cases} s_1\tilde{\mathbf{m}}_{c1} = \mathbf{P}_1\tilde{\mathbf{S}}_c = \mathbf{M}_1\mathbf{S}_c + s_{o1}\tilde{\mathbf{v}}_{o1} \\ s_2\tilde{\mathbf{m}}_{c2} = \mathbf{P}_2\tilde{\mathbf{S}}_c = \mathbf{M}_2\mathbf{S}_c + s_{o2}\tilde{\mathbf{v}}_{o2} \end{cases} \tag{7}$$

we have

$$\left[\mathbf{M}_1\mathbf{M}_2^{-1}\tilde{\mathbf{v}}_{o2}, -\mathbf{M}_1\mathbf{M}_2^{-1}\tilde{\mathbf{m}}_{c2}, \tilde{\mathbf{m}}_{c1}\right] \begin{bmatrix} s_{o2} \\ s_2 \\ s_1 \end{bmatrix} = s_{o1}\tilde{\mathbf{v}}_{o1} \tag{8}$$

where s_{o2}, s_1, and s_2 are three unknowns, while s_{o1} may be predetermined since one can always select the first view as a reference. Thus a consistent value of s_{o2} can be computed from eq.(8). The same is true for more views. □

Remark 10 *Although the consistent scalars can be computed from an arbitrary reference point in Proposition 9, it is better to select a noticeable corner point, such as the intersection of some edges, so that the point can be easily and accurately located in the images. One may choose two or more reference points and obtain more accurate estimations of the scalars via least-square fit.*

Remark 11 *The proposed algorithm recovers the projection matrix directly from the vanishing points and the image of a preassigned world origin. There is no extra constraint to the cameras of each view, and the cameras across all views may have varying intrinsic parameters. Most previous study only use the vanishing points for camera calibration, which is an essential step for the Euclidean reconstruction.*

4 Geometric Measurement and Structure Recovery

After retrieving the projection matrices, one may compute the 3D structure of any pair of correspondences that are tracked automatically or given interactively. Most man-made objects, especially architectures, are usually composed of many pieces of planar surfaces. Thus with minimal human interactions of the corners of each surface across two or more views, we can easily obtain the structure via stereo triangulation.

If we have only one view, some metric information of the structure can be recovered via the technique of single view metrology. In this section, we will show how to take geometric measurement from a single view based on scene measurement.

4.1 Single view metrology

Since three orthogonal vanishing points are known, the scenario may be taken in general as in the shape of a cuboid. Let us set the world coordinate system is on the cuboid as shown in Fig.1. Suppose the coordinates of a space plane is $\mathbf{\Pi}_i$, i.e. $\mathbf{\Pi}_i^T\tilde{\mathbf{x}} = 0$, with $\tilde{\mathbf{x}} = [x, y, z, 1]^T$. Then for an image point $\mathbf{m}_j$ on the plane, its corresponding space point $\mathbf{x}_j$ can be easily computed by the intersection of the back-projected line and the plane as:

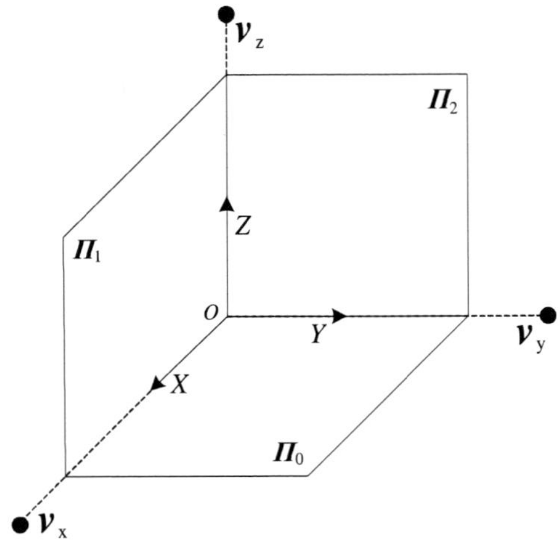

Figure 1: The world coordinate system and three orthogonal vanishing points.

$$\begin{cases} s\tilde{\mathbf{m}}_j = \mathbf{P}\tilde{\mathbf{x}}_j \\ \mathbf{\Pi}_i^T\tilde{\mathbf{x}}_j = 0 \end{cases} \tag{9}$$

Similarly, for an image line $\mathbf{l}$, its back-projection is a plane $\mathbf{\Pi} = \mathbf{P}^T\mathbf{l}$; for a conic $\mathbf{C}$ in the image, its back-projection is a view cone $\mathbf{Q} = \mathbf{P}^T\mathbf{C}\mathbf{P}$. Their corresponding space coordinates can also be computed linearly by the intersection of the back-projection and the space plane.

In Fig.1, the coordinates of plane $\mathbf{\Pi}_0$, $\mathbf{\Pi}_1$ and $\mathbf{\Pi}_2$ are obvious, while the coordinates of most other planar surfaces can be recovered from the scene constraints with respect to the three base planes [14]. Let us take the plane $\mathbf{\Pi}_0$ as a reference.

Proposition 12 *As shown in Fig.2, suppose $\mathbf{\Pi}_i$ is a plane parallel to $\mathbf{\Pi}_0$, then the coordinate of $\mathbf{\Pi}_i$ can be retrieved from a pair of vertical corresponding image points on the two planes in the direction of $\mathbf{v}_z$.*

Proof: To recover the coordinates of $\mathbf{\Pi}_i$ is equivalent to retrieving the distance z_0 between $\mathbf{\Pi}_0$ and $\mathbf{\Pi}_i$. Suppose $\mathbf{x} = [x_0, y_0, 0, 1]^T$ and $\mathbf{x}' = [x_0, y_0, z_0, 1]^T$ are the pair of corresponding points on the two planes, with three unknowns x_0, y_0, z_0, as shown in Fig.2. Their corresponding images are $\mathbf{m}_x = [u_x, v_x, 1]^T$ and $\mathbf{m'}_x = [u'_x, v'_x, 1]^T$ respectively. Then the three unknowns x_0, y_0, z_0 can be easily computed from

$$\begin{cases} s_1\mathbf{m}_x = \mathbf{P}\mathbf{x} \\ s_2\mathbf{m'}_x = \mathbf{P}\mathbf{x}' \end{cases} \tag{10}$$

Thus the coordinates of plane is recovered as $\mathbf{\Pi}_i = [0, 0, 1, -z_0]^T$. We can also use this method to compute the height of an object on the plane $\mathbf{\Pi}_0$. □

Proposition 13 *As shown in Fig.2, suppose an arbitrary plane $\mathbf{\Pi}_a$ intersect $\mathbf{\Pi}_0$ at line $\mathbf{L}$, then the coordinates of plane $\mathbf{\Pi}_a$ can be determined from the images of a pair of parallel lines on the plane.*

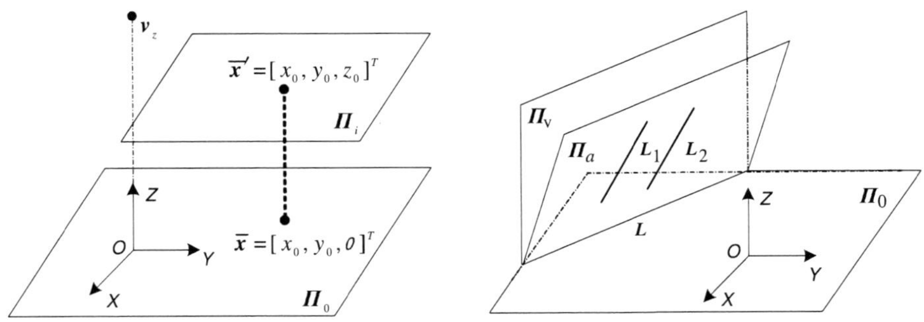

(a) (b)

Figure 2: (a) The vertical vanishing point and a pair of corresponding points between two parallel planes; (b) the relationship between the reference plane, vertical plane, and an arbitrary plane.

Proof: Since $\mathbf{L}$ lies on the plane $\mathbf{\Pi}_0 = [0, 0, 1, 0]^T$, its coordinates can be easily computed. Suppose $\mathbf{L} = [a, b, 0, d]^T$, $\mathbf{\Pi}_v$ is the plane passing through $\mathbf{L}$ and perpendicular to $\mathbf{\Pi}_0$, then $\mathbf{\Pi}_v$ must have the same coordinates as $\mathbf{L}$. All the planes passing through $\mathbf{L}$ form a pencil, and the pencil can be expressed as $\mathbf{\Pi}_a = \mathbf{\Pi}_v + \lambda \mathbf{\Pi}_0 = [a, b, \lambda, d]^T$, with λ the only unknown parameters here.

Denote the parallel lines in space and their corresponding images as $\mathbf{L}_1$, $\mathbf{L}_2$ and $\mathbf{l}_1$, $\mathbf{l}_2$ respectively, the back projection of $\mathbf{l}_1$, $\mathbf{l}_2$ form two space planes as $\mathbf{\Pi}_{b1} = \mathbf{P}^T\mathbf{l}_1$ and $\mathbf{\Pi}_{b2} = \mathbf{P}^T\mathbf{l}_2$. Suppose the normal vectors of plane $\mathbf{\Pi}_a$, $\mathbf{\Pi}_{b1}$, $\mathbf{\Pi}_{b2}$ are $\mathbf{n}_a$, $\mathbf{n}_{b1}$, $\mathbf{n}_{b2}$ respectively, then the direction vectors of $\mathbf{L}_1$, $\mathbf{L}_2$ can be computed from $\mathbf{n}_{L1} = \mathbf{n}_a \times \mathbf{n}_{b1}$, $\mathbf{n}_{L2} = \mathbf{n}_a \times \mathbf{n}_{b2}$. Thus from the parallelism of $\mathbf{L}_1$ and $\mathbf{L}_2$, λ can be easily calculated via least squares, and the coordinates of $\mathbf{\Pi}_a$ is recovered accordingly. □

Remark 14 *If some other prior information in the arbitrary plane, such as two orthogonal lines, the coordinates of a point, etc., can be retrieved from the image, the scalar* λ*, as well as the coordinates of the arbitrary plane, can also be computed in a similar way. Other geometrical entities, such as the distance between two lines, distance from a point to a plane, angle formed by two lines or two planes, angle formed by a line and a plane, etc., can also be recovered by combining the scene constraints [18].*

4.2 Optimization

The above recovered projection matrices may not be accurate since only the individual pairs of vanishing points are employed, while the vanishing points may be corrupted by imaging conditions and noise. In many cases, the feature matches across multiple views may be available, thus we can optimize the recovered projection matrices by virtue of these correspondences. Suppose we have m images, $\{\mathbf{P}^{(j)} \in \mathbb{R}^{3\times4}\}^{j=1,\ldots,m}$ are the recovered projection matrices, $\{\mathbf{m}_i^{(j)} \in \mathbb{R}^2\}_{i=1,\ldots,n}^{j=1,\ldots,m}$ are n point matches across m views, $\mathbf{x}_i \in \mathbb{R}^3$ are the reconstructed 3D points in space. Let us reproject these 3D points into the images using the estimated projection matrices and obtain the sequence of $\hat{\mathbf{m}}_i^{(j)} \in \mathbb{R}^2$. Then the projection matrices may be optimized by minimizing the image reprojection residuals.

$$f(\mathbf{P}^{(j)}, \mathbf{x}_i) = \min \sum_{i=1,\ldots,n}^{j=1,\ldots,m} d^2(\mathbf{m}_i^{(j)}, \hat{\mathbf{m}}_i^{(j)}) \tag{11}$$

where $d^2(x, y)$ stands for the squared Euclidean distance between the points x and y. The minimization process is also termed as bundle adjustment in computer vision society that can be solved via Gradient Decent or Levenberg-Marquardt algorithm [12].

5 Experiments with Synthetic data

During the simulations, we generate a cube in space, whose dimensions are $100 \times 100 \times 100$ with 100 evenly distributed points on each visible edge. As shown in Fig.3(a), the origin of the world coordinates is set at the center of the cube, and there are three parallel lines corresponding to each direction of the world axes.

5.1 Comparative results in good imaging conditions

In the simulation, we adopt three-parameter camera model, i.e. zero skew with known principal point. The image size is of 500×500, Gaussian image noise is added on each imaged point. We simulated different sets of stereo image pairs of the cube using different imaging parameters. The first set of the generated images with 1-pixel added noise is shown in Fig.4(a). The image lines are fitted via least squares from the corresponding imaged points, and the vanishing points are calculated from the intersections of each set of parallel lines as tabulated in Table 1. This is a good imaging condition, since the imaged edges of the cube have comparative lengths and the three imaged vanishing points are not very far away from the images.

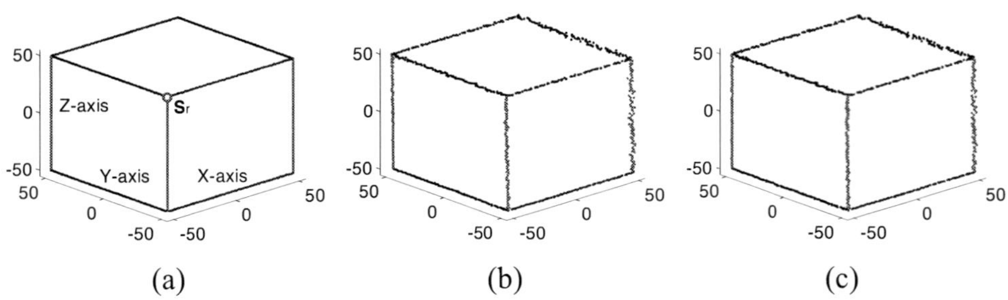

Figure 3: The ground truth and reconstruction result after registration (with 1-pixel image noise). (a) the simulated cube in the test; (b) the reconstructed cube by the proposed algorithm; (c) the reconstructed cube by stereovision technique.

We reconstruct the simulated cube by three different algorithms. The first one is the proposed algorithm, where $\mathbf{S}_0$ (as shown in Fig.3(a)) is taken as the reference point to obtain the consistent projection matrices. The second one is the optimization algorithm from the point matches which starts from the solutions of the proposed algorithm. The third one is the typical stereovision technique [12], where we utilize the normalized 8-point-algorithm

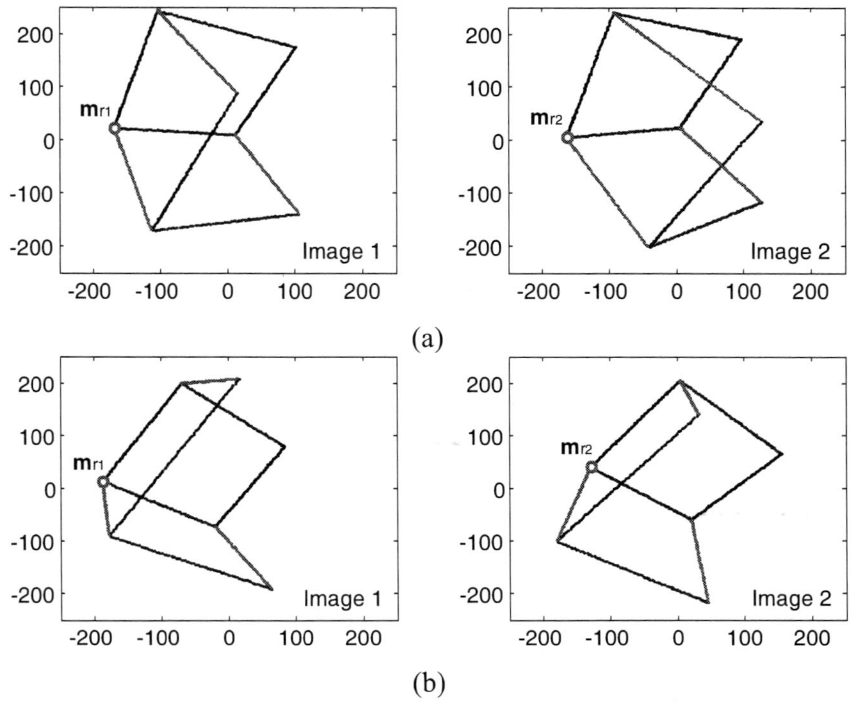

Figure 4: The obtained images in different imaging conditions (with 1-pixel image noise). (a) the first and the second images in good imaging condition; (b) the first and the second images in bad imaging condition. $\mathbf{m}_{r1}$ and $\mathbf{m}_{r2}$ are images of a reference space point.

[11] to compute the fundamental matrix from all the imaged points and use the three orthogonal vanishing points to calibrate the cameras. Since the reconstruction is defined up to a 3D similarity transformation with the ground truth, for convenience of comparison, we compute the transformation matrix by virtue of the point correspondences between the recovered structure and the associated ground truth, then register the reconstructed cube with the ground truth. The reconstructed cubes by different algorithms with 1-pixel image noise are shown in Fig.3(b), (c), and (d) respectively.

All the reconstructions are very close to the ground truth and there is not much difference visually. As stated in Section 3.2, the projection matrix is not unique if no further constraints are imposed. In order to give a more detailed evaluation, we vary the noise level from 0 to 3 pixels in step of 0.5. At each noise level we first calculate the distances between the reconstructed cubes and the ground truth (i.e. the distance between all the corresponding point pairs). Fig.5(a) shows the means and standard deviations of the distances at different noise level. The results at each noise level are evaluated by 200 independent tests so as to obtain statistically meaningful results.

One may see from Fig.5 that the proposed technique outperforms the stereovision method in the tests. This is because the proposed algorithm recovers the projection matrices directly from the vanishing points which may avoid error propagation along the computation chain. There are reports that it is unstable to compute the fundamental matrix when most of the points lie close to one or two planes [12]. The reconstruction errors are reduced greatly after optimization.

Table 1: The imaged vanishing points under different imaging conditions. 'Test-1' is in good imaging condition, 'Test-2' is in bad imaging condition, v_x, v_y, v_z stand for the imaged vanishing points of the axial directions.

Vanishing points		v_x	v_y	v_z
Test-1	View-1	[754.59, -46.52]	[-389.97, -734.41]	[-312.62, 520.16]
	View-2	[520.61, 80.13]	[-360.98, -651.02]	[-566.29, 682.80]
Test-2	View-1	[822.22, -503.42]	[-3558.04, -5294.58]	[-202.81, 185.42]
	View-2	[976.87, -695.60]	[-894.68, -911.27]	[-34.24, 297.09]

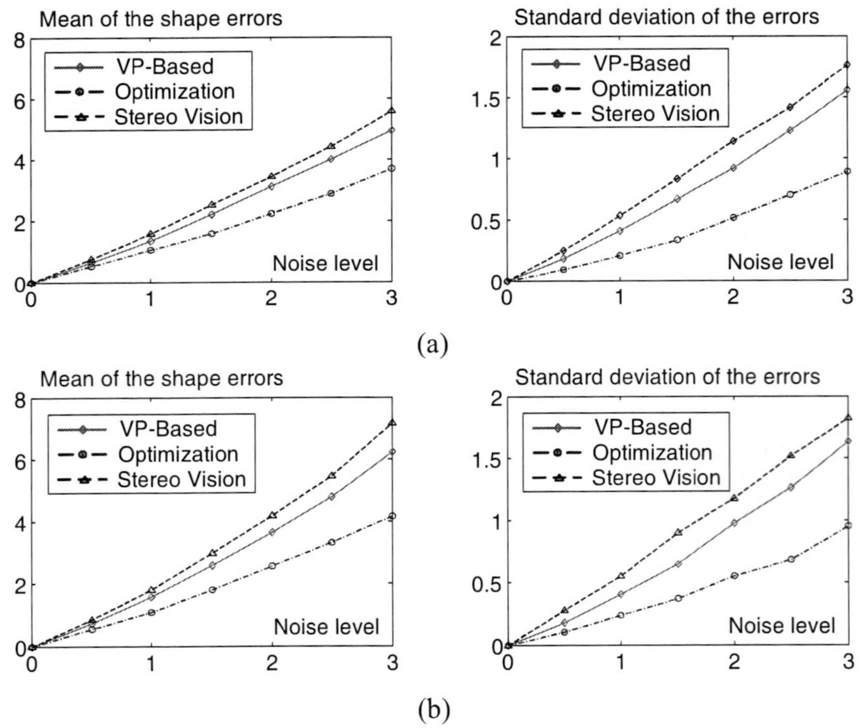

Figure 5: Some evaluation results in different imaging conditions, where 'VP-Based' stands for the proposed algorithm, 'Optimization' for the results after optimization, 'Stereo Vision' for the stereovision technique. (a) the mean and standard deviation of the errors between recovered structure and the ground truth at good imaging condition; (b) the mean and standard deviation of the reconstruction errors at bad imaging condition.

5.2 Comparative results in bad imaging conditions

In this simulation, we adopt different camera parameters and generated another set of images as shown in Fig.4(b). This is a relatively bad imaging condition compared to that of Test-1, since some of the imaged edges of the cube are short in length (see Fig.4) and some of the imaged vanishing points are far away from the images as shown in Table 1. This may cause a loss of accuracy in line fitting and vanishing point computation.

We implemented the three algorithms under the same conditions as in test 1. The reconstruction evaluations are shown in Fig.5(b). From the results we can see that the proposed algorithm outperforms the stereo vision algorithm and the optimization algorithm performs the best. While the means and standard deviations of the reconstruction errors are greater than those in good imaging conditions. However, the proposed algorithm may fail under extreme imaging conditions when the recovered vanishing points are deviated above a certain threshold. Nevertheless, the stereovision technique may also fail in these cases due to the errors introduced in calibration from these vanishing points. Besides, when the two views are in critical configuration such as with small baseline, the stereovision technique may fail due to the instability in the computation of the fundamental matrix. While this factor does not have much influence on the proposed algorithm.

6 Experiments with Real Images

We tested the proposed method on several sets of real images. Here we will report two results due to space limitation. One is the reconstruction of a single object from two images, the other is a building site of several architectures.

6.1 Reconstruction of a single object

The first test is based on two images of the Wadham College of Oxford which are downloaded from the Visual Geometry Group at the University of Oxford. As shown in Fig.6(a), the image resolution is 1024×768. We apply the Canny edge detector and orthogonal regression algorithm to fit the line segments in images [20], and compute the vanishing points from parallel lines using maximum likelihood estimation [14]. Fig.6(b) shows the detected line segments of the two images. We select the world coordinates and a pair of imaged reference points $\mathbf{m}_1$ and $\mathbf{m}_2$ as shown in Fig.6(a), then use the proposed algorithm to compute the projection matrices and reconstruct the object by interactively selecting the corner points of each planar surface. Fig.7 shows the reconstructed model with texture mapping and wireframe from different viewpoints. The results are realistic and largely consistent with the real cases.

We also carry a comparative study with the typical stereovision technique. When applying the proposed method to reconstruct the scene, we only need to seek the matches of some key corner points of each planar surface. However, for the stereovision algorithm, good initial correspondences should be established so as to obtain a stable and accurate estimation of the fundamental matrix. We adopted the method proposed by Yao and Cham [29] to establish more correspondences between the images as shown in Fig.6(c). The cameras are calibrated from the vanishing points using three-parameter-model. There are three

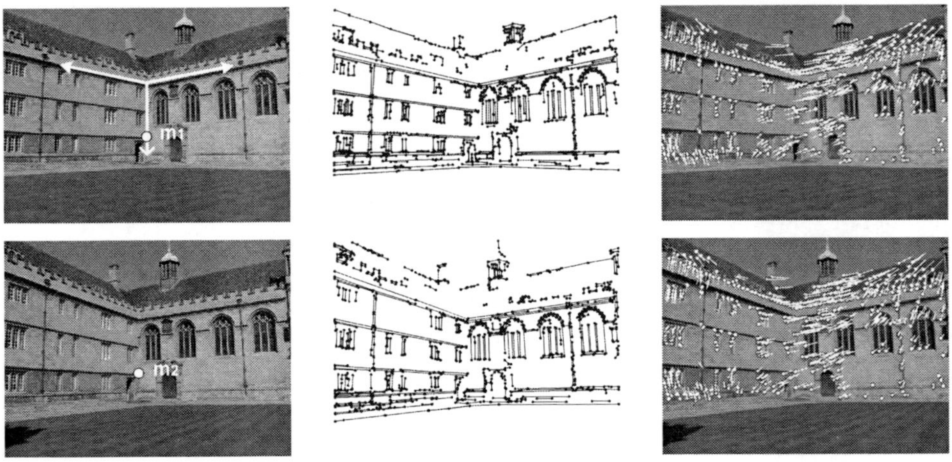

(a) (b) (c)

Figure 6: (a) Two images of the Wadham College of Oxford; (b) the corresponding detected line segments of the images; (c) the detected point matches overlaid with relative disparities.

mutually orthogonal planes in the scene, i.e. the ground plane, the left and the right walls. We take this observation as the ground truth and estimate the errors of reconstructed angles between these planes. The three errors by the proposed algorithm are $0.13°$, $0.30°$ and $0.38°$ respectively. The corresponding errors by the stereovision technique are $0.23°$, $0.35°$ and $0.33°$ respectively, two of them are larger than those of the proposed method.

6.2 Reconstruction of building site

In this section, we will present an example on structure recovery of a building site with several architectures. The site is the University Square of the Chinese University of Hong Kong, where there are four buildings around the square as shown in Fig.8(c) and (d). All images here are taken by Canon PowerShot G3 digital camera with the resolution of 1024×768. There are 16 images of the University Library and 12 images of the Sui-Loong Pao Building as shown in Fig.8(a) and (b).

We recover the structures of the two buildings separately from their own image sequence by the proposed algorithm. The reconstructed models from different viewpoints are shown in Fig.9, where the textures mapped to the model is modified slightly from their original images so as to remove some occlusions. We then use the proposed technique of visual metrology to recover the scale, orientation and relative position of the two buildings and register them to the same coordinate frame. The final model of the University Square is shown in Fig.10. Here we only reconstructed two buildings of the site and some virtual objects, such as cars, trees, flowers, square lamp, etc. are registered and inserted into the final model. Compared with the model generated by some commercial CAD softwares, the proposed algorithm only need a few human interactions and the result seems more accurate and realistic since it is directly computed from images. It should be noted that due to camera limitations and the shoot position, we do not obtain any good birdview images of the site, thus the relative scales and positions of the objects in the final model are not very accurate.

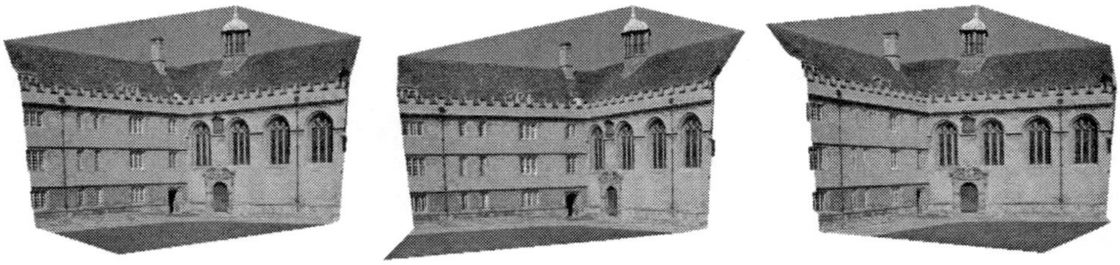

(a)

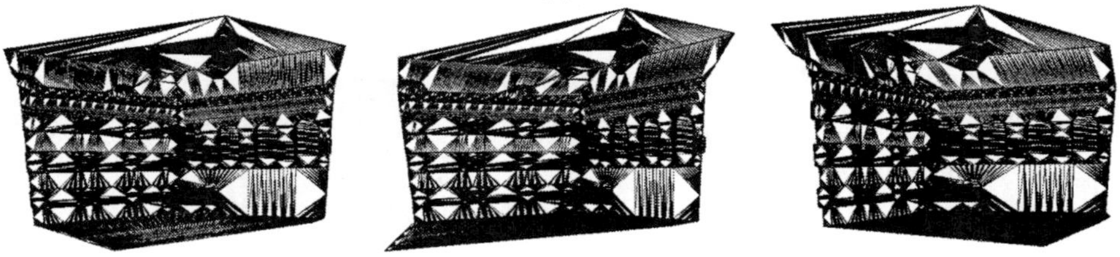

(b)

Figure 7: The reconstruction result of the Wadham College. (a) the reconstructed model by the proposed algorithm under different viewpoints with texture mapping; (b) the corresponding wireframes of the model.

7 Conclusion

In this chapter, under the assumption of three-parameter-camera model, we proved that the projection matrix can be recovered uniquely from three orthogonal vanishing points with a certain preselected world frame. We also proved that the global consistent projection matrices can be obtained by virtue of an arbitrary reference point in space. Compared with previous stereovision techniques, the method avoids the bottleneck problem of image matching and is easy to implement. Therefore a more accurate and robust result is expected. Extensive experiments on synthetic and real images validate the effectiveness of the algorithm. The proposed method is applicable to reconstruct photo-realistic and accurate model of structured scenes, especially those containing three dominate directions and some planar surfaces. However, more human interactions may be needed if one want to reconstruct more details of the scene. In practice, the method may be combined with classical stereovision technique so as to obtain better results with minimal interactions. It is obvious that the precision of the proposed algorithm depends greatly on that of the image pretreatment, such as edge detection, line fitting and vanishing point determination. Hence, it is crucial to select a robust edge detection and line fitting technique so as to increase the accuracy of measurement. The proposed method may find its use in many areas such as Augmented Reality, real estate demonstration, etc.

Acknowledgment

The work is supported in part by the Canada Research Chair program, the NSERC Discovery Grant, and the National Natural Science Foundation of China under Grant No. 60575015.

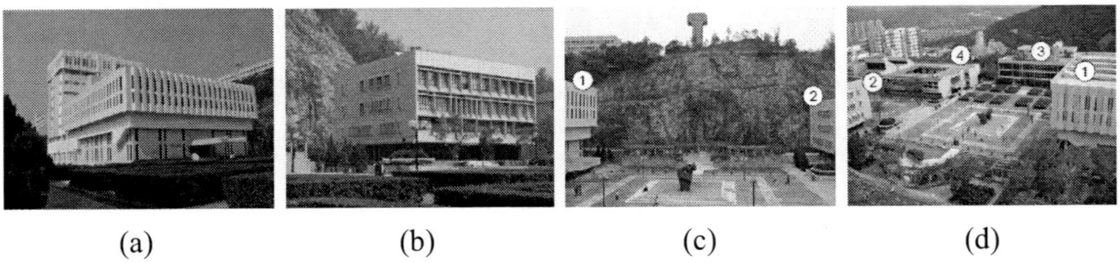

Figure 8: (a) One sample image of the University Library sequence; (b) one sample image of the Sui-Loong Pao Building sequence; (c)&(d) two birdview images of the University Square, where the building No.1 is the University Library, No.2 is the Sui-Loong Pao Building, No.3 is the University Administration Building, No.4 is the Institute of Chinese Studies.

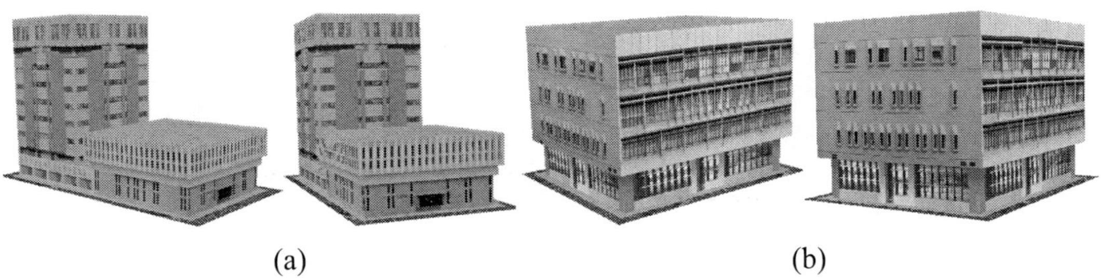

Figure 9: The reconstructed models of the University Library (a) and the Sui-Loong Pao Building (b) under different viewpoints with texture mapping.

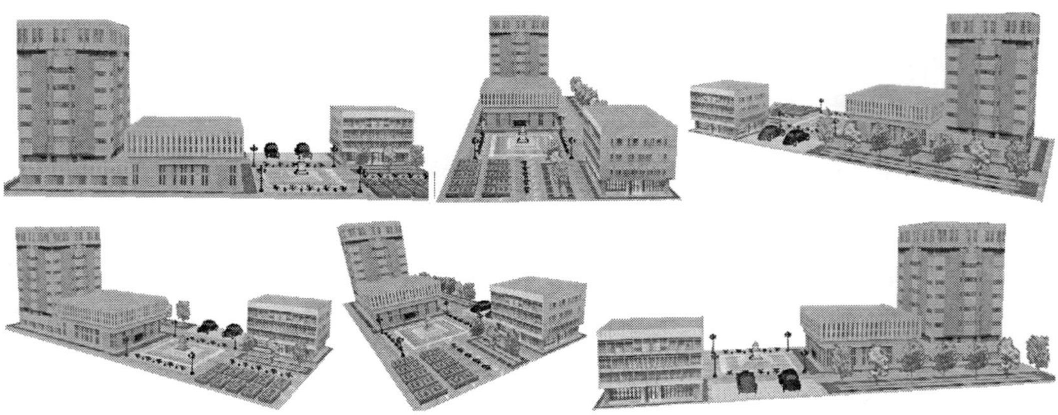

Figure 10: The reconstructed virtue model of the University Square under different viewpoints.

References

[1] Almansa, A., Desolneux, A., Vamech, S., Vanishing point detection without any a priori information, IEEE Trans. on Pattern Analysis and Machine Intelligence 25 (4) (2003) 502–507.

[2] Baillard, C., Schmid, C., Zisserman, A., Fitzgibbon, A., Automatic line matching and 3D reconstruction of buildings from multiple views, in: ISPRS Conference on Automatic Extraction of GIS Objects from Digital Imagery, IAPRS Vol.32, Part 3-2W5, 1999, pp. 69–80.

[3] Baillard, C., Zisserman, A., Automatic reconstruction of piecewise planar models from multiple views, in: Proceedings of the IEEE Conference on Computer Vision and Pattern Recognition, Vol. 2, 1999, pp. 2559–2665.

[4] Bartoli, A., Sturm, P., Constrained structure and motion from multiple uncalibrated views of a piecewise planar scene, International Journal of Computer Vision 52 (1) (2003) 45–64.

[5] Caprile, B., Torre, V., Using vanishing points for camera calibration, International Journal of Computer Vision 4 (2) (1990) 127–140.

[6] Cipolla, D., Robertson, R., Boyer, E., Photobuilder-3D models of architectural scenes from uncalibrated images, in: Proceedings of IEEE International Conference on Multimedia Computing and Systems, Vol. 1, 1999, pp. 25–31.

[7] Criminisi, A., Reid, I., Zisserman, A., Single view metrology, International Journal of Computer Vision 40 (2) (2000) 123–148.

[8] Debevec, C., Taylor, P., Malik, J., Modeling and rendering architecture from photographs: a hybrid geometry-and imaged-based approach, in: Proceedings of SIGGRAPH, 1996, pp. 11–21.

[9] Faugeras, O.D., Three-dimensional computer vision: a geometric viewpoint, MIT press, Cambridge, 1993.

[10] Grossmanna, E., and Santos-Victor, J., Least-squares 3D reconstruction from one or more views and geometric clues, Computer Vision and Image Understanding, 99(2) (2005) 151–174.

[11] Hartley, R., In defense of the eight-point model, IEEE Trans. on Pattern Analysis and Machine Intelligence 19 (1997) 580–593.

[12] Hartley, R., Zisserman, A., Multiple View Geometry in Computer Vision, 2nd Edition, Cambridge University Press, ISBN: 0521540518, 2004.

[13] Košechá, J., and Zhang, W., Extraction, matching, and pose recovery based on dominant rectangular structures, Computer Vision and Image Understanding, 100(3) (2005) 274–293.

[14] Liebowitz, D., Criminisi, A., Zisserman, A., Creating architectural models from images, in: Proceedings of Eurographics, Milan, Italy, 1999, pp. 39–50.

[15] McLean, G., Kotturi, D., Vanishing point detection by line clustering, IEEE Trans. on Pattern Analysis and Machine Intelligence, 17 (11) (1995) 1090–1095.

[16] Müller, P., Zeng, G., Wonka, P., Van Gool, L., Image-based procedural modeling of facades, ACM Transactions on Graphics (TOG), v.26 n.3, July 2007

[17] Pu, S., Vosselman, G., Automatic extraction of building features from terrestrial laser scanning International Archives of Photogrammetry, Remote Sensing and Spatial Information Sciences, vol. 36, part 5, (2006) 25-27

[18] Saxena, A., Chung, S.H., Ng, A.Y., 3-D Depth Reconstruction from a Single Still Image, International Journal of Computer Vision 76 (1) (2008) 53–69.

[19] Saxena, A. Min S. Ng, A.Y., Make3D: Learning 3D Scene Structure from a Single Still Image IEEE Trans. on Pattern Analysis and Machine Intelligence, 31 (5) (2009) 824–840.

[20] Schmid, C., Zisserman, A., Automatic line matching across views, in: Proceedings of IEEE Conference on Computer Vision and Pattern Recognition, 1997, pp. 666–671.

[21] Seo, K., Lee, J., Choi, H., An efficient detection of vanishing points using inverted coordinates image space, Pattern Recognition Letters 27 (2) (2006) 102–108.

[22] Van den Heuvel, F.A., 3D reconstruction from a single image using geometric constraints, ISPRS Journal of Photogrammetry & Remote Sensing 53 (6) (1998) 354–368.

[23] Wang, G., Hu, Z., *et.al.*, Single view metrology from scene constraints., Image Vision Comput. 23 (9) (2005) 831–840.

[24] Wang, G., Tsui, H.T., Hu, Z., Reconstruction of structured scenes from two uncalibrated images., Pattern Recognition Letters 26 (2) (2005) 207–220.

[25] Wang, G., Tsui, H.T., *et.al.*, Camera calibration and 3D reconstruction from a single view based on scene constraints., Image Vision Comput. 23 (3) (2005) 311–323.

[26] Wang, G., Tsui, H.T., Wu, Q.M.J., What can we learn about the scene structure from three orthogonal vanishing points in images. Pattern Recognition Letters 30(3): 192-202 (2009)

[27] Werner, T., Zisserman, A., New techniques for automated architecture reconstruction from photographs, in: Proceedings of the 7th European Conference on Computer Vision, Vol. 2, 2002, pp. 541–555.

[28] Wilczkowiak, E., Boyer, M., Sturm, P., 3D modeling using geometric constraints: a parallelepiped based approach, in: Proceedings of the 7th European Conference on Computer Vision, Vol. IV, 2002, pp. 221–237.

[29] Yao, J., Cham, W., Feature matching and scene reconstruction from multiple widely separated views, Technical Report, Department of Electronic Engineering, The Chinese University of Hong Kong, 2005.

In: 3D Imaging: Theory, Technology... ISBN 978-1-60876-885-1
Editors: E. H. Duke and S. R. Aguirre, pp. 293-311

Chapter 14

Structure Recovery of Nonrigid Objects under Perspective Projection Based on Power Factorization

Guanghui Wang and Q. M. Jonathan Wu
Department of Electrical and Computer Engineering,
University of Windsor,
Windsor, Ontario, Canada, N9B 3P4

Abstract

The chapter addresses the problem of estimating 3D structure and motion of non-rigid object from a monocular image sequence. Many previous methods on this problem adopt the extension technique of SVD factorization based on rank constraint to the tracking matrix, where the 3D shape of nonrigid object is expressed as weighted combination of a set of shape bases. Most solutions are based on the assumption of affine camera model which may be invalid when the object is close to the camera. The chapter makes two contributions to the problem. Firstly, we propose a constrained power factorization (CPF) algorithm that combines the orthonormal constraint and the replicated block structure of the motion matrix directly into the iteration steps of power factorization. This algorithm overcomes the limitations of previous SVD based methods. It is easy to implement and can even deal with missing data in the tracking matrix. Secondly, we propose two techniques to upgrade the solutions from affine assumption to full perspective camera model. The first algorithm updates the solutions from affine to perspective projection by linear recursive estimation. The second one is based on nonlinear optimization technique by minimizing the perspective reprojection residuals. Extensive tests on synthetic and real images validate the proposed method and noticeable improvements over previous solutions are observed.

1. Introduction

The problem of structure and motion recovery from image sequences is an important theme in computer vision. Great progresses have been made for different applications during the last two decades [14]. Among these methods, factorization based approach, for its robust behavior and accuracy, is widely studied since it deals uniformly with the data sets of all images [21, 25, 28]. The factorization algorithm was first proposed by Tomasi and Kanade [25] in the early 90's. The main idea of this algorithm is to factorize the tracking matrix into motion and structure matrices simultaneously by singular value decomposition (SVD) with low-rank approximation. The algorithm assumes an orthographic projection model. It was extended to weak perspective and paraperspective projection in [21].

More generally, Christy and Horaud [7] extended the above methods to a perspective camera model by incrementally performing the factorization under affine assumption. The method is an affine approximation to general perspective projection. Triggs and Sturm [24, 28] proposed a full projective reconstruction method via rank-4 factorization of a scaled tracking matrix with projective depths recovered from pairwise epipolar geometry. The method was further studied in [11, 15, 18], where different iterative schemes were proposed to recover the projective depths through minimizing reprojection errors. Recently, Oliensis and Hartley [20] provided a complete theoretical convergence analysis for the iterative extensions. Unfortunately, no iteration has been shown to converge sensibly, and they proposed a simple extension to give a reliable initialization to other algorithms.

The above methods work only for rigid objects and static scenes. Whereas in real world, many scenarios are nonrigid or dynamic such as articulated motion, human faces carrying different expressions, lip movements, hand gesture, and moving vehicles etc. In order to deal with such situations, many extensions stemming from the factorization algorithm were proposed to relax the rigidity constraint. Costeira and Kanade [8] first discussed how to recover the motion and shape of several independent moving objects via factorization using orthographic projection. Bascle and Blake [1] proposed a method for factorizing facial expressions and poses based on a set of preselected basis images. Recently, Li *et al.* [16] proposed to segment multiple rigid-body motions from point correspondences via subspace separation. Yan and Pollefeys [37, 38] proposed a factorization-based approach to recover the structure and kinematic chain of articulated objects.

In the pioneer work by Bregler *et al.* [4], it is demonstrated that the 3D shape of a nonrigid object can be expressed as a weighted linear combination of a set of shape bases. Then the shape bases and camera motions are factorized simultaneously for all time instants under the rank constraint of the tracking matrix. Following this idea, the method was extensively investigated and developed by many researchers, such as Brand [2, 3], Del Bue *et al.* [9, 10], Torresani *et al.* [26, 27], and Xiao *et al.* [35, 36]. Recently, Rabaud and Belongie [23] relaxed the Bregler's assumption [4] by assuming that only small neighborhoods of shapes are well-modeled by a linear subspace, and proposed a novel approach to solve the problem by adopting a manifold-learning framework.

Most nonrigid factorization methods are based on affine camera model due to its simplicity. It was extended to perspective projection in [36] by iteratively recovering the projective depths. The perspective factorization is more complicated and does not guarantee its convergence to the correct depths, especially for nonrigid scenarios [14]. Vidal and Abretske [29] proposed that the constraints among multiple views of a nonrigid shape consisting of k shape bases can be reduced to multilinear constraints. They presented a closed form solution to the reconstruction of a nonrigid shape consisting of two shape bases. Hartley and Vidal [13] proposed a closed form solution to the nonrigid shape and motion with calibrated cameras or fixed intrinsic parameters. More recently, Wang and Wu [34] proposed a quasi-perspective projection model under assumption of small camera movement. Since the factorization is only defined up to a nonsingular transformation matrix, many researchers adopt the metric constraints to recover the matrix and upgrade the factorization to the Euclidean space [2, 4, 10, 27]. However, the rotation constraint may cause ambiguity in the combination of shape bases. Xiao *et al.* [35] proposed a basis constraint to solve the ambiguity and provided a closed-form solution.

The essence of the factorization algorithm is to find a low-rank approximation of the tracking matrix. Most algorithms adopt SVD to compute the approximation. Alternatively, Hartley and Schaffalizky [12] proposed to use power factorization (PF) to find a low-rank approximation. The method is derived from the Power method in matrix computation and the sequential factorization method [19], which is actually an alternated least-square method. One noteworthy advantage of the PF algorithm is its ability to handle missing data in a tracking matrix, while SVD-based algorithm is hard to deal with incomplete tracking matrix with some entries unavailable. Vidal and Hartley [30] proposed to combine the PF algorithm for motion segmentation. Wang *et al.* extended the PF algorithm to nonrigid factorization in both metric space [32] and affine space [33]. There are many other nonlinear based studies to the missing data problem, such as Damped Newton method [5] and Levenberg-Marquardt based method [6]. Torresani *et al.* [26] proposed a Probabilistic Principal Components Analysis (PPCA) shape model and estimation algorithm to estimate the 3D shape and motion simultaneously and robustly fill-in the missing data.

Most previous nonrigid factorization methods are based on affine camera model, which is a zero-order (for weak perspective) or first-order (for paraperspective) approximation to the real imaging conditions and is only valid when the depth variation of the object is small compared to the distance between the object and the camera. Therefore, large reconstruction errors may be caused when the object is close to the camera. In this chapter, we will extend the general power factorization algorithm to nonrigid case and proposed a constrained power factorization (CPF) algorithm. The method can overcome the limitations of previous SVD based method and is easy to implement. We then extend the algorithm in [7] to the nonrigid case so as to upgrade the solutions under affine assumption to those under full perspective projection. Two kinds of algorithms, namely the linear recursive approximation and the nonlinear optimization, are proposed. Experiments demonstrate the effectiveness of the algorithms and the improvements to the final solutions. Part of this chapter was previous published in [31][32].

The chapter is organized as follows: We first introduce the SVD based nonrigid factorization method in section 2. Then the rotation constrained power factorization algorithm is elaborated in section 3. Two algorithms for upgrading the solutions from affine to perspective projection are presented in section 4. Some simulation and comparison results are illustrated in section 5, followed by the experiment results on real image sequences in section 6. Finally, a conclusion is given in section 7.

2. Background on Nonrigid Factorization via SVD

Suppose the camera is calibrated and we are working with normalized image coordinates. Given a sequence of m video frames and n tracked feature points across the sequence. Let

$\{\mathbf{x}_i^{(j)} \in \mathbb{R}^2\}_{i=1,\ldots,n}^{j=1,\ldots,m}$ be the normalized coordinates of these features. The aim is to recover the shape $\mathbf{S}^{(j)} \in \mathbb{R}^{3\times n}$ (i.e. the corresponding 3D coordinates of the features) and the motion $\mathbf{R}^{(j)} \in \mathbb{R}^{3\times 3}$ that correspond to each frame.

As described by Bregler *et.al.* [4], the nonrigid shape can be represented as weighted combination of k shape bases, i.e. $\mathbf{S}^{(j)} = \sum_{l=1}^{k} \omega_l^{(j)}\mathbf{S}_l$, where, $\mathbf{S}_l \in \mathbb{R}^{3\times n}$ is one of the shape bases, $\omega_l^{(j)} \in \mathbb{R}$ is the deformation weight (a perfect rigid object would correspond to the case of $k = 1$ and $\omega_l^{(j)} = 1$). Under the weak perspective assumption, we have:

$$[\mathbf{x}_1^{(j)}, \mathbf{x}_2^{(j)}, \cdots, \mathbf{x}_n^{(j)}] = \mathbf{R}_w^{(j)}\Big(\sum_{l=1}^{k}\omega_l^{(j)}\mathbf{S}_l\Big) + \mathbf{T}_w^{(j)}, (j = 1, \cdots, m) \tag{1}$$

where, $\mathbf{R}_w^{(j)}$ stands for the first two rows of the rotation matrix corresponding to the jth frame. $\mathbf{T}_w^{(j)}$ is the corresponding translation of the camera. If we register the coordinates of all image features to their centroid in each frame, then the translation term can be eliminated, and we can obtain the factorization expression of the tracking matrix by stacking all equations in (1) for each frame.

$$\mathbf{W}_{2m\times n} = \begin{bmatrix} \mathbf{x}_1^{(1)} & \cdots & \mathbf{x}_n^{(1)} \\ \vdots & \ddots & \vdots \\ \mathbf{x}_1^{(m)} & \cdots & \mathbf{x}_n^{(m)} \end{bmatrix}_{2m\times n}$$

$$= \begin{bmatrix} \omega_1^{(1)}\mathbf{R}_w^{(1)} & \cdots & \omega_k^{(1)}\mathbf{R}_w^{(1)} \\ \vdots & \ddots & \vdots \\ \omega_1^{(m)}\mathbf{R}_w^{(m)} & \cdots & \omega_k^{(m)}\mathbf{R}_w^{(m)} \end{bmatrix}_{2m\times 3k} \begin{bmatrix} \mathbf{S}_1 \\ \vdots \\ \mathbf{S}_k \end{bmatrix}_{3k\times n} \tag{2}$$

The above equation can be written in short as $\mathbf{W}_{2m\times n} = \mathbf{M}_{2m\times 3k}\mathbf{B}_{3k\times n}$. It is easy to see from the right side of (2) that the rank of the tracking matrix $\mathbf{W}$ is at most $3k$ (usually $2m$ and n are larger than $3k$ respectively). By performing singular value decomposition (SVD) on the tracking matrix and imposing the rank constraint, $\mathbf{W}$ may be factored as $\mathbf{W}_{2m\times n} = \tilde{\mathbf{M}}_{2m\times 3k}\tilde{\mathbf{B}}_{3k\times n}$. However, the decomposition is not unique since it is only defined up to a non-singular $3k\times 3k$ linear transformation as $\mathbf{W} = \mathbf{M}\mathbf{B} = (\tilde{\mathbf{M}}\mathbf{G})(\mathbf{G}^{-1}\tilde{\mathbf{B}})$. If the transformation $\mathbf{G}$ is known, the shape bases can be recovered from $\mathbf{B} = \mathbf{G}^{-1}\tilde{\mathbf{B}}$, while the rotation matrix $\mathbf{R}_w^{(j)}$ and the weighting coefficient $\omega_l^{(j)}$ may be recovered from $\mathbf{M} = \tilde{\mathbf{M}}\mathbf{G}$ by Procrustes analysis, such as sub-block factorization [2][4] or a further iterative optimization step proposed in [27].

The computation of the transformation matrix $\mathbf{G}$ is a very important step here. Many researchers [2][4] utilize the rotation constraint to the motion matrix. Let $\mathbf{Q} = \mathbf{G}\mathbf{G}^T$, which is a positive definite symmetric matrix with $(9k^2 + 3k)/2$ unknowns, then from $\mathbf{M}\mathbf{M}^T = \tilde{\mathbf{M}}\mathbf{G}\mathbf{G}^T\tilde{\mathbf{M}}^T$ we have:

$$\tilde{\mathbf{M}}_{2i-1:2i}\mathbf{Q}\,\tilde{\mathbf{M}}_{2j-1:2j}^T = \sum_{l=1}^{k}\omega_l^{(i)}\omega_l^{(j)}\mathbf{R}_w^{(i)}(\mathbf{R}_w^{(j)})^T, (i, j = 1, \cdots, m) \tag{3}$$

where, $\tilde{\mathbf{M}}_{2i-1:2i}$ stands for the ith two-row of $\tilde{\mathbf{M}}$. Expanding (3) and considering the orthonormality of $\mathbf{R}_w^{(i)}$ may yields the following linear constrains on $\mathbf{Q}$.

$$\begin{cases} \tilde{\mathbf{M}}_{2i-1}\mathbf{Q}\,\tilde{\mathbf{M}}_{2i-1}^T = \tilde{\mathbf{M}}_{2i}\mathbf{Q}\,\tilde{\mathbf{M}}_{2i}^T = \sum_{l=1}^{k}\left(\omega_l^{(i)}\right)^2 \\ \tilde{\mathbf{M}}_{2i-1}\mathbf{Q}\,\tilde{\mathbf{M}}_{2i}^T = \tilde{\mathbf{M}}_{2i}\mathbf{Q}\,\tilde{\mathbf{M}}_{2i-1}^T = 0 \end{cases} \tag{4}$$

It appears that if we have enough features and frames, there will be enough constraints and the matrix $\mathbf{Q}$ can be solved linearly by stacking all the equations in (4). However, as proved in [35], only the rotation constraints may be insufficient when the object deforms at varying speed, since most of the equations in (4) are redundant. Another drawback of using only rotation constraint is that there has no constraints on the deformation weights, thus the recovered shape bases may not correspond to some reasonable shapes, since one may recover a large shape basis with small corresponding weight or a small basis with large weight and achieve the same reconstruction from their combination.

To solve the ambiguity in computing the correct transformation, Xiao *et.al.* [35] introduced the basis constraint, whose main idea is to select k frames that includes independent shapes and take them as a set of bases. For example, suppose the first k frames are independent on each other, then we may take their corresponding shapes as the bases, and the corresponding weighting coefficients can be determined as:

$$\begin{cases} \omega_i^{(i)} = 1, \ (i = 1, \cdots, k) \\ \omega_i^{(j)} = 0, \ (i, j = 1, \cdots, k \ and \ i \neq j) \end{cases} \tag{5}$$

However, it is not easy to select the set of bases automatically in practice. Since any k frames may seem to be numerically independent under noisy measurements, even though they are indeed mutually dependent. A false selection of the bases may cause large errors to the recovered shapes.

After the matrix $\mathbf{Q}$ is obtained, the transformation $\mathbf{G}$ can be recovered via eigen decomposition [2] or Choleskey decomposition [14]. However, in norigid case, the recovered matrix $\mathbf{M} = \tilde{\mathbf{M}}\mathbf{G}$ usually does not conform to the replicated block structure of the motion matrix in (2), thus a Procrustes analysis as in [4] [27] is needed so as to obtain the rotation matrices and the deformation weights from the motion matrix. The process may introduce additional errors to the final results. Another problem of the method is that the recovered matrix $\mathbf{Q}$ may not be positive definite in some situations due to image noise, thus it is impossible to decompose the correct $\mathbf{G}$ from it except for some approximation methods as given in [2].

3. Rotation Constrained Power Factorization

The general power factorization method (PF) in [12] was proposed to find a low-rank approximation of a tracking matrix of static scene. Suppose $\mathbf{W} \in \mathbb{R}^{2m\times n}$ is the tracking matrix, we wish to find two rank-r matrices $\mathbf{A} \in \mathbb{R}^{2m\times r}$ and $\mathbf{B} \in \mathbb{R}^{n\times r}$ such that $\left\|\mathbf{W} - \mathbf{A}\mathbf{B}^T\right\|_F$ is minimized. The method starts with an initially random selected $2m \times r$ matrix $\mathbf{A}_0$ and iterates as follows:

$$\begin{aligned} \mathbf{B}_t &= \mathbf{W}^T\mathbf{A}_{t-1}\left(\mathbf{A}_{t-1}^T\mathbf{A}_{t-1}\right)^{-1} \\ \mathbf{A}_t &= \mathbf{W}\mathbf{B}_t\left(\mathbf{B}_t^T\mathbf{B}_t\right)^{-1} \end{aligned} \tag{6}$$

until the product $\mathbf{A}_t\mathbf{B}_t^T$ converges. As stated in the study [12], the above iteration process converges quickly to the global minimum solution provided that $\mathbf{W}$ is close to have rank r.

Compared with the SVD based method, the power factorization algorithm is very simple and computational cheap, since it only involves the multiplication and inverse of matrix. One noteworthy point of the method is that it allows us to deal with the tracking matrix with incomplete data, since each update in (6) is equivalent to solving a linear least squares problem that can be done only with the existing entries of the tracking matrix.

In the case of nonrigid factorization, our objective is to recover the motion matrix $\mathbf{M} \in \mathbb{R}^{2m\times 3k}$ and the shape matrix $\mathbf{B} \in \mathbb{R}^{3k\times n}$ as shown in (2). Intuitively, this is similar to the above case for rigid and static scene, and the power factorization method may be employed directly here. However, the recovered motion matrix by (6) does not observe the replicated block structure of the motion matrix in (2), thus it is defined up to a correction matrix $\mathbf{G}$ that is not easy to compute as explained in the previous section. In the following, we will introduce a constrained power factorization algorithm (CPF) to solve this problem. Let us denote the motion matrix of (2) into two parts:

$$\mathbf{M} = \mathbf{\Omega} \otimes \mathbf{\Phi} = \begin{bmatrix} \omega_1^{(1)} & \cdots & \omega_k^{(1)} \\ \vdots & \ddots & \vdots \\ \omega_1^{(m)} & \cdots & \omega_k^{(m)} \end{bmatrix} \otimes \begin{bmatrix} \mathbf{R}_w^{(1)} & \cdots & \mathbf{R}_w^{(1)} \\ \vdots & \ddots & \vdots \\ \mathbf{R}_w^{(m)} & \cdots & \mathbf{R}_w^{(m)} \end{bmatrix} \tag{7}$$

where $\mathbf{\Omega}$ denotes the weighting part, $\mathbf{\Phi}$ denotes the rotation part, $'\otimes'$ stands for the element-by-element multiplication. Then the algorithm can be summarized as follows.

Algorithm 1 (Constrained power factorization). Given the tracking matrix $\mathbf{W} \in \mathbb{R}^{2m\times n}$, initial rotation part $\mathbf{\Phi}_0 \in \mathbb{R}^{2m\times 3k}$ and initial shape matrix $\mathbf{B}_0 \in \mathbb{R}^{3k\times n}$. Repeat the following 3 steps until the product of $(\mathbf{\Omega}_t \otimes \mathbf{\Phi}_t)\mathbf{B}_t$ convergence.

1. Given $\mathbf{\Phi}_{t-1}$ and $\mathbf{B}_{t-1}$, find $\mathbf{\Omega}_t$ that minimize $\|\mathbf{W} - (\mathbf{\Omega}_t \otimes \mathbf{\Phi}_{t-1})\mathbf{B}_{t-1}\|_F$;

2. Given $\mathbf{\Phi}_{t-1}$ and $\mathbf{\Omega}_t$, find $\mathbf{B}_t$ that minimize $\|\mathbf{W} - (\mathbf{\Omega}_t \otimes \mathbf{\Phi}_{t-1})\mathbf{B}_t\|_F$;

3. Given $\mathbf{\Omega}_t$ and $\mathbf{B}_t$, find $\mathbf{\Phi}_t$ that minimize $\|\mathbf{W} - (\mathbf{\Omega}_t \otimes \mathbf{\Phi}_t)\mathbf{B}_t\|_F$, subject to the constraint that $\mathbf{\Phi}_t$ is a block replicated rotation matrix.

In the above algorithm, step 3 is the most important step, since the orthonormal property of the rotation matrix and the block structure of the motion matrix are explicitly involved into the minimization scheme. Here we will give the computation details of this step. For simplicity, the iteration times (i.e. the subscripts t) will be ignored in the following analysis.

Suppose $\mathbf{W}^{(j)} \in \mathbb{R}^{2\times n}$ is the jth two-row of $\mathbf{W}$, which is composed of the tracked features in the jth frame. Then we have:

$$\mathbf{W}^{(j)} = \mathbf{R}_w^{(j)}\mathbf{S}^{(j)}, \quad \mathbf{S}^{(j)} = \sum\nolimits_{l=1}^{k} \omega_l^{(j)}\mathbf{S}_l \tag{8}$$

where $\mathbf{R}_w^{(j)}$ is the first two rows of the rotation matrix corresponding to the jth frame, $\mathbf{S}^{(j)}$ is the corresponding affine shape of this frame, $\omega_l^{(j)}$ is the deformation weight that can be obtained from $\mathbf{\Omega}_t$ in step 1, $\mathbf{S}_t$ is the shape basis that can be obtained from $\mathbf{B}_t$ in step 2. Therefore, $\mathbf{R}_w^{(j)}$ may be computed via least squares as:

$$\mathbf{R}_w^{(j)} = \mathbf{W}^{(j)}(\mathbf{S}^{(j)})^T\left(\mathbf{S}^{(j)}(\mathbf{S}^{(j)})^T\right)^{-1} \tag{9}$$

The so recovered rotation matrix, however, may not be a true rotation matrix. Thus the orthonormal constraint should be enforced afterward. Suppose the SVD decomposition of $\mathbf{R}_w^{(j)}$ is $\mathbf{U}\mathbf{\Sigma}\mathbf{V}^T$, where $\mathbf{\Sigma}$ is a 2×3 matrix made of the two singular values of $\mathbf{R}_w^{(j)}$. Thus we may obtain the best approximation to the rotation matrix from

$$\mathbf{R}_w^{(j)} = \mathbf{U}\begin{bmatrix} 1 & 0 & 0 \\ 0 & 1 & 0 \end{bmatrix}\mathbf{V}^T \tag{10}$$

since a rotation matrix should have unit singular values. Straightforwardly, the matrix $\mathbf{\Phi}_t$ can be recovered.

The main difference of the proposed algorithm with general power factorization is that we divide the computation of $\mathbf{M}$ into two steps (i.e. the computation of weighting part $\mathbf{\Omega}$ and that of the rotation part $\mathbf{\Phi}$). This makes it simple and efficient to combine the rotation constraint and the repeated block structure of the motion matrix into the computation. Nevertheless, as one may see from the experiments, this kind of process will not affect the convergence property of the algorithm. Suppose s_i is the ith largest singular value of $\mathbf{W}$, then the convergence is closely related with the property of $\mathbf{W}$, i.e. $(s_{3k+1}/s_{3k})^{2t}$, the initial values of $\mathbf{B}_0$ and $\mathbf{\Phi}_0$. However, the convergence speed may be somewhat slower than that of the process of (6) due to the enforcement of orthonormal constraint to the rotation matrix.

Determination of the convergence: There are several methods to determine the convergence of the algorithm. The most feasible way is to check the variation of the reprojected tracking matrix. Suppose $\mathbf{W}_t = (\mathbf{\Omega}_t \otimes \mathbf{\Phi}_t)\mathbf{B}_t$ is the reprojected tracking matrix at the tth iteration, then the variation can be defined as the Frobenius norm of the difference with previous iteration:

$$\delta = \left\|\mathbf{W}_t - \mathbf{W}_{t-1}\right\|_F \tag{11}$$

The algorithm will converge ($\delta \to 0$) usually after about 5 iterations when reasonable initial values are provided.

Selection of initial values: In nonrigid case, the expected shape of the object is expressed as the weighted combination of a set of shape bases. This kind of expression is not unique if no constraints are enforced to the bases. Therefore, during the implementation of the CPF algorithm, it is crucial to provide reasonable initial values of $\mathbf{B}_0$ and $\mathbf{\Phi}_0$ so as to achieve better solutions of the problem and speed up the convergence rate at the same time. In our applications, we first take the object as a rigid one and utilize the weak perspective rank-3 factorization method [21][25] to factorize the tracking matrix into $\mathbf{W} = \hat{\mathbf{M}}\hat{\mathbf{B}}$, where $\hat{\mathbf{M}} \in \mathbb{R}^{2m\times 3}$ is the rigid motion matrix that contains m two-row rotation matrices $\hat{\mathbf{R}}_w^{(j)}$ corresponding to all the frames, $\hat{\mathbf{B}} \in \mathbb{R}^{3\times n}$ is the rigid affine shape of the n tracked features. Then we may set the first shape basis $\hat{\mathbf{S}}_1 = \hat{\mathbf{B}}$, other shape bases $\hat{\mathbf{S}}_l$ $(l = 2, ..., k)$ as $\hat{\mathbf{B}}$ with randomly added small noise such that they are independent with each other. Thus the initial values may be constructed as:

$$\mathbf{\Phi}_0 = [\hat{\mathbf{M}}, \cdots, \hat{\mathbf{M}}] = \begin{bmatrix} \hat{\mathbf{R}}_w^{(1)} & \cdots & \hat{\mathbf{R}}_w^{(1)} \\ \vdots & \ddots & \vdots \\ \hat{\mathbf{R}}_w^{(m)} & \cdots & \hat{\mathbf{R}}_w^{(m)} \end{bmatrix}, \quad \mathbf{B}_0 = \begin{bmatrix} \hat{\mathbf{S}}_1 \\ \vdots \\ \hat{\mathbf{S}}_k \end{bmatrix} \tag{12}$$

The reasons for doing so are based on two observations: First, most nonrigid object may be approximated by a rigid one, and the motions recovered by rigid factorization are usually very close to the real solutions, this is why we update the rotation part at the last step in the algorithm, though the order of these steps can be exchanged. Second, all shape bases of the same nonrigid object should have almost the same size in 3D space, the above selection of $\mathbf{B}_0$ can avoid the worse situation that one may recover a small basis with a large deformation weight as discussed in previous section.

Working with missing data: As one may have noticed, each minimization step in algorithm 1 is equivalent to solving a set of equations by least squares. This can allow us to deal with the tracking matrix with some entries unavailable in a similar way of general power factorization [12]. In case of missing data, the cost function in the algorithm can be modified as:

$$\sum_{(i,j)\in\mathcal{A}} \left| W_{ij} - \left((\mathbf{\Omega} \otimes \mathbf{\Phi})\mathbf{B}\right)_{ij} \right|^2 \tag{13}$$

where W_{ij} denotes the (i, j)th element of the tracking matrix, $\mathcal{A}$ stands for the set of available entries of (i, j) in the tracking matrix. Thus we can update $\mathbf{\Omega}$, $\mathbf{B}$ and $\mathbf{\Phi}$ via least squares only using the available features in $\mathbf{W}$ according to (13). This is a very important attribute of the algorithm, since it is hard to have all the features been tracked across the whole sequence due to self-occlusion in real applications. While it is difficult to deal with missing data in SVD factorization.

4. Upgrading from Affine to Perspective Projection

Previous SVD based algorithms in section 2 and the proposed CPF algorithm are all based on the assumption of affine camera model. This is a zero-order (for weak perspective) or first-order (for paraperspective) approximation of the perspective camera model. The assumption will become invalid and cause large reconstruction errors when the object is close to the camera. In this section, we will introduce two algorithms to upgrade the solutions from affine to perspective projection.

4.1. Linear Recursive Estimation

Under perspective projection, the mapping between a space point $\mathbf{X}_i \in \mathbb{R}^3$ and its normalized image $\mathbf{x}_i \in \mathbb{R}^2$ can be modeled as:

$$s_i\tilde{\mathbf{x}}_i = \mathbf{R}\mathbf{X}_i + \mathbf{T} \tag{14}$$

where, $\tilde{\mathbf{x}}_i = [\mathbf{x}_i^T, 1]^T$ is the homogeneous form of $\mathbf{x}_i$, $\mathbf{R} = [\mathbf{r}_1^T, \mathbf{r}_2^T, \mathbf{r}_3^T]^T$ is the rotation matrix with $\mathbf{r}_i$ the ith row of the matrix, $\mathbf{T} = [t_x, t_y, t_z]^T$ is the translation vector of the camera, and s_i is a non-zero scalar. Suppose the normalized image coordinates of $\mathbf{x}_i$ is $[u_i, v_i]^T$, then we have:

$$\begin{cases} u_i = \frac{\mathbf{r}_1\mathbf{X}_i + t_x}{\mathbf{r}_3\mathbf{X}_i + t_z} = \frac{\mathbf{r}_1\mathbf{X}_i/t_z + t_x/t_z}{1+\mathbf{r}_3\mathbf{X}_i/t_z} = \frac{\mathbf{r}_1\mathbf{X}_i/t_z + t_x/t_z}{1+\varepsilon_i} \\ v_i = \frac{\mathbf{r}_2\mathbf{X}_i + t_y}{\mathbf{r}_3\mathbf{X}_i + t_z} = \frac{\mathbf{r}_2\mathbf{X}_i/t_z + t_y/t_z}{1+\mathbf{r}_3\mathbf{X}_i/t_z} = \frac{\mathbf{r}_2\mathbf{X}_i/t_z + t_y/t_z}{1+\varepsilon_i} \end{cases} \tag{15}$$

Under weak perspective assumption, the depth variation of the object is small compared with the distance to the camera, This is equivalent to a zero-order approximation ($\varepsilon_i = 0$) of perspective projection. Let $\lambda_i = 1 + \varepsilon_i$, then the relationship between the perspective and weak perspective projections can be modeled as $\hat{\mathbf{x}}_i = \lambda_i \mathbf{x}_i$. For the features in the jth frame, the relationship can be expressed as:

$$\hat{\mathbf{x}}_i^{(j)} = \lambda_i^{(j)} \mathbf{x}_i^{(j)}, \; \lambda_i^{(j)} = 1 + \varepsilon_i^{(j)}, \; (i = 1, \cdots n, \; j = 1, \cdots, m) \tag{16}$$

Let us define a weighted tracking matrix as:

$$\hat{\mathbf{W}} = \begin{bmatrix} \hat{\mathbf{x}}_1^{(1)} & \cdots & \hat{\mathbf{x}}_n^{(1)} \\ \vdots & \ddots & \vdots \\ \hat{\mathbf{x}}_1^{(m)} & \cdots & \hat{\mathbf{x}}_n^{(m)} \end{bmatrix}_{2m\times n} = \begin{bmatrix} \lambda_1^{(1)}\mathbf{x}_1^{(1)} & \cdots & \lambda_n^{(1)}\mathbf{x}_n^{(1)} \\ \vdots & \ddots & \vdots \\ \lambda_1^{(m)}\mathbf{x}_1^{(m)} & \cdots & \lambda_n^{(m)}\mathbf{x}_n^{(m)} \end{bmatrix}_{2m\times n} \tag{17}$$

then if the scalars $\{\lambda_i^{(j)} \in \mathbb{R}\}_{i=1,\ldots,n}^{j=1,\ldots,m}$ are recovered consistently with (16), then the shape and motion obtained by factorization of the weighted tracking matrix $\hat{\mathbf{W}}$ just correspond to the solutions of perspective projection. Here we adopt a similar method as [7] (which is for rigid case) to estimate the scalars iteratively. The algorithm is summarized as follows:

Algorithm 2 ((Linear recursive estimation with perspective projection)). Given the tracking matrix $\mathbf{W} \in \mathbb{R}^{2m\times n}$, construct the weighted tracking matrix $\hat{\mathbf{W}}$ according to (17) and set the initial value of $\lambda_i^{(j)} = 1$ for $i = 1, \cdots, n$, $j = 1, \cdots, m$. Repeat the following 3 steps until the convergence of $\lambda_i^{(j)}$.

1. Update the weighted tracking matrix according to (17)*;*

2. Recover the shape and motion via CPF from $\hat{\mathbf{W}}$ according to section 3*;*

3. Estimate the new value of $\lambda_i^{(j)}$ according to (15) and (16)*;*

Convergence property of the algorithm: A theoretical proof of the convergence of this algorithm is unavailable. However, as stated by Christy and Horaud [7], this kind of recursive algorithm converges fast, even the expected value of each $\lambda_i^{(j)}$ is quite different with its initial value. Thus the convergence may be guaranteed by most imaging conditions as demonstrated by our experiments. One convenient way to determine the convergence of the algorithm is to check the scalar variations. Let us arrange all the scalars at the tth iteration into a matrix $\mathbf{\Lambda}_t = [\lambda_i^{(j)}]_{m\times n}$. The scalar variation is defined as the Frobenius norm of the difference of the scalar matrix.

$$\delta = \left\|\mathbf{\Lambda}_t - \mathbf{\Lambda}_{t-1}\right\|_F \tag{18}$$

The algorithm will converge ($\delta \to 0$) usually after 4 to 5 iterations.

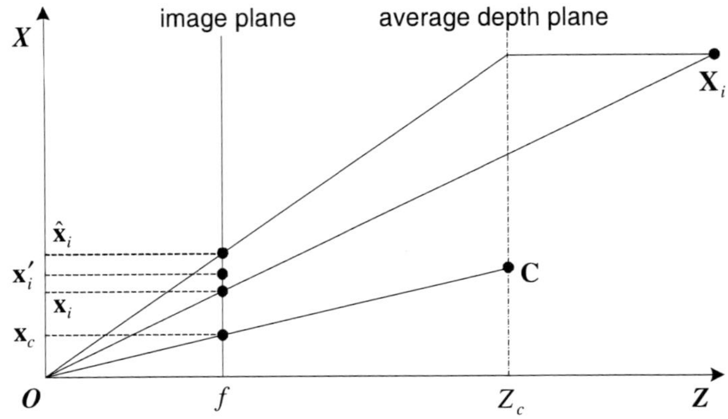

Figure 1. Cross-sectional view of perspective approximation from weak perspective projection. Where $\boldsymbol{O}$ is the optical center, with $\boldsymbol{Z} = f$ the image plane. $\mathbf{C}$ is the centroid of the object, $\boldsymbol{Z}_c$ is the average depth plane, $\mathbf{X}_i$ is a point on the object, $\mathbf{x}_i$ is the image under perspective projection, $\hat{\mathbf{x}}_i$ is the image under weak perspective projection.

Dealing with the reversal ambiguity: Due to the inherent property of the affine camera model, a reversal ambiguity remains for the recovered shapes and motions. As one may see from (2), if we denote $(\mathbf{S}^{(j)}, \mathbf{R}^{(j)})$ as "positive" solution, then a "negative" solution $(-\mathbf{S}^{(j)}, -\mathbf{R}^{(j)})$ is also hold true to the algorithm. The ambiguity may be easily handled in the algorithm. After recovering the shape and motion in step 2, we can reproject the "positive" and the "negative" solutions to each frame and form two new tracking matrices, say $\mathbf{W}^+$ for the "positive" and $\mathbf{W}^-$ for the "negative". Check the Frobenius norms of $\|\hat{\mathbf{W}} - \mathbf{W}^+\|_F$ and $\|\hat{\mathbf{W}} - \mathbf{W}^-\|_F$. The one with the smaller error would be the correct solution.

Geometrical explanation of the algorithm: The geometrical illustration of the algorithm is very clear as shown in Figure 1. The initial tracking matrix is composed of the image point $\mathbf{x}_i$, which is actually formed by perspective projection. The weighted tracking matrix of (17), which may be composed of the point $\mathbf{x}'_i = \lambda_i \mathbf{x}_i$, varies in accordance with the updated scalars of step 3. Upon convergence, the image points are modified to $\hat{\mathbf{x}}_i$ such that they fit the weak perspective projection. Thus, the process of the algorithm is to recursively adjust the image coordinates from the position of perspective projection to that of weak perspective by adjusting the value of $\lambda_i^{(j)}$. While the image of the centroid $(\mathbf{x}_c)$ remains untouched during iterations.

It should be noted that the algorithm takes the weak perspective projection as an example. Nevertheless, it can also be applied to upgrade the solutions from paraperspective to perspective projection, and the only difference lies in the computation of $\lambda_i^{(j)}$.

4.2. Nonlinear Optimization Algorithm

One may see from Figure 1 that the solution obtained by the linear recursive algorithm is just an approximation to the fully perspective projection. Here we will give a nonlinear optimization algorithm to upgrade the reconstruction from affine to perspective projection.

Suppose the camera rotation, translation, shape bases and deformation weights under perspective projection are $\mathbf{R}^{(j)}$, $\mathbf{T}^{(j)}$, $\mathbf{S}_l$ and $\omega_l^{(j)}$, respectively. Our goal is to recover these parameters by minimizing the image reprojection residual.

$$f(\mathbf{R}^{(j)}, \mathbf{T}^{(j)}, \mathbf{S}_l, \omega_l^{(j)}) = \left\|\mathbf{W} - \bar{\mathbf{W}}\right\|_F^2 = \sum_{i=1,\ldots,n}^{j=1,\ldots,m} \left\|\tilde{\mathbf{x}}_i^{(j)} - N(\tilde{\bar{\mathbf{x}}}_i^{(j)})\right\|_F^2$$
$$s_i^{(j)}\tilde{\bar{\mathbf{x}}}_i^{(j)} = \mathbf{R}^{(j)} \sum_{l=1}^{k} \omega_l^{(j)} \mathbf{S}_l + \mathbf{T}^{(j)} \tag{19}$$

where $\bar{\mathbf{W}}$ denotes the reprojected tracking matrix, $\tilde{\mathbf{x}}_i^{(j)} = \left[(\mathbf{x}_i^{(j)})^T, 1\right]^T$ is the homogeneous form of the initial tracked features, $N(\bullet)$ denotes the normalization of a homogeneous vector so as to make its last element unit, $\tilde{\bar{\mathbf{x}}}$ is the homogeneous form of the reprojected image point under perspective projection, $s_i^{(j)}$ is a non-zero scalar. The minimization process is also termed as bundle adjustment in computer vision society that can be solved via Newton iteration or other gradient descent methods. Here we employ the sparse Levenberg-Marquardt iteration method as given in [14]. During computation, the rotation matrix is parameterized by three parameters $\mathbf{l}^{(j)} = \left[l_1^{(j)}, l_2^{(j)}, l_3^{(j)}\right]^T$ using the exponential map as:

$$\mathbf{R}^{(j)} = \exp \begin{bmatrix} 0 & l_3^{(j)} & -l_2^{(j)} \\ -l_3^{(j)} & 0 & l_1^{(j)} \\ l_2^{(j)} & -l_1^{(j)} & 0 \end{bmatrix} \tag{20}$$

The method presented here is similar to that in [10]. However, the work in [10] is designed to optimize the solutions of affine reconstruction, while ours is to minimize the perspective reprojection error and take the affine solutions as the initial values of iteration. In this chapter, we assume the camera is calibrated. However, the camera parameters can also be optimized if we combine these parameters into the minimization process of (19). Suppose $\mathbf{K}^{(j)}$ is the camera matrix of the jth frame, $\tilde{\mathbf{m}}_i^{(j)}$ is a feature point in the frame in homogeneous form measured in pixels, $\tilde{\mathbf{x}}_i^{(j)}$ is the corresponding normalized image point, then we have:

$$\tilde{\mathbf{x}}_i^{(j)} = N\left(\left(\mathbf{K}^{(j)}\right)^{-1}\tilde{\mathbf{m}}_i^{(j)}\right) \tag{21}$$

where $N(\bullet)$ has the same meaning as in (19). Compared with the linear recursive algorithm, the nonlinear method may converge to a more accurate solution of perspective projection, since the algorithm minimizes a geometrical meaningful cost function. Nevertheless, the nonlinear method may lead to a local minimum solution when good initial values are not guaranteed. In practice, we can combine the two algorithms together, use the linear method to obtain initial values and then further optimized by the nonlinear method, or we may start with the solutions provided by paraperspective assumption since this assumption is a first-order approximation of the perspective projection. The nonlinear algorithm is usually computational intensive compared with the linear recursive algorithm, readers may refer to [7][14] for a comparison of their complexities.

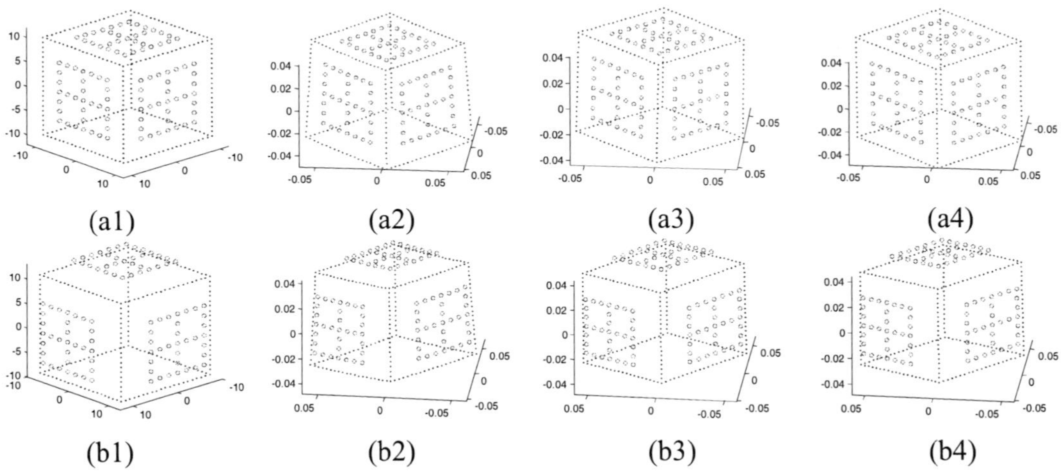

Figure 2. Synthetic data and reconstruction results of different algorithms. (a1)&(b1) the first and the 10th generated 3D shapes of the synthetic cubes (in dot) and the three sets of moving points (in circle); (a2)&(b2) the corresponding recovered affine shapes by the CPF algorithm; (a3)&(b3) the upgraded perspective shapes by the linear recursive algorithm; (a4)&(b4) the upgraded shapes by the nonlinear optimization algorithm.

5. Experiments with Synthetic Data

During the simulations, we generate a cube in the space, whose dimension is $20 \times 20 \times 20$ with 21 evenly distributed points on each side. The origin of the world coordinate system is set at the center of the cube. There are three sets of points (33×3 points) on the adjacent three surfaces of the cube that move along the axes at constant speed toward outside as shown in Figure 2. We generate 30 cubes (together with the three moving parts) in space with randomly selected poses, then project each cube to an image by perspective projection. For each frame, the distance of the camera to the object is set at about 14 times of the object size such that the imaging condition is close to weak perspective projection. There are 351 points (252 points belong to the cube and the rest 99 points belong to the three moving parts) in each frame.

Reconstruction results: We recover the shape and motion corresponding to each frame using CPF and then upgrade the solution from affine to perspective projection according to the proposed algorithms. Figure 2(a) and Figure 2(b) shows the recovered 3D shapes of two frames. We can see from the results that both the linear recursive and the nonlinear algorithms can achieve very good results that are almost the same as the ground truths visually. But the errors of affine reconstructions are obvious, as we can see from Figure 2(a2) and Figure 2(b2), the reconstructed shapes are not exactly cubes and the reconstructed lines are curved a little bit due to the perspective effect, although the camera setup in the simulation is very close to weak perspective assumption. If we move the camera close to the object, the reconstruction error would increase accordingly. At the same time, the proposed upgrading algorithms may not converge to the correct solutions when the error increases to a certain extent. We also find that the nonlinear method is more sensitive to the initial values than the linear recursive algorithm.

Convergence property of CPF algorithm: We test the algorithm in three conditions: First, we utilize the CPF algorithm to recover the 3D shape and motion from all the points in 30 frames. At each iteration, we record the variation of the reprojected tracking matrix defined in (11) and the relative reprojection error which is defined as:

$$Err = \|\mathbf{W} - \mathbf{W}_t\|_F / \|\mathbf{W}\|_F \times 100\ (\%) \tag{22}$$

where, $\mathbf{W}$ is the initial tracking matrix, $\mathbf{W}_t$ is the reprojected tracking matrix at the tth iteration. The results are shown in Figure 3(a) and Figure 3(b) respectively. Then, we randomly delete 20% entries from the initial tracking matrix and perform the CPF using the remaining data, the relative reprojection error of the available data at each iteration is given in Figure 3(c). In the third situation, we add Gaussian noise (the noise level is equivalent to 2 pixels) to the initial tracking matrix and do the test again, the relative reprojection error is shown in Figure 3(d). It can be seen from these tests that the convergence speed of the CPF algorithm is fast, even with some missing data and measurement errors. The missing data seems to have no influence to the convergence rate and solutions at this experiment. However, the algorithm may fail when the proportion of missing entries increases to a certain level as that has been demonstrated by Hartley [12]. One may also find that a small residual error still exists when there is no added noise, this is because the images are produced by perspective projection rather than affine projection. The residual error will increase as well with that of the noise level.

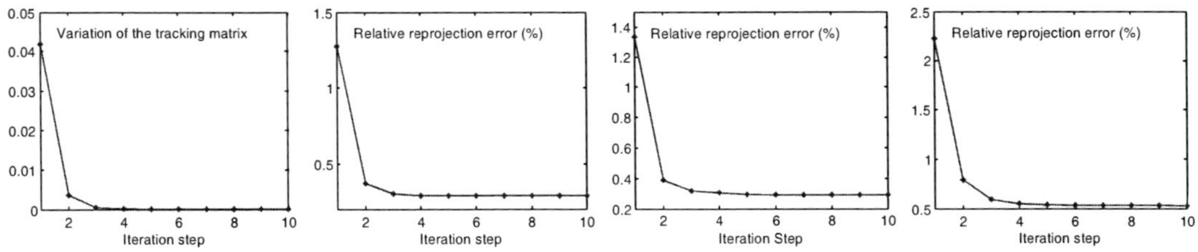

(a) (b) (c) (d)

Figure 3. The convergence property of the CPF algorithm. (a) the variation of the reprojected tracking matrix at each iteration step; (b) the relative reprojection errors of the algorithm *vs.* iteration steps; (c) the relative reprojection errors with 20% missing data *vs.* iteration steps; (d) the relative reprojection errors with 2 pixels added noise *vs.* iteration steps, note the increase of the residual error.

Comparative study with SVD+RB based method: We first carry some comparative tests on the reconstruction accuracy between the CPF and the algorithm based on SVD factorization and the rotation and basis constraints (SVD+RB) given in section 2. Here, we use all the data from 30 frames and vary the noise level from 0 to 3 pixels with a step of 0.5 during the test, and take 100 independent tests at each noise level so as to give a statistically meaningful results. The means and standard deviations of the relative reprojection errors by the two algorithms are shown in Figure 4(a) and Figure 4(b) respectively, where the solutions of the CPF algorithm are evaluated at the 20th iteration. The results show that the solutions by CPF outperform those by SVD+RB. The main reason is that the motion matrix M obtained by the SVD+RB algorithm does not strictly conform to the block structure of (2), so a Procrustes analysis should be performed in order to obtain the values of $\omega_i^{(j)}$ and $\mathbf{R}_w^{(j)}$, The process may introduce additional errors to the final solutions. While the CPF algorithm can assure this block structure and orthonormal constraint at each step of iterations.

We then compare the processing time of the two algorithms. In this chapter, all algorithms are implemented in Matlab 6.5 on Dell PC with Intel Xeon 2.6GHz CPU. Figure 4(c) shows the actual computation time of the two algorithms with respect to the data size (here we only change the frame numbers with fixed amount of features in each frame), where the time for CPF is taken only in one iteration. It is clear that the computation time of the SVD+RB increases faster than that of the CPF, while for small tracking matrix, such as the case in this study, the SVD+RB based algorithm is faster than the CPF algorithm.

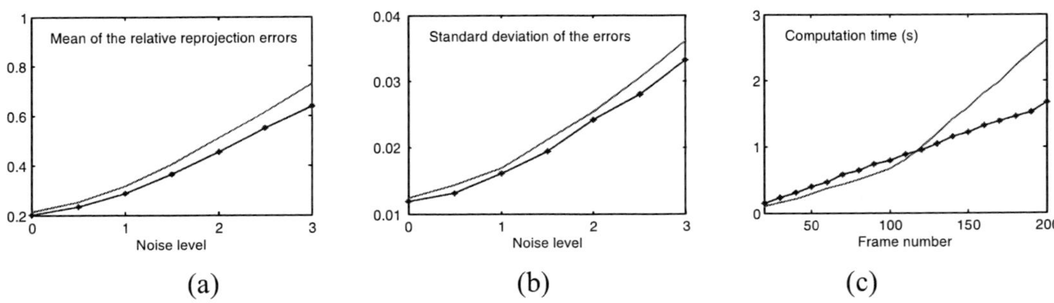

Figure 4. Comparative study between the CPF based algorithm (curves with asterisk markers) and the SVD+RB based algorithm (curves without marker). (a) means of the relative reprojection errors at different noise level; (b) standard deviations of the relative reprojection errors at different noise level; (c) the actual computation time (seconds) with the increase of frame numbers.

Performance of the upgrading algorithms: Figure 2 has shown the improvements of the two upgrading algorithms to the affine reconstruction results. During iterations, we record the scalar variations defined in (18) and the relative reprojection errors at each iteration step. The results are shown in Figure 5, from which we can see that the linear recursive algorithm converges quickly, while the nonlinear method converges a little bit slower. The reprojection error of the affine reconstruction corresponds to that at the first iteration as shown in Figure 5(b) and Fig.5(c). The error is reduced greatly by the proposed algorithms. Their residual errors after convergence are 0.12% for the linear recursive algorithm and 0.07% for the nonlinear one.

6. Experiments with Real Sequences

We tested the proposed methods on several real image sequences. Here we will only report the results Franck sequence due to space limitation. The sequence is downloaded from the

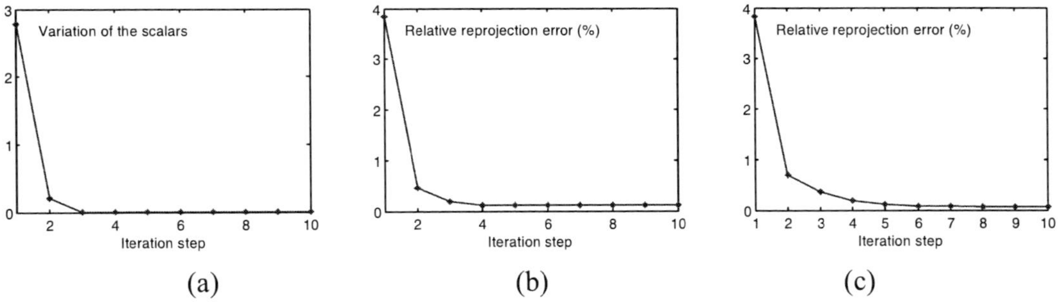

Figure 5. Performance of the two upgrading algorithms. (a) the scalar variations of the linear recursive algorithm with respect to the iteration steps; (b) the relative reprojection error of the linear recursive algorithm at each iteration; (c) the relative reprojection error of the nonlinear optimization algorithm at each iteration.

European working group on face and gesture recognition (www-prima.inrialpes.fr/FGnet/). We select 60 frames with various facial expressions for the experiment. The tracking data, which contain 68 automatically tracked feature points using the active appearance model (AAM) method, are also downloaded from the site. In this test, we use a simplified camera model with square pixel and the principal point at the image center, the intrinsic parameters of the camera is assumed to be constant during shooting. The only unknown parameter (i.e. the focal length) is estimated by the method proposed by Pollefeys *et.al* [22].

Figure 6 shows the reconstructed VRML models with texture mapping and the triangulated wireframes corresponding to five frames, which are obtained by CPF and then upgraded by the linear recursive algorithm with 10 iterations. The reconstruction results by other methods are omitted here, since there is no much difference visually. For a comparison, the relative reprojection errors of the CPF algorithm, the linear recursive and the nonlinear optimization algorithm are 6.28%, 0.25%, 0.17%, respectively. The improvements of the proposed upgrading algorithms are obvious.

We may see from the results that the models at different frame, as well as the different facial expressions, are correctly recovered. The results are useful for normal purposes such as visualization and recognition. However, the positions of some reconstructed points may be not very accurate. This is mainly caused by the errors of the tracked features and the camera parameters.

7. Conclusion

In this chapter, under the assumption of affine camera, we have introduced a rotation constrained factorization algorithm to recover the shapes and motions of nonrigid object from a monocular image sequence. The algorithm is more accurate than previous SVD based methods and easy to implement. It can deal with a tracking matrix with missing data and overcome some limitations of the SVD based methods. These features make the algorithm more practical. We also propose two algorithms to upgrade the above nonrigid factorization results from affine to a full perspective camera model. Experiment results with synthetic data and real sequences validate the proposed algorithms and show the improvements over

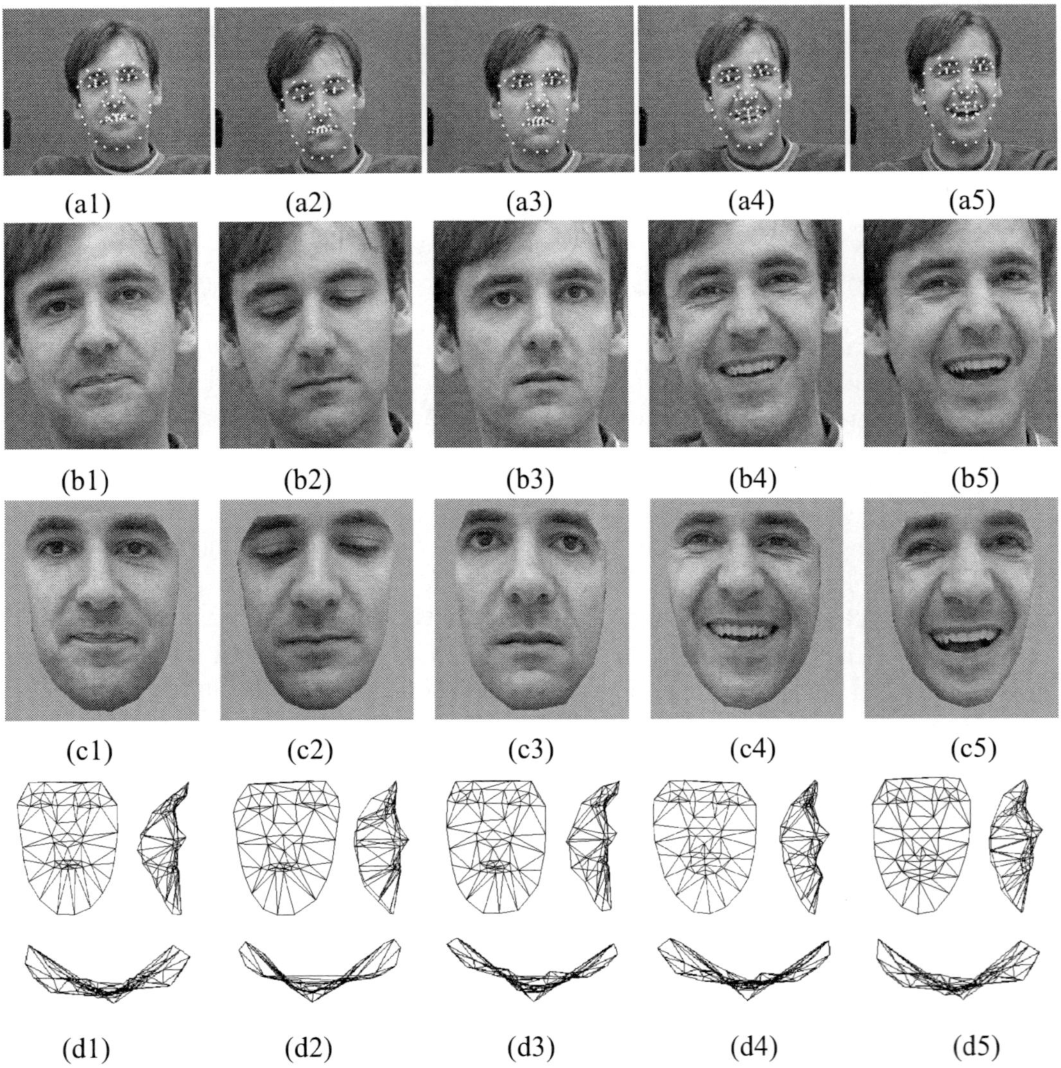

Figure 6. Reconstruction results of five frames with different facial expressions from the Franck sequence. (a1)-(a5) five key frames from the sequence overlaid with 68 tracked feature points, the image resolution is 720×576; (b1)-(b5) the enlarged facial parts of the original frames corresponding to (a1) through (a5); (c1)-(c5) the front views of the corresponding reconstructed VRML models with texture mapping; (d1)-(d5) the front, side and top views of the corresponding triangulated wireframe models.

previous methods. Some further extension is possible to more challenging cases that usually happen in practice. These include the problems of how to deal with the outliers and the uncertainty in image measurement, and how to accurately self-calibrate the cameras from nonrigid sequences.

Acknowledgment

The work is supported in part by the Natural Sciences and Engineering Research Council of Canada, and the National Natural Science Foundation of China under grant no. 60575015.

References

[1] B. Bascle and A. Blake. Separability of pose and expression in facial tracing and animation. In *Proc. of the International Conference on Computer Vision*, pages 323–328, 1998.

[2] M. Brand. Morphable 3D models from video. In *Proc. of IEEE Conference on Computer Vision and Pattern Recognition*, volume 2, pages 456–463, 2001.

[3] M. Brand. A direct method for 3D factorization of nonrigid motion observed in 2d. In *Proc. of IEEE Conference on Computer Vision and Pattern Recognition*, volume 2, pages 122–128, 2005.

[4] C. Bregler, A. Hertzmann, and H. Biermann. Recovering non-rigid 3D shape from image streams. In *Proc. of IEEE Conference on Computer Vision and Pattern Recognition*, volume 2, pages 690–696, 2000.

[5] A. M. Buchanan and A. W. Fitzgibbon. Damped newton algorithms for matrix factorization with missing data. In *Proc. of IEEE Conference on Computer Vision and Pattern Recognition*, volume 2, pages 316–322, 2005.

[6] P. Chen. Optimization algorithms on subspaces: Revisiting missing data problem in low-rank matrix. *Int. J. Comput. Vision*, 80(1):125–142, 2008.

[7] S. Christy and R. Horaud. Euclidean shape and motion from multiple perspective views by affine iterations. *IEEE Trans. Pattern Anal. Mach. Intell.*, 18(11):1098–1104, 1996.

[8] J. Costeira and T. Kanade. A multibody factorization method for independent moving objects. *Int. J. Comput. Vision*, 29(3):159–179, September 1998.

[9] A. Del Bue, X. Lladó, and L. de Agapito. Non-rigid metric shape and motion recovery from uncalibrated images using priors. In *Proc. of IEEE Conference on Computer Vision and Pattern Recognition*, volume 1, pages 1191–1198, 2006.

[10] A. Del Bue, F. Smeraldi, and L. Agapito. Non-rigid structure from motion using nonparametric tracking and non-linear optimization. In *IEEE Workshop in Articulated and Nonrigid Motion ANM04, held in conjunction with CVPR2004*, pages 8–15, June 2004.

[11] M. Han and T. Kanade. Creating 3D models with uncalibrated cameras. In *proc. of IEEE Computer Society Workshop on the Application of Computer Vision (WACV2000)*, December 2000.

[12] R. Hartley and F. Schaffalizky. Powerfactorization: 3D reconstruction with missing or uncertain data. *Australia-Japan Advanced Workshop on Computer Vision*, 2003.

[13] R. Hartley and R. Vidal. Perspective nonrigid shape and motion recovery. In *ECCV (1), Lecture Notes in Computer Science*, volume 5302, pages 276–289. Springer, 2008.

[14] R. Hartley and A. Zisserman. *Multiple View Geometry in Computer Vision*. Cambridge University Press, second edition, 2004.

[15] A. Heyden, R. Berthilsson, and G. Sparr. An iterative factorization method for projective structure and motion from image sequences. *Image Vision Comput.*, 17(13):981–991, 1999.

[16] T. Li, V. Kallem, D. Singaraju, and R. Vidal. Projective factorization of multiple rigid-body motions. In *IEEE Conference on Computer Vision and Pattern Recognition*, 2007.

[17] Q. Luong and O. Faugeras. Self-calibration of a moving camera from point correspondences and fundamental matrices. *International Journal of Computer Vision*, 22(3):261–289, March 1997.

[18] S. Mahamud and M. Hebert. Iterative projective reconstruction from multiple views. In *IEEE Conference on Computer Vision and Pattern Recognition*, volume 2, pages 430–437, 2000.

[19] T. Morita and T. Kanade. A sequential factorization method for recovering shape and motion from image streams. *IEEE Transactions on Pattern and Analysis and Machine Intelligence*, 19(8):858 – 867, August 1997.

[20] J. Oliensis and R. Hartley. Iterative extensions of the sturm/triggs algorithm: Convergence and nonconvergence. *IEEE Trans. Pattern Anal. Mach. Intell.*, 29(12):2217–2233, 2007.

[21] C. Poelman and T. Kanade. A paraperspective factorization method for shape and motion recovery. *IEEE Transactions on Pattern and Analysis and Machine Intelligence*, 19(3):206 – 218, March 1997.

[22] Pollefeys, M., Koch, R. and Van Gool. L. Self-calibration and metric reconstruction in spite of varying and unknown intrinsic camera parameters. *International Journal of Computer Vision*, 32(1):7–25, August 1999.

[23] Rabaud, V. and Belongie, S. Re-thinking non-rigid structure from motion. In *IEEE Conference on Computer Vision and Pattern Recognition*, 2008.

[24] Sturm, P. F. and Triggs, B. A factorization based algorithm for multi-image projective structure and motion. In *European Conference on Computer Vision (2)*, pages 709–720, 1996.

[25] Tomasi, C. and Kanade, T. Shape and motion from image streams under orthography: A factorization method. *International Journal of Computer Vision*, 9(2):137–154, November 1992.

[26] Torresani, L., Hertzmann, A. and Bregler, C. Nonrigid structure-from-motion: Estimating shape and motion with hierarchical priors. *IEEE Trans. Pattern Anal. Mach. Intell.*, 30(5):878–892, 2008.

[27] Torresani, L., Yang, D. B., Alexander, E. J. and Bregler, C. Tracking and modeling non-rigid objects with rank constraints. In *IEEE Conference on Computer Vision and Pattern Recognition*, volume 1, pages 493–500, 2001.

[28] Triggs, B. Factorization methods for projective structure and motion. In *Proceedings of the IEEE Conference on Computer Vision and Pattern Recognition, San Francisco, California, USA*, pages 845–851, 1996.

[29] Vidal, R. and Abretske, D. Nonrigid shape and motion from multiple perspective views. In *European Conference on Computer Vision (2)*, *Lecture Notes in Computer Science*, volume 3952, pages 205–218. Springer, 2006.

[30] Vidal, R., Tron, R. and Hartley, R. Multiframe motion segmentation with missing data using powerfactorization and GPCA. *International Journal of Computer Vision*, 79(1):85–105, 2008.

[31] Wang, G., Tsui, H.-T. and Hu. Z. Structure and motion of nonrigid object under perspective projection. *Pattern Recogn. Lett.*, 28(4): 507-515, 2007

[32] Wang, G., Tsui, H.-T. and Wu, J. Rotation constrained power factorization for structure from motion of nonrigid objects. *Pattern Recogn. Lett.*, 29(1):72–80, 2008.

[33] Wang, G. and Wu, Q. J. Stratification approach for 3D euclidean reconstruction of nonrigid objects from uncalibrated image sequences. *IEEE Transactions on Systems, Man, and Cybernetics, Part B*, 38(1):90–101, 2008.

[34] Wang, G. and Wu, Q. J. 3D Quasi-perspective projection model: theory and application to structure and motion factorization from uncalibrated image sequences. *International Journal of Computer Vision*, in press (2009) DOI: 10.1007/s11263-009-0267-4

[35] Xiao, J., Chai, J. and Kanade, T. A closed-form solution to non-rigid shape and motion recovery. *International Journal of Computer Vision*, 67(2):233–246, April 2006.

[36] Xiao, J. and Kanade, T. Uncalibrated perspective reconstruction of deformable structures. In *Proc. of the International Conference on Computer Vision*, volume 2, pages 1075–1082, 2005.

[37] Yan, J. and Pollefeys, M. A factorization-based approach to articulated motion recovery. In *IEEE Conference on Computer Vision and Pattern Recognition* (2), pages 815–821, 2005.

[38] Yan, J. and Pollefeys. M. A factorization-based approach for articulated nonrigid shape, motion and kinematic chain recovery from video. *IEEE Trans. Pattern Anal. Mach. Intell.*, 30(5):865–877, 2008.

INDEX

A

B

C

H

I

M

N

O

P

Q

R

T

U

V

W

X